South of the desert

KATHY JACKSON AND OKEY ABOSI

South of the desert

A TEACHER GUIDE TO CHILD DEVELOPMENT IN SUB-SAHARAN AFRICA

UNIVERSITY OF SOUTH AFRICA
PRETORIA

First edition, first impression

ISBN 1-86888-327-2

Published by Unisa Press, University of South Africa, PO Box 392, Unisa, 0003
Editing: Liz Stewart
Design, layout and typesetting: Thea Bester-Swanepoel
Printed by Pinetown Printers, Pinetown

Contents

Africa's own identity requires self-awareness

A. A. Mazrui

List of tables

Preface

Children do not grow up in a vacuum; rather they grow in a series of overlapping contexts, each of which influences the kind of person they will be at maturity. For the great majority of African children the physical context is a rural one, in which traditional values and practices have changed relatively little as a consequence of modernisation. African children are still largely socialised to act in ways that maintain the wellbeing of the group above the personal satisfactions of the individual. They learn their culture's expectations with regard to eating, playing, working and studying. They learn how boys should behave and ways in which girls' behaviour differs from that of their male peers. They learn what emotions can be expressed towards whom. They experience good health and learn to cope with poor health in ways that are influenced by poverty and tradition. They learn these things in their families, communities and schools, a series of contexts each of which influences the others. This book is about these many and varied influences on child development in sub-Saharan Africa.

The idea that we might write this book arose out of frustration. Trying to teach African teachers about child development using information based on research into the socialisation and experiences at school of more privileged children from other continents felt like a waste of time and was perceived as such by the students. Thus, the material in the book draws on information from countries across sub-Saharan Africa. African research is included in preference to research done elsewhere, and the majority of the studies cited included at least one African among the research team. Other studies, done by outsiders, are evaluated critically if they give uninformed explanations for events.

We chose quite deliberately to take a broad approach to this material. As we point out in Chapter One, we believe that an African is more like another African than he or she is like a Chinese or an American. The broad sweep of the material is presented so that African teachers can learn about their own Africanness as well as that of their students. We hope that this broader view of themselves and their students will help teachers to accept ethnic group difference within their classroom and community and also to accept the differences in children's abilities, values and beliefs. Well-educated teachers who value the children in their classrooms are well placed to enhance their development. We hope that this book will assist in this process in sub-Saharan Africa.

Although the book is primarily designed for use by teachers and teacher trainees, other professionals who work with children may also find its contents useful in their work. This book contains material on parental behaviours and their influence on development during the child's early years, information about maternal and child health from the pre-natal period through to adolescence, material on the impact of sensory and physical disabilities on development, and on the potential for harm that occurs during times of social disruption such as war. Such information will be useful to social workers and health professionals who are working with children.

A first attempt at something new like this book will always have room for improvement. Suggestions from readers as to what we might include or ways in which we might improve the presentation will be very much appreciated by us, should a revised or second edition be possible.

Kathy Jackson **Okey Abosi**

Chapter One

Introduction and overview

Introduction

Growing up is not just a physical experience, nor is it entirely biologically or genetically determined. Children's understanding of the world and their place in it develops and changes throughout their early years, with special growth and change in understanding and behaviour during adolescence. The growth in cognitive skills, in social and emotional skills is studied by psychologists and others interested in child development. This book focuses on the psychology of African child development.

Why study the psychology of African child development?

The study of psychology provides a basic way of understanding human behaviour and the mental processes of human beings. One major gap in the huge amount of research in psychology concerns the influence of the beliefs and culture of a given group of people on the development of children born and raised within the group. Psychology has always maintained that no two people or children are exactly alike. The same may be said for groups of people from different ethnic and cultural backgrounds – people from different cultures may react differently to the same situation.

It is clear that a line can be drawn within psychology between the patterns of child development that cut across all ethnic groups and cultures and other aspects of development that reflect the influence of environment, beliefs and values. Patterns of development that are universal are almost certainly genetically determined, but where development varies between groups some cultural influences have had an effect. As a result there are almost certainly some unique patterns of behaviour and mental processes in each of the many cultures of the world. These identify members of that group as separate and unique from other groups.

As Akinboye (1996) has pointed out, Africans have certain characteristics, patterns of behaviour, and mental processes that identify them as Africans. Akinboye outlines some of the unique patterns of behaviour that manifest in Africans' thought processes about the world, people, their environment, marriage and family life, education, religions, politics and economics. Other uniquely African thought processes that he outlines include ideas about the dead and the living, interests, creativity and achievements, character and values, norms, growth and development, progress, normality and abnormality, bargaining, relating, negotiating, happiness and sadness, and success and failure. Importantly, he stated that Africans have special skills in 'reading' or comprehending the patterns of behaviour and feeling generated by these unique thought patterns in other people in their group.

It is not always possible to separate the genetic or biological differences from differences that arise as a result of differences in culture. As Worthman (1999) points out, cultural and biological processes interact to shape human development. Worthman, Akinboye (1996) and others (e.g. Graber, Brooks-Gunn and Petersen 1996) maintain that to divorce the study of physical development and other variations in the biological state of individuals from the study of enculturation and social process is to miss a cultural dynamic that must be central to more complete explanations of human development.

The study of adolescent development provides a good example of an interaction between biology and culture. Much attention has been given to the biological developments of puberty and to the implications and management of developmental differences in adolescents in northern hemisphere populations. In contrast, little is systematically known about the biology of adolescent development in other regions or about what other societies do about differences while achieving their specific cultural agenda for social maturation.

Tanner (1989) and Berk (2000) have pointed out that chronological age is a poor predictor of individual developmental states during puberty. This is recognised in Africa, where age does not always determine participation in rites of puberty; rather, maturation is the determinant of participation. The development of a young girl's breasts is seen as an indication that she is ready for marriage or mature enough to have babies, irrespective of her chronological age, for example. The concept of the 'age group' that is recognised in Africa and has formed the basis for grouping people according to a combination of age and maturity also allows considerable flexibility in dealing with young people while biologically determined development towards maturity takes place.

More generally, cultural prescriptions cover material and non-material aspects of all human needs such as shelter, sex, safety, marriage and love. Cultural prescriptions contribute to beliefs, values and attitudes, to a people's religion, forms of marriage and family, youth culture, environment, sexual behaviours, beliefs about reproductive health, pregnancy, birth control, and gender relations. Cultural myths are created that reinforce social structural inequalities, taboos and behavioural patterns in each of these areas of life. But culture is learned and shared with people from the same group, so it is amenable to change. It is thus dynamic and can change when new needs develop through exposure to different influences. Change can occur at the behavioural or cognitive level of a cultural system. Individuals or groups who benefit from certain traditional or long-standing cultural practices and the status quo tend to resist change when it threatens their power and influence.

Briefly, psychological research shows that the significance of socio-cultural factors lies in their central role in socialising individuals and determining their beliefs, values and behavioural patterns pertaining to all aspects of life within their group. Understanding both traditional and more modern African cultural influences on development helps one to understand African psychology and the behaviour patterns of Africans. An African is not American or European or Asian and cannot be. An African is unique in every aspect of his or her life and development, hence the need to study the psychology of African child development as it occurs within the various socio-cultural environments that exist across the continent.

Why use other sources of information?

Research findings from other social sciences and from health, history and literature all provide additional information about cultural factors and personal experiences that influence child development outcomes. The study of epidemiology, for example, provides information about infant and maternal mortality rates and about the rates of various illnesses. Additionally, epidemiological studies are important because they may show that patterns of disease vary from one region of the country to another. Thus, health planners can put additional resources into areas where a disease is more common in their attempts to overcome it. Teachers, too, need to be aware of variations in rates of disease so they can be alert to diseases that are especially common in the region where they are working.

Studies of the past, such as those reported by historians, can contribute to understanding of present-day difficulties and strengths. Anthropologists provide information about both traditional and modern cultures found in Africa, throwing further light on some of the current influences on children. Sociologists and other researchers all study societies and social change. Knowledge from these fields of study contributes to a fuller picture of the environment in which African children are growing up today. Thus, information from a wide range of sources has proved useful when considering African child development.

Overview of the material in this book

This book has the following general aims:

- To provide African teachers and trainee teachers with culturally relevant material about child development
- To provide teachers with an opportunity to gain deeper knowledge about child development so that they develop a truly professional understanding about the various influences on young people during childhood
- To help teachers become aware of the many factors that contribute to children's success and failure at school
- To help teachers recognise commonalities in culture in different groups in Africa, while assisting them as they try to cope with differences between cultures
- To encourage teachers to recognise that knowledge from outside Africa can be adapted to the African context and that using this knowledge can enhance their teaching practice.

Although the book is not divided into separate parts, the focus changes from culture and family as influences on child development outcomes to child development itself, and then to health issues affecting the growth and development of African children. In the final three chapters teachers and trainee teachers are asked to think about how their own beliefs about themselves and about children are reflected in their behaviour in the classroom. These chapters ask teachers to consider what they need to do to create a classroom environment in which children's development is optimised in all areas – physical, social-emotional and intellectual.

This book focuses on aspects of African child development that are most likely to be different from child development in other parts of the world. For this reason most of the material concerns social and emotional change, cognitive development, physical wellbeing and illness. Physical growth, the growth of motor skills, and the physical changes at adolescence are not discussed unless growing up in Africa means they differ in some way from the physical development of children in other parts of the world. Thus, for example, the development of vision and hearing are not described because this is biologically determined, but common visual impairments and the high rate of ear infection among African children are discussed because they have negative implications for children's school learning.

The book consists of 11 chapters, including the present one. Most chapters follow a similar pattern. Traditional knowledge and ideas are presented first, because they still influence child development in most African families to a greater or lesser extent. Modern knowledge from any research in Africa is presented next, usually in a section of the chapter that follows immediately after the information about tradition. African teachers, like teachers everywhere, need to use modern knowledge if they are to be most effective in their work. But teachers in Africa need to find a way of adapting the research findings from other parts of the world to fit in with their circumstances and values. Where possible, some suggestions as to how teachers might do this are offered.

Chapters One to Three provide the basic understandings necessary for later chapters. As is already evident, Chapter One provides a brief introduction to the importance of various fields of knowledge that contribute to knowledge about child development in Africa. It emphasises the importance of social and cultural influences on the way children develop. The second chapter picks up on the suggestion that the culture that surrounds the child is an important influence on his or her development. The chapter outlines briefly some cultural values and ways of behaving that have been important in many parts of Africa. It then goes on to present material from recent psychological research into culture-related behaviours and shows how African cultures can be examined using a modern framework. Chapter Three moves closer to the child, showing how different forms of family life, along with parents' beliefs and behaviours, can modify the way each child develops.

Chapters Four and Five describe the normal development of children from infancy through to adolescence. The chapters focus more on children's social, emotional, speech, and cognitive development than on physical development because normal physical development is the same for children and adolescents around the world. African children's attendance at school is influenced by some important cultural values; the impact of these is explored in chapter Five.

Unfortunately, many children in Africa suffer from preventable and non-preventable ill health, and from sensory and psychological disorders that affect their general development and their progress at school. Chapters Six to Eight discuss these problems. The chapters also provide some guidelines as to what teachers might do to reduce the negative impact of health problems on children's development.

The last three chapters, Chapters Nine to Eleven, ask teachers to consider their own behaviours, values and attitudes, because what teachers think and do also have a major impact on the development of the child during his or her school years. These chapters challenge teachers to review and revise some of their beliefs about child development and learning, and to think about how they might change their behaviours with a goal of becoming effective and professional in their work with the children in their care.

Because only a limited amount of information about African children is available, the book uses examples from across the region. Some readers may react by saying 'This is not what happens in my country, group, or culture.' Such a reaction shows the beginning of an awareness of the need to think about their own culture more deeply. Exercises presented at the end of Chapters Two to Eleven offer an opportunity for teachers to extend their knowledge of their own community and to explore their own values, beliefs, attitudes, and behaviours and those of others in greater depth than is possible in a book such as this one.

Chapter Two

Culture as an influence on development

Introduction

The important traditional values, beliefs, practices and ways of thinking that were outlined briefly in Chapter One continue to influence African child development today. These values, beliefs and practices may be more evident in rural communities, but they also influence children living with well-educated parents in large urban areas in ways that African teachers and parents may take for granted. The aim of the present chapter is to increase teachers' conscious awareness of the impact of culture on child development. To achieve this goal the chapter outlines some traditional cultural values in more detail. It then defines some terms that are currently used when educators, child psychologists, anthropologists and others discuss culture in modern research. Finally, the chapter shows how African cultures can be understood using this framework.

Teachers and trainee teachers may wonder about the relevance of knowledge about culture to what they do in the classroom. They need to realise that the same features of community life that influence child development have also influenced the teacher. So the cultures of both the teacher and the child indirectly and directly influence interactions in the school. Educational texts such as that of Hollins (1996:2) state quite explicitly that,

> Schools, like other social institutions, are shaped by cultural values and practices . . . As a classroom teacher, you bring your own cultural norms into your professional practice. The extent to which your teaching behavior will . . . incorporate the cultures

of the students you teach may be influenced by your perceptions of the relationship between culture and school practices, political beliefs and conceptualisations of school learning.

If teachers are unaware of the impact of their culturally determined beliefs and values on teaching, they may not be able to achieve the goal of helping children to develop socially, emotionally, physically, and intellectually.

Traditional African values and behaviours

Although groups in various parts of Africa differ in the way they express certain values, the values themselves appear to be very widespread in the cultures of different groups across the continent. Some key values that may influence child development are discussed briefly in this section. In some instances long-held values are still important. In other instances new behaviours and values have had a marked influence on behaviours.

Family and kinship

Most societies in Africa were traditionally patriarchal and they still are. Power and authority are held by the male household head until his death. Then, brothers or male offspring take over. Ownership and control over economic resources as well as decision-making are the right and responsibility of the males in the lineage or family line. Women are valued mainly for their ability to produce sons who can perpetuate the lineage and its economic interests. Agriculture and the drudgery of household production benefit considerably from child labour, and hence a large number of children are considered essential to the family economy.

The patriarchal family organisation gives rise to unequal and paternalistic social relationships between men and women. Such practices as widow inheritance (where a man's widow is inherited by his brother), denial to women of inheritance or custody of children and lack of rights to own property or enter into legally binding agreements without the consent of husbands demonstrate the low status of women. Women are thus legal minors, permanently dependent on fathers, husbands and sons for their social status and economic welfare in the home and community. On a positive side, the family commonly includes the extended family relations. Relatives beyond one's immediate nuclear family (parents and siblings) occupy a central role in a family's social and economic planning. There is mutual social, economic and emotional support among extended family members. Thus, the care of the elderly, children and economically or socially stranded members of the extended family are burdens that are normatively shared, making the family a strong and positive force for the wellbeing of its members and of the broader society.

It is important to note, however, that in recent times the family has been subjected to disruptive changes. There is increasing evidence that the traditional social support systems are overwhelmed by high levels of poverty, AIDS victims, orphans, and people displaced by political and civil strife. In general discussions, some people assert that donor relief packages and government subsidy schemes have disrupted traditional family organisation and values. Communal or lineage land is being sold, thus rendering many family members landless. Other changes are also occurring. In Botswana, for example, minority ethnic groups such as Basarwa are reported to be experiencing loss of hunting land owing to the encroachment of other ethnic and cultural groups (Seboni, Dambe and Abosi 1999).

In some countries the need for employment has had a disruptive effect on family life. A UNICEF (1993) study showed that in Botswana, for example, migration to South Africa and rural-urban migration have created an unprecedented level of female-headed households, amounting to 47% of the households in the country. In most cases women in these households are single or live in consensual unions in which there is marginal paternal investment or economic contribution. While women have assumed additional burdens of economic support to the family, they are, in some instances, deprived of the principal sources of wealth and livelihood such as land and cattle. In 1991, the Botswana Ministry of Agriculture made a survey of 79 000 households and found that 62% of female-headed families had no cattle, compared with 32% of male-headed ones (UNICEF 1993). This situation is unique to Botswana, where there are more women than men, but the pattern of male migration for work is widespread across Africa and families in many countries are adversely affected by the absence of adult males.

Gender hierarchy

Apart from the biologically based capacities for reproduction, such as pregnancy, childbirth and breast-feeding, all other roles in society can be performed by both men and women. African society has generally based the division of labour on the 'comparative advantage' that men and women hold in performing certain tasks. For example, men's superior physical strength traditionally meant that they were the people who did especially heavy work, such as felling trees. Advances in science and technology, however, have reduced or eliminated most of or all of the arguments in support of traditional division of labour because physical strength is no longer the criterion for successful performance of many tasks. Thus the division of labour between men and women is now based on socio-cultural expectations. These expectations constitute the 'gender system'. The gender system is a hierarchy because power, prestige and wealth are attached to the roles performed by men in contradistinction to those that are performed by women.

In traditional African society the woman was seen as the man's personal property. Her rights were based on the interests of the man. Nare (1995) has observed that this obstacle to the full development of women in Africa remains. Nare maintains that it is the result of deeply rooted prejudices that emphasise the 'natural' inferiority of girls and women. Another obstacle for women is the cultural valuing of distinct distribution of roles and status to each sex. These prejudices, of course, find their basis in the African traditional image of the woman. Where men and women continue to hold traditional beliefs about their relative status, the development of girls is especially likely to be limited. Today progress towards greater equality may be seen. Some women are able to move from one social class to another, depending on their ability and education. However, as Mullei (1995) points out, the pattern of female movement from one social class to another varies between countries, depending on the indigenous culture, religion and economic status.

Marriage

Marriage in Africa is important and is regarded as an institution. But it is obvious that there will be non-marital sexual relationships in countries where women outnumber men and where polygyny (also called polygamy) is outlawed. In general, though, the marriage process is largely the same across the continent. Marriage is usually between the two communities involved, the boy's on one side and the girl's on the other.

Dowry is very important. It is demanded throughout Africa and it is paid by the men. It is evidence both that the man appreciates the marriage and that a marriage has, in fact, taken place. It also binds the families together and reduces the likelihood that couples will divorce, because divorce involves breaking the bond between the families and returning the dowry, and often this is not easy, even impossible. Where differences in marriage patterns do exist between ethnic groups, they often involve variations in dowry payments. In some cultures men pay dowry in the form of money, others in cattle or goods and gifts.

Early marriage for girls was traditionally common across the many tribes and religions of Africa, although the actual age at marriage varied from culture to culture. Men are still generally several years older than their first wife. In Botswana, for example, Seboni et al. (1999) found that women typically married in the age range 13–25 years and men in the range 21–35 years. The determining factor in male age at marriage is that the man must show he is able to look after a family before he is allowed to marry. Naturally, where polygyny continues to be practised, the husband may be many, many years older than later wives, especially if he has to accumulate sufficient wealth to provide dowry payments for the second or third wife.

Sexuality

Closely related to concerns about kinship and marriage are concerns about sexual knowledge and expression. Beliefs, values, and practices surrounding sexuality in Africa have implications for sexual health, sexual and social relationships. Traditionally, selected older people taught adolescents how to behave in their relationships with members of the opposite sex, usually in the context of initiation rites around the time of puberty. This education took place in isolation from the general community, where there were strong taboos against discussion of sexual matters (Caldwell, Caldwell and Quiggin 1994). Boys and girls received this teaching in separate groups.

It is worth noting that the taboos against discussing sexual matters remain strong today, despite the high prevalence of sexually transmitted diseases in African communities. Common sexually transmitted diseases, sexual problems and disorders are health issues that are shrouded in cultural mystique, stigma and taboos. Hence they are usually endured in silence. Africans attempting to inform young people about sexuality and sexually transmitted diseases struggle to face up to their own beliefs, and against cultural taboos about discussing these matters (Seboni et al. 1999).

The pregnancy of a married woman has always been highly valued. The African cultural value system gave, and continues to give, strong emotional and social support to pregnant women. But some traditional practices are more negative, such as female genital mutilation, and are aimed at controlling women's sexuality. The traditional perception and treatment of menstruation, infertility and miscarriage as polluting and mythical exposes women to isolation and neglect, and prevents constructive approaches to handling these problems using modern medical knowledge.

Other erroneous or harmful beliefs and practices documented in studies in Botswana include objections to modern practices such as episiotomy. In this procedure a small cut is made in the wall of the vagina during the birth of an infant. The procedure reduces the risk of random and irregular tearing of the vaginal wall, which can be difficult to repair and may heal badly (Ball 1988; Seboni 1993). Beliefs about male sexuality may also be harmful. Men in many parts of Africa fear the effects of using contraceptives because of myths and misunderstandings about the consequences of introducing new practices in their relationships with women (Sekgoma 1994; SIAPAC AIDS Unit 1994).

Tradition and child development

The very brief review of some features of African cultures that has been presented in the previous section shows that traditional cultural practices, values and beliefs continue to influence the behaviour of adults in Africa. A moment's thought will reveal that, as a result, most of these socio-cultural dimensions also seriously affect the way in which African children are brought up today and hence they influence the children's development. Children learn what people should do and how they should do it in their physical and cultural environment. The ideas and rules presented by adults become internalised by the children (are absorbed into children's thought processes) and influence their behaviours.

This process is referred to as 'enculturation' and begins at birth. Thus, the development of a typical African child is influenced by the culture and values of the African environment. For example, a child brought up in a Christian or Muslim environment will develop the norms and values of Christianity or Islam. Older traditional influences also continue to affect child development. Even today people may attribute some health problems to witchcraft. School failure may also be blamed on witchcraft. These kinds of beliefs impair children's development because parents embark on an outward instead of an inward search for causes of problems impairing the development of their children.

As this book explains in more detail in later chapters, socialisation practices in the home and in schools tailor girls and boys along stereotypical paths via unequal treatment. This is achieved through control of privileges, assignment of duties, access to health care and educational opportunities. Girls are mostly socialised to be obedient and pay deference and respect to men and elders. As a result, they do not develop the skills in asserting themselves and competing against others that are essential for social mobility in occupational and educational settings. Boys, on the other hand, are socialised to be independent and assertive, while also being taught to be respectful and obedient to elders.

Nare (1995) claims that although education is meant to bring about a change in the thinking in any given society, traditional African society does not seem to be ready for this change. Rather, he says, the influence of sexist cultural stereotypes in girls' access to school, and their retention once there, is very important. He notes that during the entire process of acquisition of knowledge in places such as Senegal and Burkina Faso, girls face a hostile environment of discrimination because the societies are primarily concerned with the success of boys. In Nigeria, too, cultural factors determine who goes to school. Although the economic status of the country allows boys and girls equal chances of attending school, in real practice the situation is different. Enrolment rates for girls in Nigeria's Christian south equal those of boys, while in the Muslim north, female enrolments are very low (Mullei 1995). (This problem is discussed in more detail in later chapters.)

Conclusion

Although it is easy to assume that traditional ideas and practices have little effect on the development of children in Africa in the twenty-first century, it is obvious that traditional ideas are still strong and that they continue to influence child development outcomes. Traditions are important to children's sense of who they are and where they belong, that is, in the development of their identity. Teachers need to recognise this. They should not assume that all influences from the past have been lost as they and the children they teach develop the skills and knowledge necessary for modern times. So, a more detailed exploration of the impact of the environment on child development is needed. This is presented in the following sections of the chapter.

Environment at the broadest level

Culture-wide values with regard to marriage and family, sexuality, and the status of women developed as people across Africa tried to understand and deal with problems that arose in their physical and social environment. But many other aspects of modern environment have an impact on the overall development of African children. Each child lives in a country or nation, and is a member of a particular ethnic group that has its own culture. Some people prefer to think that differences between groups and between individuals within groups are best explained by referring to nationality or ethnic group, so it is important to consider these terms. Another term that is often used by people when trying to explain why others behave in certain ways is *race*. The terms *traditional* and *modern* may also be used on occasion. These terms are included in the discussion in the present section.

The nation

A nation, country or state is a political entity and has fixed boundaries. It is often believed to consist only of people from one ethnic group, for example only Shona or only Xhosa. But this is clearly inaccurate. Most nations of the world, including those in Africa, have people in their total population who have different religious beliefs, eat different foods, live in differently shaped houses and generally have different traditions; in short, they think of themselves as belonging to different groups. Thus, a person from the Yoruba tribe has different beliefs and social practices from an Ibo person, whose beliefs and behaviours are different again from Hausas, and from those of other tribal groups in the same country, Nigeria. Within any one nation, therefore, there is usually considerable diversity. Trying to explain differences between people based on nationality is not helpful because of this diversity. It is not possible to say with any accuracy that all people in Nigeria have the same values and beliefs, because members of the different tribal groups may think quite differently about the same issues.

Race

Within a nation there are also likely to be people who are identified as belonging to different races. The word *race* refers to observable physical differences that are believed to be genetically based. It is used to divide people into very broad groupings, for example Caucasian, Asian and African. More informally, the words *white* and *black* serve the same purpose. Recent research in this area has used special tests called DNA tests to find out how similar various groups of people are genetically. These tests have shown that the word *race* describes only superficial physical difference such as skin and eye colour or nose shape. These differences are rather trivial, and hide the much greater genetic similarity between members of different *races*. In fact, people of all different colours, shapes and sizes are so closely related that the term *race* is no longer used by scientists. From this, it is evident that explaining differences in behaviour in terms of race is not useful either, although social use of the term currently persists. According to common use, then, people who seem to belong to the same *race* may belong to different groups. The groups may have quite different histories, values, beliefs and behaviours. Thus, Caucasians, or whites, from Sweden, Switzerland and the United Kingdom do not resemble each other very much except that they are all light skinned.

Ethnic group

Some people use the terms *ethnicity* or *ethnic group* as an explanation for differences between groups. When people talk about their ethnic group, they mean something more than just their race. Berry, Poortinga, Segall and Dasen (1992) state that ethnicity is usually believed to consist of two facets, one more objective and one subjective. From the objective point of view, there is an expectation of both biological and cultural continuity that can be observed and recorded. Biological continuity implies that one's ancestors were of the same ethnic group. At the cultural level, there is evidence that present-day culture is derived from earlier forms and practices, although specific practices may have changed over time. Subjectively, there is the sense of attachment to the same group, and identification with that group, referred to as ethnic or social identity (Tajfel 1978).

Khoo and Price (1996:2) define the term *ethnic* as referring 'to groups of families and persons who . . . feel themselves, or are felt by others, to be a separate people'. This feeling of separateness may be based on history, language, culture, religion or other shared characteristics. In Africa a person's ethnicity is usually defined in terms of tribal affiliation. A person will state that he or she is a Motswana (member of the Tswana tribe) or a Yoruba, and this sense of belonging to the group may be a source of psychological strength. On the other hand, it may not help in nation building and it is not helpful when one person is trying to understand another's behaviour. This is because many different experiences contribute to each person's sense of belonging or ethnicity. It is not possible to identify any one of these experiences as the one that causes a person to behave or think in a particular way.

Tradition and modernity

Besides belonging to an ethnic group within their nation, people in Africa live in a variety of environments that may also influence beliefs and behaviours. Most Africans live in rural areas in villages or small rural communities where they mix with members of their own clan and tribe. They continue to practise subsistence farming, although they may also sell some goods at the market. Their lives are frequently contrasted with the lives of those who live in bigger towns and cities. The terms *traditional* and *modern* are used to describe differences in lifestyle, behaviours and values between rural and urban dwellers. These two terms are not well defined. Generally, though, a person whose lifestyle is traditional behaves in ways that have been practised in a community or tribe over a long period. These behaviours developed in response to problems in the immediate environment some time in the past and have not been influenced by ideas or behaviours from other parts of the world. For example, a person building a new house using the kinds of materials and techniques that were used by members of the community when building houses in times past is showing a traditional behaviour.

Modern behaviours, in contrast, are those that have been influenced by ideas and practices from other countries, typically the technologically advanced countries of the northern hemisphere. A modern approach to house building might involve using concrete bricks and corrugated iron roofing or building a square house instead of the round one that used to be the preferred style in the community. People using a modern approach to problems can see that there are sometimes advantages in using information from outside their traditional culture. These people have more choice about the way they live, often because they are better educated than those who continue to live in a traditional style. They also have the opportunity to consider their values and beliefs from different perspectives and make a choice about which aspects of tradition they want to keep and which aspects of introduced ideas and practices they will adopt either completely or in some modified form.

The behaviour and practices of almost all people in Africa have been influenced by modernity to some degree. Village people or those living in rural communities may have experienced the least change in behaviours and values. People who live closer to the bigger towns and markets have experienced more change. (The term *peri-urban* is sometimes used to describe these people's experience and place of residence.) People living in major towns and big cities have probably experienced the greatest amount of change. However, even these categories are too simple. For example, a young adult who has recently moved to the city from a rural or peri-urban area has probably had less education, or lower-quality education, than a person who has had the advantage of going to a better-funded school in the city. The person from the rural background will have values and beliefs that are more influenced by traditional ways than a person who has grown up in an educated family in the city. But it is also possible for well-educated city people to over-emphasise the extent to which they have separated themselves from the past and given up old values. Well-educated Africans often feel some conflict about how they should behave, for example, when visitors arrive unexpectedly. The traditional obligation to provide hospitality may cause financial difficulties, but the urban dweller will often feel that despite these difficulties it is important to meet social obligations that have been taught since childhood.

So, the situation is more complex than it seems. Drawing a contrast between traditional and modern behaviours is too simplistic, because what a person does may reflect aspects of both tradition and modernity. It would be quite possible for a well-educated person to build a modern-style house using traditional materials, or to build a traditionally round house using modern materials such as concrete bricks and corrugated iron. Alternatively, a person whose values and lifestyle are almost entirely traditional might choose to have corrugated iron on his or her house rather than a thatched roof. Some people who have only recently been exposed to ideas and values from other cultures feel confused about whether they should retain traditional ways or adopt modern ones. For a few of these, the solution appears to lie in rejecting traditional values entirely. This can result in a loss of culture that is harmful to individuals and communities.

Conclusion

Ideas about nations or races cannot be used to explain the behaviour of groups of people because there is so much variability in behaviours of people from the same nation or the same race. The same problem arises in relation to modern or traditional behaviours; many behaviours are a mixture of the two. Another way of explaining differences in behaviour between different ethnic groups is needed. Differences in culture may result in differences in behaviour. This is discussed in detail in the following section.

Culture as environment

Culture is an important aspect of the total environment into which each child is born. Modern definitions of culture (e.g. Berry et al. 1992; Brislin 1990; P. B. Smith and Bond 1993) used by psychologists and others studying human behaviour in different ethnic groups typically come from definitions developed by anthropologists. Tylor's (1871, as cited in Berry et al. 1992) first definition described culture as the 'complex whole which includes knowledge, belief, art, morals, laws, customs and any other capabilities and habits acquired by man as a member of society'. Herskovits (1948:17) described culture simply as 'the man-made part of the environment'. This definition is still used, but it should be noted that this 'man-made' environment does not just consist of the material culture, houses, churches, mosques, fences and so on. It also includes ways of viewing the world, religious and other beliefs and values, and ways of thinking, interacting with others, and solving problems.

The culture of an ethnic group is not fixed, but changes in response to changes in the physical environment and in the social and political situation. Williams (1980) states that at any given moment the dominant culture of a community contains residual and emergent features. Residual features of culture are left over from earlier practices and beliefs. These practices continue to be effective in the present. For example, a mother who treats her child's sore throat with a herbal remedy that her own mother and grandmother found to be effective is using some cultural information from the past in her modern family. If she did not want to use old practices, she could visit the health clinic and obtain some more recently developed syrup, produced and tested by scientists in laboratories, perhaps in another country altogether.

Culture is also influenced both by extremely new features of the environment and by extremely old beliefs. New meanings, values and practices that are just being incorporated into the culture form the emergent features of that culture. A class of schoolchildren learning to use a computer are incorporating new behaviour into their lives and into their culture. Farmers using new technologies are also introducing new practices into the culture. Changes in their beliefs about technology and its relation to their lives introduce new meanings into their culture. In contrast, extremely old influences on current culture are called 'archaic' (Jayasiruya 1993). These archaic features of culture relate to past patterns and core values. They make up the historical tradition of a people and are often conveyed to children in folk stories, tales of travelling storytellers, and through traditional dance and rhyme. Children are likely to be exposed to residual, emergent and archaic aspects of their culture in the process of socialisation.

Modern developments in understanding the influence of culture

A close assessment of the relationship of culture to behaviour was made by Hofstede (1980). Hofstede's attempt to find out about some of the characteristic values of people with different cultures led him to conclude that there were marked differences in values across cultures. Hofstede's work has had a major influence on research into the relationship between culture and behaviour over a period of more than twenty years. It has generated huge amounts of research into all aspects of human behaviour. Although Hofstede was concerned with adult values and behaviours, his ideas have also been used in the study of children from various ethnic groups. These ideas are worth considering in some detail, because they will be referred to many times in the remainder of this book.

Hofstede (1980) described the preferred patterns of behaviour of people in various relationships and decision-making contexts. His study drew on information from a sample of over 100 000 employees at all levels of a multinational company in 39 of these countries and employees in another firm in the same industry in the fortieth country. From his data he identified four dimensions along which cultures varied. He also concluded that certain psychological traits occur more commonly in cultures in which specific values are widespread. The values themselves are as follows:

Individualism-collectivism

Hofstede (1980) describes cultures as individualist or collectivist according to the extent to which members of each culture are group-focused. More collective cultures are ones in which there is concern for the wellbeing of a clearly identified group. This involves taking account of others before the self, and being willing to live with a larger group and to work as a group. Members of individualistic cultures are more concerned with their own wellbeing and development. They have more flexible membership of a number of groups that they join and leave as they wish.

Uncertainty avoidance

Uncertainty avoidance refers to the extent to which members of a culture are comfortable with uncertainty. People in cultures where there is a high need to avoid uncertainty experience discomfort when rules are not clear. They tend to live in societies where job stability is valued, and to have rather high levels of stress. High scores on this dimension are likely to be associated with high scores on masculinity, another of the cultural dimensions. People with low uncertainty avoidance are more comfortable with risk-taking and are less rule-bound. As a group they are less likely to experience the psychological symptom of stress.

Masculinity-femininity

This describes the extent to which men and women value having clearly defined male roles. In high *masculinity* societies the psychological characteristics of independence and decisiveness are valued and people aspire to success. Societies identified as *feminine* allow more role flexibility for males. (Hofstede did not consider women's roles, despite the label.) Hofstede suggested that an alternative name for this set of values might have been 'Career versus social orientation', with 'social' replacing 'feminine'.

Power distance

This label describes the gap in personal power and influence between higher status people and those with lower status, for example the power difference between an employer and his or her employee. It is the employee's sense that there is a gap in power that is important. The more powerful people in any relationship tend to try to maintain or increase the interpersonal distance between themselves and others who are less powerful. In contrast, the less powerful try to reduce this gap between themselves and their superiors. *High power distance* commonly occurs in societies in which there are marked inequalities across a number of areas of life, for example wealth, rights and privileges. In high power distance cultures, people feel unable to challenge authority figures and may feel humble as a result. *Low power distance* is typical of more egalitarian, less hierarchical cultures.

Conclusion

Considering some aspects of the culture of different groups can provide general background knowledge about what makes people behave the way they do. The model developed by Hofstede (1980) has proved useful over time. It has contributed to a greatly increased understanding of the relationship between culture and behaviour.

Using a modern framework to study African cultures

Among many others, Rodney (1982) and Nsamenang (1992a) have pointed out that there was considerable variation between the experiences of different ethnic groups in Africa in the period prior to the arrival of the Europeans. The range of physical environments and climatic conditions, from tropical rain forest to savannah to desert, low to moderate to high rainfall falling seasonally as in the monsoon areas, or more generally throughout the year in other regions, resulted in widely different types of plants and animals. The problems that any one group had to solve in order to survive were quite different from those of people who lived in a region with another kind of climate and geography. But the material presented in the section 'Traditional African values and behaviours' in the early part of this chapter shows that the core cultural values were more similar than we might have expected. In many instances the core values were just expressed differently.

The differences and similarities between the traditional cultures of different ethnic groups in Africa can be examined using ideas from psychology, such as the framework developed by Hofstede (1980). Core cultural ideas change slowly. They influence patterns of interaction within the group over long periods. Wu (1996) has suggested that parental child-rearing practices change even more slowly than some other aspects of culture. This means that the way children are raised and the psychological characteristics they develop are very likely to have been influenced by the past. It is therefore important to consider the nature of traditional African societies in order to develop some understanding of the goals of African child-rearing today. Only limited amounts of published material about African cultures are available, so the conclusions presented in the following few pages are necessarily tentative.

Collectivism as a feature of traditional African cultures

It seems probable that the cultures of African ethnic groups in traditional societies were generally collective in Hofstede's (1980) sense. Most authors (e.g. Rodney 1982; Mazrui 1986) who have described African cultures in the past discuss the 'communalism' that was widespread. This refers to the concern for the maintenance and wellbeing of the group, to training children to be group-oriented and to the structures put in place to maintain harmony in relations with other group members. Features of language that emphasise sharing (e.g. sharing one's shade, sharing one's smiles) that are still widely used possibly provide additional evidence of concern for the wellbeing of the group that is the basis of collectivism.

Masculinity as a feature of traditional African cultures

The clear separation of roles based on gender in traditional African cultures, and the value both men and women place on this separation, is also widely reported in the anthropological and historical literature. In these masculine cultures (to use Hofstede's term), beliefs about the responsibility of one gender for specific tasks are strong. Taboos often prevent members of the other gender from undertaking defined tasks. At the most general level it is believed that women should collect water, do planting and weeding, cook and raise young children. They should continue to teach girls until their daughters reach maturity. Men teach boys the necessary skills for male work (herding cattle, fishing, going to war, hunting) once boys reach a minimal level of independence. More specific rules about who does what and when they do it vary between ethnic groups. So, although roles may be fixed within any one ethnic group, not all roles are, or were, fixed across the continent. For example, in a few communities men make the pots they use and women make the ones they use (Barley 1994), although in most parts of Africa women have always been the potters. Weaving is another task that was allocated to men in some ethnic groups and to women in others (Barley 1986).

This separation of roles and tasks has been attributed to the widespread warrior tradition in Africa (Mazrui 1986). Women were excluded from roles as warriors with only occasional exceptions during the pre-colonial period (Boulding 1992; Mazrui 1986). However, Mackey (1981) has offered another explanation. Mackey assessed patterns of interaction between the genders in subsistence economies in parts of the world outside Africa. He defined a 'plowman-protector complex' and says that the complex develops in communities where there is a perceived on-going threat to survival. The threat can come through aggression from outsiders, from the large animals that are herded for food, or from wild animal attack. Mackey states that in such communities men and boys spend more time together, and boys are taught to protect the women and girls from harm. Even in mixed social settings boys and men group together more than in cultures where there is less concern about physical safety. In addition, women and children associate less with men and more with other women in cultures where the male plowman-protector role is well established. The separation of men and boys from women and girls clearly favours the development of separate roles. It may also have contributed to the development of masculine cultures in many parts of Africa.

High and low power distance in the past

There may have been considerable variability in power distance in traditional cultures in Africa. Formal political structures varied across the continent from early times. Rodney (1982) notes that by the 1500s some African ethnic groups had already formed states with fixed boundaries, while others were organised more loosely. Statehood had developed to varying degrees. In some instances, states were rather weak, with a ruling class that was not very powerful and that had little impact on the daily lives of the people, except for occasional demands for taxes or tribute. However, some larger states had more powerful rulers and stronger political structures. These states already had a sort of class system, with a ruling class that was interested in obtaining luxury and prestige items, and a privileged class who were interested in promoting trade and manufacturing. In these systems a large labouring class was encouraged to supply produce surplus to their own needs, in order to permit more privileged classes to meet their own goals (Onwuejeogwu 1975; Rodney 1982).

Societies without fixed boundaries and formal political structures are referred to as 'stateless.' Statelessness was not necessarily associated with lack of complexity in social and political matters. Stateless societies in Africa were characterised by the absence of a class structure. They did not have formally recognised power figures. In the smaller units of family and village life, informal – but at times highly complex – social structures ensured that the wellbeing of the group was successfully maintained. These societies sometimes had relatively advanced material and non-material cultures (Rodney 1982). Onwuejeogwu (1975) mentions many examples of successful stateless societies across Africa, including the Tiv and Yako peoples of Nigeria and the Nandi in East Africa. Rodney (1982:47) mentions the Kikuyu of Kenya and the Ibo, noting that both of these ethnic groups had 'sophisticated systems of political rules based on clans and, in the case of the Ibo, on religious oracles and "secret societies"'.

In modern psychological language the differences in the extent to which societies had formal power structures and associated social classes reflect probable differences in power distance between ethnic groups. Where some group members had many more privileges and much more power than others, a culture would be more likely to value larger power distance between the more powerful and the less powerful. In contrast, the so-called stateless societies were more likely to value a small power distance between members of the community. In this regard they may have had more egalitarian values. These stateless societies included tribes of nomadic herders (Mazrui 1986).

High and low uncertainty avoidance in the past

Uncertainty avoidance is another dimension of culture that probably also varied quite a lot between ethnic groups in the past. In particular, there may have been general differences between farmers and herders in the extent to which uncertainty or risk taking was acceptable. For example, a farmer who suddenly decides to plant maize at a different time of year from the one that had been established over the years is at risk of having crop failure and of facing starvation in the subsequent year as a result. The need to behave in the same way as others in the past may perhaps be associated with a general preference for uncertainty avoidance in the culture. Onweujeogwu (1975) has provided evidence from anthropological studies that independent behaviours were required of herders who met change and variety as they cared for their animals.

These cultures probably expected a greater tolerance for uncertainty than was valued in farming communities.

African cultures today

The peoples of Africa have experienced rapid and continuous change in recent times and there appear to have been dramatic shifts in the cultures of the many ethnic groups who live on the African continent. Some might argue that traditional characteristics of culture have been eroded or lost. Once again, it is useful to consider Hofstede's (1980) work. Unfortunately, he obtained data in only one country in Africa and that was South Africa. He reported that, as a group, South Africans were fairly egalitarian and tolerated uncertainty. They were rather individualistic, but not highly so, and scored fairly highly on measures of masculinity.

Hofstede's (1980) data were gathered during the apartheid regime. It is therefore difficult to know how representative of the peoples of South Africa his findings were, because of the skewed selection of whites to positions of authority, while indigenous Africans were restricted to less powerful positions. On the other hand, Hofstede did discuss some other research that relates to the four dimensions of culture he had identified. His data, which suggest that African cultures are likely to be characterised by high power distance and uncertainty avoidance, collectivism and masculinity, are supported by evidence about where and when these characteristics occur today. Some of this material is shown in table 1.

Within the general values of the culture, there is room for considerable variation in practices. Ejiofor (1981) showed how individualism is valued within the Ibo family in Nigerian villages. In this ethnic group each member of the family is expected to express an honest opinion about a problem in the process of reaching a family agreement about it. But if the problem is also to be discussed in a community meeting, the family is expected to function as a collective group, adhering to the consensus that has been privately reached.

Both Mazrui (1986) and Onwuejeogwu (1975) describe cultures in which this pattern of private individualism and public collectivism occurs. This mix of individualism and collectivism, depending on context, needs to be further explored in Africa. (On the surface, it appears to be different from the kind of collectivism found in Asia, the region where collectivism has been most widely studied to date. In Asia subordinate members of the family commonly try to discover, by indirect means, the solution to the problem that older members of the family prefer. Then they offer that solution. Clearly, the young African and the young person in Asia are developing in different ways, although cultures in both regions are described as collectivist.)

Table 1 Features of society associated with different dimensions of culture

Cultural characteristic	Features of society
High power distance	More frequent in tropical and subtropical climates Traditionally low levels of technology used More traditional farming, less urbanised population Little wealth or wealth concentrated in hands of few Government unstable, autocratic or oligarchic, subject to rapid change by revolution Elected governments right wing, not interested in egalitarianism
High uncertainty avoidance	Occurs where life felt to be under continuous threat Aggression believed to be outcome of competition, consensus preferred Aggression against self or others more common than in low uncertainty avoidance cultures Occurs in 'younger democracies' with inherited system of laws Religious intolerance, emphasise hereafter, sinfulness Leaders of advanced age
Collectivism	Group decisions considered better than individual People thought of in terms of in-groups and out-groups Social relations predetermined in terms of in-groups
Masculinity	Men should behave assertively and women should care Sex roles should be clearly differentiated Men should dominate in all settings

Source: Adapted from Hofstede (1980)

It is possible, too, that there are other dimensions of culture that are not explored when Hofstede's model is applied to African cultures. This has already been found in another non-Western culture, that of the Chinese, where a fifth dimension of culture called the 'Confucian work ethic' is commonly reported (Chinese Culture Connection 1987). Some work by Schwartz (1994) on personal, rather than culture level values has suggested that Africans' personal values include what might be called 'spiritual values'. In this regard Africans' personal values differed from those of people from the other 43 countries where Schwartz obtained data. This suggests the possibility that, as in the Chinese culture, core values in African cultures may include an extra dimension.

Some authors have argued that cultures become less collectivist and more individualist as they modernise. It is true that many well-educated city-dwelling people in Africa describe themselves as behaving in more individualistic ways, such as making decisions about jobs, places of residence and so on without the traditional reference to their larger group that is characteristic of those with more collectivist values. However, Kagitcibasi (1996) has assessed the changing patterns of relationships in a number of developing economies. She identifies a pattern whereby the close relationships valued in traditional collective cultures are maintained when educated, financially independent city dwellers in developing countries no longer need material support (e.g. money, food) from the group. Thus, pleasure in relationships with, and obligations to, members of the extended family or clan may remain even when these educated people no longer expect their family to help with children's school fees, housing costs, or daily provision of food.

Conclusion

Culture has often been used to explain behaviour and is clearly important since it allows us to consider general preferences for ways of behaving within groups. Studies of the values of a large number of ethnic groups have shown that using Hofstede's model of culture level values provides one way of thinking about culture and cultural difference. It seems likely that this approach can also be useful when considering African cultures. To date, however, conclusions about culture level values rely mostly on information about the past. An interesting finding, that Africans are concerned with spirituality to a degree that it may be a core value, merits further investigation.

A limitation to the usefulness of studying culture is that it still does not explain the behaviour of any one individual on one specific occasion. Hofstede (1980) himself recognised that the dimensions he identified are culture-wide characteristics so that they contribute mainly to our understanding of general preferences for interactions with others in the group. It is also possible, as Schwartz (1996) has pointed out, for apparently contradictory values to co-exist in the same culture. For example, in a culture in which high power distance is valued, humility is also valued. Workers interacting with employers are expected to show humility, whereas the employer is haughty. Should the worker be promoted, he or she will also express haughtiness in interaction with subordinates. Thus, the capacities to express haughtiness and humility co-exist in members of the culture and both are valued. These opposing values result in differing sets of behaviours, depending on the relative status of the individual. To learn about individual behaviour and the way it develops, it is necessary to look more closely at how these culture level values influence children's development.

Culture and child development

To understand how culture level values influence child development it is necessary to consider what happens in the child's family and local community. Naturally, this includes patterns of interaction between parents and children and between teachers and children during the child's school years. Psychologists and anthropologists have developed a number of theories about how the environment influences what children learn.

Bronfenbrenner (1979, 1988) described a hierarchy of four systems, each of which influences child development. He named these systems the microsystem, mesosystem, exosystem and macrosystem. The microsystem is closest to children and has the most direct influence. This includes events that occur at home, in the classroom, and in the playground. Children are interacting directly with others in these settings. Obviously, this means that when parents act in a way that is consistent with the general values in their culture, they pass some information about these values to the child. For example, if parents live in a high power distance culture they will act in ways that teach their children to behave respectfully towards powerful people in the community.

Events in the next system, the mesosystem, still influence the child, although their effects are more indirect. The mesosystem consists of the links between the various settings that directly influence the child. So the quality of the relationship between home and school is a mesosystem influence that is still quite close to the child. In high power distance cultures, these links may be quite distant and formal, whereas in low power distance cultures there may be more egalitarian relationships between parents and teachers.

The last two systems are further from the child. The exosystem includes events that the child is not directly involved in, but that still influence his or her development, such as the parents' work. Finally, the broadest influences on child development, at the macrosystem level, are the social institutions in the society, for example the ways in which political events and decisions alter family life and experiences.

Bronfenbrenner (1988) believes that it is not really possible to understand child development without taking all these influences into account. The extent to which parents hold traditional beliefs and behave in traditional ways influences how the child develops, so do their beliefs about schooling and about how much they should be involved in school-related activities. Teachers' beliefs about tradition and modernity and the extent to which they encourage parents to be involved in their children's schooling will also alter the child's development. An old study that is still widely cited (Kohn 1969) has shown that the nature of the parents' work, whether they are able to be independent decision-makers or are more likely to be instructed as to what they should do, is associated with differences in what they teach their children. The stability of political systems, the quality of local government decisions, and the degree of support for struggling families add the final influences to child development outcomes.

A second view of influences on child development is that of Super and Harkness (1986). These authors used the term *developmental niche* to refer to the broad environment in which children develop. They are concerned with three major subsystems. These are, first, the physical and social settings in which the child lives; second, the 'culturally regulated customs of child care and child-rearing' (p. 552); and third, the psychology of the caretakers. These authors emphasised the very personal nature of the environment. For example, a child who is born first in the family enters a different environment from that into which the second child is born, since the first-born is without siblings, at least during the early part of his or her life, while the second-born does not have this experience.

Similarly, variations in the physical world mean that children born in different years experience a different environment. Children born in a time of drought have different early experiences from those of children who are born when there is adequate food and water. This difference is not just in terms of how much food is available, but is associated with different levels of caregiver distress and time spent away from home seeking supplies. Thus, caregivers may be both psychologically and physically less available to children during times of drought than when food is plentiful. Older children in the family may be able to cope with this unavailability, but very young children may be less likely to obtain the kind of care that optimises their development.

A detailed model of how the environment influences the behaviour and psychological characteristics of individuals was first proposed by Berry (1976; 1994) in relation to adult behaviours and characteristics. It has now been developed further (Berry, Poortinga, Segall and Dasen 2002). The model, shown in figure 1, incorporates major background factors such as the physical environment or ecological context and the socio-political context. According to the model, biological adaptations to the environment and cultural adaptations to the socio-political situation combine to influence the genetic material and cultural information that is transmitted to subsequent generations. Together with other influences this results in differences in both the observable behaviours and the inferred characteristics of members of a group. Although Berry et al. discuss their model in relation to cross-cultural interactions, it can be a useful aid when considering child development. The only box that would be modified in this instance is the one labelled 'Acculturation'.

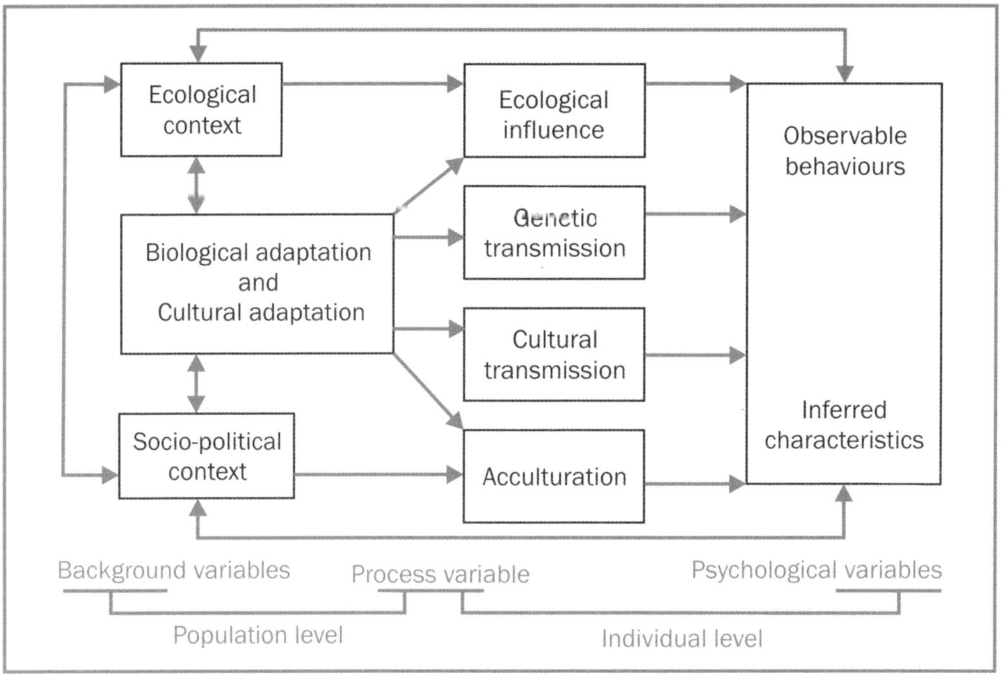

Note: For developing children, the word 'acculturation' can be replaced by 'enculturation' without changing the meaning of the table.
Source: Berry, Porrtinga, Segall and Marshall (2002:11).

Figure 1 An ecocultural framework of relationships among classes of variables employed in cross-cultural psychology

Ogbu (1981, 1988) has proposed a model that relates directly to child development. This model, shown in figure 2, recognises the initial impact of the environment in determining what tasks are required. According to the model, members of the community develop certain motor, cognitive, language, and social-emotional skills and characteristics as they find ways of coping with the environment. Certain patterns of social organisation also develop and become valued in the culture. Adults who show the required characteristics for task completion and group survival become models of success.

Parents and others in the community develop theories about what they should do when raising their children to produce a new generation of adults with desired competencies. Parents then try to instil these characteristics in their children during the process of child-rearing. They do this by using child-rearing techniques that they think will bring the desired result. Children in the group develop in ways that are similar. All develop skills that will ensure the continued survival of the group.

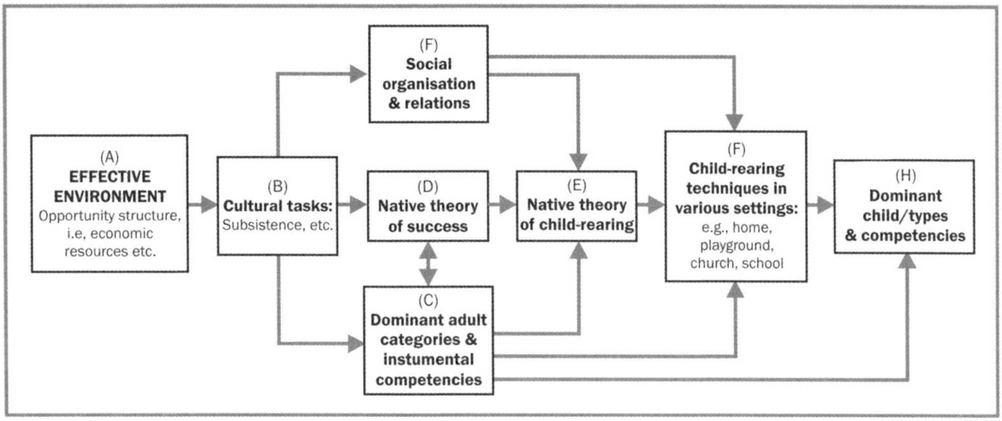

Source: Ogbu (1981:422)

Figure 2 A cultural-ecological model of child-rearing

These authors all acknowledge that behaviour is influenced by both the physical and social environment. They recognise that besides growing up in the man-made environment that constitutes their culture, children are developing in a physical environment. The man-made environment is not independent of the physical environment. Children are taught the ways of behaving, as well as the values and attitudes that prevail in their community in the process of enculturation, and adults who move away from their country of birth show some psychological changes as their environment changes.

Parents' beliefs and child-rearing

It is clear that these theorists agree that parents' beliefs and values have an impact on what they do when they are raising children, on what they tell their children, and on how they interpret or understand their children's behaviours. So it is important to consider parental beliefs more closely. Parental beliefs are based on commonsense rather than factual evidence and are seldom discussed. They are seen as being so obviously true that there is no point in talking about them. Everyone in the community will agree. For example, almost all parents in many countries agree that children should help with household chores. When they talk about children doing household chores, they do not ask 'Is it necessary for children to do chores?' but 'What is a reasonable amount of help to ask my child to give?' Parental beliefs can have a powerful impact on how adults go about raising or teaching their children.

Psychologists and others have only recently begun to study the ideas and beliefs that adults in different parts of the world have about how best to live in their group or community. They use the terms *folk theory*, *naive theory* or *ethnotheory* to refer to the kind of knowledge that ordinary people in each community have about what is important, how to do things, how to teach things, and so on. Such knowledge is not scientific, but is powerful, because it is implied in what is done. It is also procedural. This means it is knowledge about how to do things. This kind of knowledge contrasts with more explicit, formalised (declarative) knowledge that comes from study in science and other fields of research (Sigel and Kim 1996). Ethnotheory, as it relates to children, includes beliefs that parents have about being a parent, about child development, and about child-rearing (Shaver, Schwartz, Carson, and O'Connor 1987; K. D. Smith 1995). These beliefs have been called *parental beliefs* (Sigel and Kim 1996), *parents' cultural beliefs* (Harkness and Super 1996) or *parental ethnotheories* (Super et al. 1996).

Parental beliefs are generalisations that influence what parents do when raising their children. In turn, parents' beliefs are influenced by their child's responses to that behaviour (Harkness, Super and Keefer 1992). Parental beliefs tell parents what children are like and what they can be expected to do (Valsiner and Litvinovic 1996). They almost certainly include beliefs about children's abilities, for example 'girls are better at sewing than boys', 'boys are better at mathematics than girls', and beliefs about the experience and expression of emotion such as 'boys express anger physically' or 'girls express sadness by crying'. They include timetables for development, including development of motor skills, cognitive skills, social skills and emotional control (e.g. Hess, Kashiwagi, Azuma, Price and Dickson 1980; Goodnow, Cashmore, Cotton and Knight 1984).

Parents' beliefs probably include ideas about how children learn, what they should learn, and how it should be taught. In addition, parents probably have certain beliefs about the influence of the physical environment on child development. For example, they may believe that eating certain foods helps keep children healthy, while other foods will make them ill even where there is no proof that these foods have such effects. Or they may believe that certain activities are harmful for girls, again without any evidence that this is the case. These beliefs cover all aspects of development and underpin socialisation practices used by parents with their offspring throughout childhood (Super et al. 1996).

The school as cultural environment

Schools reflect the culture of the community. Where the culture of the community is collective, the school will generally teach ways of behaving that are consistent with collective values. Where the culture has clearly defined and different roles for men and women, the school will generally also have separate roles for male and female staff and will teach pupils how to behave in ways consistent with their gender. This is also true of the other two dimensions of culture – uncertainty avoidance and power distance.

But the extent to which this is true in African schools is unclear. Children in many schools lack the opportunity to work as a group, the preferred style of work in collective cultures. This is almost certainly an outcome of the introduction of formal schooling to Africans by Europeans in the nineteenth century. In European schools at that time children sat in rows, recited aloud, and were punished rather severely for minor misdemeanours. Some of these practices became incorporated into African cultural beliefs about how children learn in school and are still practised today.

In addition there is the lasting influence from nineteenth-century and early twentieth-century missionary education. Missionaries were interested in educating African children so that they would become good Christians, and colonial administrators wanted the mission schools to teach Africans enough to be able to perform low-level clerical tasks (Makulu 1971). In this context Africans developed ideas about the reasons that schooling was worth having. Makulu stated that,

> Some of the tribesmen who converted (to Christianity) came for the fascination of the white man's knowledge and promise of a better life rather than because of faith and understanding of Christian teaching. Education, more than anything else, was the compelling factor, since education was seen as the white man's key to success (1971:8).

Education permitted the individual to remove himself from tribal controls and get away from manual work.

Makulu (1971) claimed that the outcome of this pragmatic view of education was that the psychological and social development of the child was neglected in African schools, that children were growing up with a limited knowledge of their own culture and that they believed that solutions to problems came from outside Africa. A Ninga chief in Cameroon, who said to a visiting European anthropologist that 'white men and black men are brothers, it's just that white men are cleverer' (Barley 1986) also expressed such a mistaken view more recently.

Besides reflecting these general cultural beliefs to some degree, schools have their own explicit and implicit beliefs and cultures. An explicit belief is one that is clearly stated. An implicit belief is a hidden belief that affects what happens in the school. An example of the explicit culture concerns regulations with regard to punishment. In most countries now there are regulations that prevent teachers from using corporal punishment. Some teachers will agree with these regulations and some will not, but all are required to obey them. Among teachers, some understand that excessive physical punishment produces such high levels of anxiety in pupils that they cannot learn. These teachers develop a set of beliefs about punishment that support not using the strap or cane when punishing children. They learn to work within the explicit framework for education laid down by the head teacher or the educational administrators in the country. In this instance, the culture of the school may be quite different from that of the community, where parents probably believe that it is all right to beat their children.

But the implicit culture of the school may remain powerfully in favour of using the cane. This implicit, unspoken, or hidden culture may influence the teachers' actions. Teachers who disagree with regulations forbidding caning may stop using the strap or cane to punish children, but may replace these means of punishment with pinching or hair-pulling, justifying these practices to themselves as culturally acceptable and not specifically forbidden in the regulations. Their cultural valuing of physical punishment means that they continue to use it in their classrooms. Their behaviour is based on a naïve theory about what helps children to learn. Such teachers have not developed the understanding of psychology in the classroom that is required for truly professional management of children.

Other parts of the implicit culture of the school are concerned with whose culture is being conveyed to the pupils. Generally, this is the culture of the dominant or majority group in the country. Where minority group children are required to behave in ways consistent with the majority culture, their learning can be reduced. These children will find it difficult to learn in a situation where their natural ways of behaving are criticised and misunderstood. But the majority group teacher who is working with children from a minority ethnic group may not even realise that he or she reacts negatively to some of their behaviours. Problems such as these are more likely to occur with increasing urbanisation. Teachers in towns are perhaps more likely than rural teachers to be working with children drawn from the more mixed ethnic and social environments of the larger towns and cities. Teachers can reduce or eliminate the negative impact of assuming that their way is the 'normal' way, but they can do this only if they understand and accept cultural difference as a normal part of life.

Conclusion

Differences between ethnic groups and nations provide some of the information that is needed for understanding the ways in which adults and children behave.

But a great deal of information is lost if these are the only clues that are used. Adults' cultural values provide some additional clues as to the preferred behaviours of the group as a whole, but again do not yield much information about individuals or about how young children become socialised. It is clear, however, that African teachers can use information about children's physical, social and cultural environment as a starting point in their search for understanding how children develop. Parental beliefs about how children develop are important, as are the beliefs held by teachers themselves. Teachers need to gain knowledge of these kinds of beliefs if they are to become effective in the classroom.

In your community (one)

This chapter has made very general statements about cultural influences on values and behaviours. To explore your own culture further, complete some of the following activities:

1. List ways of behaving that most people in your ethnic group think are important. Note beside each behaviour whether men or women (or both) think this behaviour is important. Then indicate whether the behaviours are only important to old people, middle-aged and younger, or whether this behaviour is still strongly valued at all age levels. What does this tell you about culture change?
2. Talk to an elderly person in your ethnic group about what he or she thinks are important values for the group. Do you agree, or do you have some different values? What has contributed to your values?
3. Read an anthropological study of your ethnic group, if one has been done at any time. Can you see evidence of any of these behaviours, values, beliefs in yourself? In others in your ethnic group?
4. Talk to a person of your own age group but from a different ethnic group about values and behaviours. Discover common values, perhaps expressed in different behaviours.
5. Think about your own family. Sometimes the behaviours and values of a family are different from those held by the majority of the same ethnic group. List family values or ways of behaving that are atypical for your group. Comment on whether you think your family's ways are better or worse than those of the majority of the group, or just different.

Chapter Three

Family and community influences on child development

Introduction

Parents' beliefs and values influence children's psychological and social development because beliefs and values influence the ways parents behave as they raise their children. But the family does not exist in a vacuum. As Bronfenbrenner (1988) has pointed out, the broader social system and events in the working world of parents also influence child development. The present chapter describes some beliefs about child development, some child-rearing practices, and ways in which characteristics of the family life and society influence the development of African children.

Beliefs about development

African parents, like parents everywhere, have learnt about child development in their ethnic group through observation, listening and discussion, and experience. Because family networks include many children, young African parents have also probably had more practice in dealing with children than is common today among the small families of the northern hemisphere. Because of their experiences, new parents have developed beliefs about child development such as those described in this section.

Belief in the existence of innate psychological characteristics

Traditional African beliefs and modern scientific research both affirm that some characteristics of the child are determined before birth. This is implicitly recognised in cultures where children are seen as reincarnations of ancestors. Nsamenang (1992a), for example, has reported that among the Nso of Cameroon there is much discussion about the probable characteristics of the neonate (newborn) and that this discussion includes reference to characteristics of his or her ancestors. Similarly, Zeitlin (1996) points out that various groups of Yoruba in Nigeria may use divination in the first few days of an infant's life to discover what its psychological characteristics will be. The conclusions reached may have long-term effects on child-rearing practices that are then put in place, with special efforts being made to overcome potential flaws in character. Finally, Barley (1986) states that the Dowayo in Cameroon believe that bad character may be passed from one generation to the next. They put special ritual procedures in place to prevent this from happening.

Modern research shows that the genetic inheritance of the child is determined at the moment of conception. At this time the newly formed embryo receives genes from both mother and father who, at the moment when they were conceived, had themselves received genes from both their parents. Genes determine many of the characteristics of the potential person (Berk 2000). In this way, modern knowledge confirms and expands on traditional African awareness that infants had characteristics that had been present in earlier generations. This happens in the same manner in all pregnancies, and is described in a great deal of detail in many existing child development texts.

A belief that development progresses by stages

Like parents everywhere, African parents hold culturally valued beliefs about the various phases or stages through which children pass as they develop. These are reflected in the widespread traditional practice of holding initiation ceremonies to mark the changes in status that accompany changes in physical and social maturity. LeVine et al. (1996) and Nsamenang (1992a) have outlined stages of development. Since these authors describe stages as perceived by ethnic groups at opposite sides of the continent, it is worth comparing their descriptions. Table 2 (on page 38) shows the developmental stages identified by these different authors. Stages that are conventionally presented in texts on human development are also shown.

Nsamenang (1992a) reports that the various stages of child development identified in West Africa generally approximate the stages that are referred to in modern child development texts, although in the West African belief system the periods before birth and after death are included as stages in the life cycle. Prior to birth each individual is believed to exist in the spiritual plane and after death in the ancestral plane. The inclusion of these two phases of life reveals a belief in the continuity of life from the past, through the present, to the future.

In addition to these two stages, Nsamenang identifies seven stages or phases in the part of the life cycle that occurs between the birth of a child and his or her death in old age. In each stage the main developmental task is a social one. Among the Nso of Cameroon, for example, the period of the newborn, which ends with the naming ceremony a few days after birth, is a period in which the future development of the child is predicted by members of the family and broader community group who meet and discuss his or her characteristics. Traditionally, the name chosen was one that fitted with expectations for the child's future development, although the modern tendency is to choose names for other reasons, often simply because of the parents like a particular name.

The third stage in the West African belief system is the period of social priming. It is concerned more with physical development (e.g. development of social smiling, sitting up), but teaching for culturally determined socially acceptable behaviours also begins at this early stage. This is followed by a period of social apprenticeship, which begins when the child learns to walk, and continues throughout childhood. At this time children are expected to begin to recognise, to learn about, and to practise their various social roles in the household, kinship network, and public spheres. During adolescence young people are formally introduced to the knowledge and behaviours required in adulthood, they gain social entry into the adult world and are given opportunities to practise new skills. This period, therefore, is seen as one of social induction or social internship. The seventh phase, adulthood, commences when the young person marries, and the eighth at the onset of old age.

LeVine et al. (1996) show that the life stages of Gusii men and women, although similar, are not identical. In Gusii culture circumcision rites mark the transition from childhood into early adulthood. LeVine et al. state that 'men and women want children, worldly goods, and spiritual safety and immortality' (p. 81). There is a recognised timetable for achieving these goals, social recognition for their early attainment, and stigma if they are not reached at culturally acceptable times. Although these authors did not include the spiritual realm in their table, they recognise that it is important for the Gusii. Individuals move from one stage to the next when they have reached the physical and social maturity that fits them for the next stage. Thus, it is clear that there is quite a lot of similarity in ideas about child development between the Gussi and the Nso, despite the large geographical distance between them.

Table 2 Stages of development according to different models

West African stages of social development	Gusii life stages		Conventional developmental stages*
	Female	Male	
Spiritual self-hood			Prenatal stage
Period of the newborn	Infancy	Infancy	Neonatal stage
Social priming			Infancy
Social apprenticing	Uncircumcised girl	Uncircumcised boy	Childhood
Social entrée			Puberty
Social induction/ internship	Circumcised girl	Circumcised boy warrior	Adolescence
Adulthood	Married woman	Male elder	Adulthood
Old age/death	Female elder		Senescence/death
Ancestral self-hood			--?--

* = as described in northern hemisphere research
Source: Adapted from Nsamenang (1992:148) and LeVine et al. (1996:81)

Beliefs that certain outcomes are desirable

Socialisation has been defined as the process 'through which children acquire the beliefs, values, and behavior considered appropriate for people in their society and culture' (Berndt 1992:429). Besides valuing obedience and responsibility, parents across much of Africa traditionally wanted children to learn to show respect towards elders, to control expression of emotion in public, and to develop strategies for resolution of conflict that avoided direct confrontation (Kayongo-Male and Onyango 1984; Kilbride and Kilbride 1983). Even where physical fighting between children was permitted or encouraged, as in some groups in which a warrior class was important, respect for elders, obedience, and other values that were common elsewhere were still required (P. Mayer and I. Mayer 1970; Ryback, Sanders, Lorentz, and Koestenblatt 1980; Nsamenang 1992a).

These sorts of outcomes are still widely valued in modern Africa, as Nsamaneng (1992a; 1992b) confirmed. Nsamenang interviewed 347 Nso parents in Cameroon, asking about the goals of socialisation practices used with their children. A total of 66% of parents said that they had responsibility for instilling good character, 53% said they should encourage a willingness to work and 50% wanted their children to make good progress at school. They expected that their children would be obedient (35%) and wanted them to develop properly (25%) and to become competent in some vocational skill (20%). In their old age they expected that their children would provide financial support (7%) and give them a decent burial when the time came (12%).

Different expectations may arise when mothers have received some schooling. Lloyd (1970) interviewed Yoruba mothers (and some fathers) of children aged 5 to 6 years in Ibadan. She compared the expectations of 30 traditional market women with 30 women who had had a minimum of four years secondary schooling. The educated women were typically married to well-educated men who held high-ranking positions or were wealthy merchants. They were, therefore, part of a small elite group in the city at that time. As table 3 shows, some expectations with regard to children's behaviour varied in conjunction with different levels of education.

Table 3 Expectations concerning the well-behaved child (% of responses)

Group	Behaviours shown by child					
	Obedience	Errands	Household chores	Self-reliance	Sociability	Intellectual achievement
Market women	20	41	9	7	11	11
Elite women	18	10	15	22	22	11

Source: Adapted from Lloyd (1970:85)

Women in the elite group were less likely than traditional women to demand instant obedience, although mothers in both groups expected obedience from their children. Mothers' responses to questions about running errands or doing household chores might also provide information about expectations for obedience, because mothers might insist on immediate completion of tasks or accept that the child would do them when he or she is ready. Lloyd suggested that when expectations about obedience and about errands, which imply a demand for obedience, were taken together, there was evidence that elite mothers made fewer demands for obedience than traditional mothers. However, it is possible that elite mothers made fewer demands for work because they had other adult caregivers in the home who could do errands and household chores, rather than because they had different expectations about obedience.

Mothers expected their 5- to 6-year-old children to be responsible as well as obedient. Lloyd believed that running errands, doing household chores, being self-reliant and sociable, and working hard towards intellectual achievements were all responsible behaviours. As is evident in table 3, there was some variation between the more traditional and the elite group on some of these dimensions. The lack of evidence that elite mothers valued intellectual achievement more than traditional mothers is perhaps puzzling. But other data showed that 14% of elite mothers mentioned intellectual achievement first when describing their expectations as compared with only 6% of traditional mothers. This suggests the possibility of a difference in values with regard to this aspect of development. Elite mothers also prioritised sociability (mentioned first by 31%) while fewer traditional mothers did so (15%). Instead, 55% of traditional mothers mentioned children's ability to run errands first, compared with only 3% of elite mothers. Again, this might reflect the demands of daily life among traditional families.

Beliefs that boys and girls should be treated differently

As in other cultures around the world, parents in Africa have traditionally believed that boys and girls should be socialised differently. In the past, boys in traditional environments were increasingly separated from girls during middle childhood and later, spending constantly increasing amounts of time with their fathers and with other men. Boys were taught to break in new land for farms and learned some specific trades, such as black-smithing. They were taught skills required for success in public life, and learned to hunt and fight. Girls spent more time with other girls and women and traditionally learned the skills required to be successful wives, mothers and producers of food. Today, many parents still think it is desirable for boys and girls to learn different behaviours, although husbands and wives may disagree over this issue (Palmer 1993). The strength of this belief may vary with education and religion. For example, in better-educated urban families a more egalitarian attitude may mean that differences in treatment of boys and girls is less evident. Moslem parents may continue to value differences between boys and girls strongly.

Subtle differences in the way mothers respond to their children from the first few months of infancy have been reported in Africa, as elsewhere. Goldberg (1977) observed urban Zambian mothers interacting with their infants. She found that mothers were likely to vocalise around the same time as their daughters cried or made some sound, but did not respond much to them as they moved about. In contrast, they were more likely to touch their sons when they moved about than to respond to vocalisations. Studies from the field of behaviourism (e.g. Kazdin 1989) show that these maternal responses would increase the frequency with which girls made sounds and the boys moved about rather than making sounds.

These differences in treatment remain evident throughout the children's lives. Parents in many parts of Africa are less likely to send their daughters to school than they are to send their sons (UNICEF 2000a), a choice which reflects the value placed on sons as future providers for the family. When they do go to school, daughters may be expected to do more chores after school (Kayongo-Male and Onyango 1984). The lack of opportunity to do homework can have an adverse effect on girls' progress at school, resulting in loss of motivation and feelings of low self-esteem that further impede learning. Girls from Moslem families are less likely than their brothers or girls of other faiths to go to school. The high value placed on female chastity and honour in the Moslem faith means that girls marry at a young age (Mathews, Everett, Binedell and Steinberg 1995). Again, this reflects cultural ideas about the different ways boys and girls should be raised.

Conclusion

Differences in beliefs are associated with differences in the decisions parents make about what is best for their children and the ways they behave towards them. Some of these responses are made consciously, with certain goals in mind, but in many instances parents do not think much about what they are doing. They act in certain ways because these actions are consistent with beliefs that are widespread in their community and ethnic group.

General socialisation practices

Like parents everywhere, African parents begin to socialise children towards desired behaviours during their first year. Traditionally, the process of teaching children the desired behaviours involved all members of the broader community. Children were believed to belong to everyone, not just their parents (Kayongo-Male and Onyango 1984). More recently there has been some erosion of this belief. However, because values that relate to goals of child-rearing appear to change slowly, it is likely that this value continues to influence adults as they raise children in their community to some extent, even today.

Infants in traditional settings in Africa live in a dense social environment, although ethnic group differences have been reported in just how much social interaction goes on around the child. These differences relate in part to the way the housing compound is laid out. LeVine et al. (1996) described differences between the crowded compound life of Yoruba infants in Ibadan, Nigeria, and the lives of women and children among the Gusii of Kenya in the mid-1950s and early 1960s.

At that time, women in both ethnic groups lived in polygynous marriages, following their traditional lifestyle. Among the Yoruba, a co-wife had her own hut within a shared compound. Visitors were common and interacted with everyone in sight. Cultural norms required cheerful interaction, lengthy and hilarious conversation, and expressions of concern for the wellbeing of others. LeVine et al. (1996) point out that similar, very social arrangements have been reported among the Giriama of Kenya and the Fulani of Burkina Faso. In contrast, a Gusii co-wife in the study had her own yard and received only occasional personal visitors. They believed that excessive sociability was dangerous and lived by a general code of restraint. Visitors to the compounds elicited quite different responses from the children. Gusii children reacted with fear, while Yoruba children were interested in what was going on. Although lifestyles may have changed in recent times, it is likely that differences in child-rearing remain.

In this social setting the infant is never alone. LeVine et al. (1996), for example, made detailed records of patterns of care among the Gusii in Kenya. In the first nine months at least one or two people were within 1,5 metres (5 feet) of the infant for over half the time. About 20% of the time three or four adults or older female siblings were within this distance of the child. The infant was most likely to be more than 1.5 metres from any other person only when placed on a mat, sleeping. Fathers were rarely near the infant at this age, and male children were only occasionally nearby. Female children were often even more likely to be present than the mother.

In the first few months infants in traditional settings are in physical contact with their mother or some other adult for 70% or more of the times they are observed. Bril and Zack (1989, as cited by Rabain-Jamin 1989) found that in West Africa infants were held as much as 90% of the time at the age of six months. Konner (1977) reported that !Kung mothers in his study held their infants for 70% to 80% of the time during their first year. In contrast, Efe infants aged 18 weeks who were studied by Tronick, Morelli and Winn (1987) in the Democratic Republic of Congo were held by someone who was not their mother for 60% of the time.

The extent to which individual others are involved in infant care varies from one ethnic group to another. Mulder and Milton (1985) reported that Kipsigis fathers were traditionally excluded from seeing their infant in the first few months. Although this custom is now breaking down, it is still rare for Kipsigis adult and adolescent males to interact with infants. Tronick, Morelli and Ivey (1992) found that Efe fathers were more involved with very young infants than the Gusii were in studies LeVine et al. (1996) reported. But fathers still only held their infants during about 6% of times they were observed. Efe infants were frequently passed from one caregiver to another. At four months they were held by about eight different people per hour (Tronick, Morelli and Winn 1987). At five months, they were held by their mothers about 50% of the time, by other adults, excluding the father, about 18% of the time, and by other children during 29% of the observations (Tronick, Morelli and Ivey 1992).

Patterns of infant care change rapidly after about six months, but the change is mainly in the amount of time the child is not interacting with anyone, and in the amount of time other children are caring for him or her. Among the Efe, for example, the amount of care provided by fathers and other adults remains fairly constant, but by three years children are with their mothers only about 21% of the time, and spend 62% of time with other children (Tronick, Morelli and Ivey 1992). A similar shift towards increasing time spent with other children, often older female siblings, is reported for the Gusii (LeVine et al. 1996).

In traditional settings, older infants and very young children are cared for in mixed-gender, mixed-age groups, with children aged about 8–10 years on average having responsibility for care of these very young ones. In some instances caregivers might be as young as six years (Harkness and Super 1985). When children in the age group 6–10 years attend school they are obviously not available to care for toddlers and preschoolers. The mother may need to expand her role from being the person who ensures the physical wellbeing of the infant to one in which she also has a much greater responsibility for its cognitive and social-emotional growth (Leiderman and Leiderman 1974).

Wealthier and better-educated mothers who are employed outside the home may hire a substitute caregiver. This can create problems if the substitute caregiver comes from a different ethnic group from that of the family. Such a person may not have a good command of the language or culture of the host family. This can reduce her capacity to provide the kind of cognitive and socialisation experiences that the child might have obtained from older siblings, or from older women within the family's ethnic and cultural group (Kayongo-Male and Onyango 1984).

Reward and punishment

Traditionally, parents across Africa believed that physical punishment was needed when children did not behave well. They used this form of punishment to establish required levels of obedience and courtesy in social interactions. There are sayings in many languages that reflect both the parents' concern for their child and the need to punish that child if it is to develop well. For example, the Yoruba say 'When we use the right hand to flog him, we use the left hand to draw him back to ourselves' (Zeitlin 1996), and the Baganda state that 'To beat a child is not to hate him' (Kilbride and Kilbride 1990).

Both these sayings clearly recognise the use of physical punishment within a loving relationship. All adults in traditional communities can expect any child to obey their instructions and requests, and may punish them if they do not comply. Similarly, older children have the right to expect obedience from younger siblings. They may even be encouraged to punish younger children as required (Kayongo-Male and Onyango 1984). But within each ethnic group there are probably some adults who think punishment should start quite early, and others who think it should be introduced quite a lot later. This kind of difference has sometimes been found in studies from other parts of the world (e.g. Qasem, Mustafa, Kazem and Shah 1998).

Physical punishment is still commonly used when children do not show required skills or social behaviours (Nsamenang 1992a; Zeitlin 1996), although this reduces when parents are better educated. Lloyd (1970) reported that only one of her elite group of 30 well-educated women said she used physical punishment when her child had irritated her 'just a little'. In contrast, 12 of the 30 traditional market women hit children who had been mildly irritating. But this significant difference between traditional and better-educated women disappeared if the child had done something more seriously wrong. More recently, the personal experience of the authors suggests that there may be more widespread tolerance of physical punishment in some communities than in others. (A Malawian gardener, for example, was adamant that 'You don't hit children' while university students in Botswana reported that they had often been hit for minor misdemeanours.)

Besides learning to meet desired standards of behaviour towards adults, children and adolescents have to learn socially accepted ways of interacting with their siblings and peers. Some of this learning comes from the way parents respond when they observe their children's socially unacceptable behaviours. Only Lloyd's (1970) study addresses this issue. Mothers in this study said they always intervened if they found their child teasing or fighting with another child. They chose to intervene in order to prevent physical harm to children and so that social relationships with families in their compound or community would not be harmed. Market women were more likely to intervene when children were teasing another child, but the great majority of both traditional and more educated women intervened when physical aggression was occurring. Other research into African parents' management of socially unacceptable interactions is greatly needed to enhance understanding of African child development.

African parents have been reported as being less likely to reward 'good' behaviour because of fears that reward will make a child proud (Nsamenang 1992a). However, Nsamenang argues that this emphasis on punishment might have been overstated, perhaps because parents who have responded to interviews do not have the same concept of reward as researchers. He points out that West African parents 'entice children to perform tasks or services with food, favors, other objects, and sometimes with Western toys' (p. 151). If children are given these things immediately *after* they have done the required task, the criteria for 'reward' as defined in northern hemisphere research have clearly been met.

Conclusion

Socialisation towards high levels of involvement with others in the family and community begins almost immediately the infant has been born. From the first few days onwards the child is cared for by a range of people of varying ages, although in most ethnic groups men and boys are less involved in socialising very young children than women and girls. Generally, parents want their children to develop social skills that will enable them to become effective members of the social group. Traditionally, they have used quite a lot of physical punishment as a tool when teaching their children how to behave in acceptable ways. This use of punishment decreases with increased education.

Family structure and characteristics

The general ideas about child development and the parenting practices that follow from these ideas are applied by parents who may be in polygynous or monogamous marriages. Children may also be raised by women who have never been married, who have been divorced or widowed, or by women whose husbands are away from the family home for long periods working as migrant labourers. The social and financial situations of families in these varying circumstances all influence the development of the child in direct and indirect ways.

Polygynous marriage

Polygynous marriage (also called polygamous marriage) was the traditional form of marriage across most of Africa. In areas where polygyny is still a cultural norm, a man expects to have more than one wife during at least some part of his adult years, although his opportunity to acquire additional wives might be restricted by poverty. Historically, though, the rate of polygynous marriage varied widely among different ethnic groups. P. L. and J. C. Kilbride (1990) note, for example, that 50 years ago the Babukusu were more likely than the Marogoli, both of Western Kenya, to be polygynously married and the difference remains today. The Samia, also of Kenya, still have many polygynous households, some with as many as 15 wives.

In the past, relationships within polygynous marriages varied among ethnic groups. For example, Wilson (1977, as cited in Kayongo-Male and Onyango 1984) reported quite marked differences between Xhosa and Nyakyusa polygynous marriages. Among the Xhosa the husband mediated between his wives and allocated their work, and co-wives generally had a close relationship.

When there was conflict, it was expressed through witchcraft. In contrast, the more powerful mother-in-law mediated between wives and allocated their jobs in Nyakyusa polygynous marriages, the relationship between wives was less close, and witchcraft was not used in situations of conflict. It is not known whether these kinds of differences in practice continue to influence family life in different ethnic groups today.

Both monogamously and polygynously married men and women are able to list the advantages of polygyny. When P. L. and J. C. Kilbride (1990) asked Nzoia and Samia adults (n = 41, about half of whom were women) about polygyny, most respondents described its economic advantages. Polygynous families are large, so there are plenty of workers to produce sufficient food for both home consumption and for marketing, without the cost of hiring labour. The second most common response concerned personal and political power – by having many children one became well known and perhaps politically influential. More children meant a greater probability that one of the offspring would become powerful and rich and be able to support other members of the family.

Psychological and social advantages of polygyny were mentioned less frequently. Men thought that having several wives protected them from the loneliness and child-care responsibilities that might otherwise arise if one wife died. Women felt that the larger group in the family compound provided additional security against theft and attack by outsiders. Other responses referred to easy access to child-care in times of need, co-wives balancing each other's strengths and weaknesses, and better intertribal communication if wives came from different tribal backgrounds.

The rate of polygynous marriage across the continent has been falling in more recent times. Adult males still widely value this kind of marriage, but adolescents, and many women, are likely to reject the practice (Kilbride and Kilbride 1990; Timaeus and Graham 1989). This may reflect changes in culture and the law, but the change is also related to the costs of polygyny in the modern world. Some respondents in the Kilbrides' study reported that poorer husbands with several wives and children were often unable to pay the children's school fees. Where economics meant that the husband was unable to treat all his wives and children in the same way (e.g. buying a radio for only one wife instead of one for each wife, buying new clothes for only some children), jealousy, envy and anger disrupted life in the compound and accusations of witchcraft might be made. If frequent, these strong negative emotions on the part of their mothers can have an adverse effect on children's wellbeing.

To some extent children's experience of polygyny varies according to when they were born and to which wife. The first child of the first wife is born into a setting that is different from that of his or her later born siblings. Children born to second and later wives are never without siblings and, from birth, are answerable to more authority figures than early born children of the first wife. While the effects of these differences in position in the family are not well understood, there is some research that suggests that birth order is associated with differences in psychological characteristics (e.g. Jefferson, Herbst, and McCrae 1998; Wilson, Mundy-Castle and Panditji 1990). This implies that the relationship of birth order to child development outcomes in polygynous households could be worth investigating.

Children who have grown up in polygynous households do report practical advantages that occur in association with polygyny. For example, if co-wives live in different parts of the country, such as when a man has a wife in the city and one in his home village, children are sometimes sent to live with a co-wife who is not their mother, perhaps to give them access to better schooling. Sometimes this placement is successful, but some children are badly treated by the alternative mother figure, especially if there is hostility between co-wives (Kilbride and Kilbride 1990).

Monogamous marriage

Monogamous marriage exists when a man has only one wife and has no expectation that he would take additional wives if he could afford to do so. Although there have always been poor men who had only one wife, the desire to live in a monogamous marriage is a modern one in sub-Saharan Africa. It can be seen as a result of the teachings of Christian missionaries in the period after European contact. As expected, therefore, monogamous marriage is more common among Christians. It is also associated with modernity in education and values. In addition, patterns of land use may have led to variation in the rate of acceptance of monogamy, as Timaeus and Graham (1989) have suggested. These authors argued that the early move towards monogamy in Botswana and Lesotho occurred because there was no real economic advantage in having more than one wife farming the poor-quality land in the region.

Monogamous marriage in Africa does not limit the number of people in the home to husband and wife and their children, as it typically does in the nuclear family of the northern hemisphere. In urban areas especially, there are often other relations and sometimes even strangers living with the family as these can help with daily living costs. Children must learn to interact successfully with these adults. Thus, to some degree at least, they are still living in a relatively dense social environment.

Monogamous marriage may result in family life that has some characteristics that do not promote good psychological health among the children. Arguments between parents are reportedly very common. They reflect changing ideas about parental roles and responsibilities, money and the husband's right to have girl-friends or 'outside' wives (mistresses) towards whom he also has financial responsibilities (Kayongo-Male and Onyango 1984; Timaeus and Graham 1989). Studies in northern hemisphere countries have shown that children are distressed when parents argue in front of them, becoming anxious, angry or sad. They show this distress in their interactions with others. While some arguments are inevitable in a modern nuclear family, frequent high-intensity arguments, especially those involving physical violence between parents, have been repeatedly shown to have long-term detrimental effects on children's wellbeing (Cummings 1987; Cummings, Pellegrini, Notarius and Cummings 1989).

Female-headed households

Across Africa about 30% of African households in which children are growing up are headed by women who are without resident partners (Kayongo-Male and Onyango 1984; Munroe and Munroe 1992). This can vary significantly, however, depending on the local availability of work for men and whether many men have had to go to war in recent times. Besides being raised by widows, children may be raised by women who have never married, those who have been divorced once or more often, and those where the children's father works away from the family home for long periods of time. The developmental and social difficulties that children from these single-parent homes sometimes experience are often said to be the result of not having a resident father. But the disruption to children's development is likely to come from events that co-occur with living in a female-headed household. In particular, divorced and widowed women may be in poor economic circumstances, especially if they live in a city some distance from their extended family. As a result, they are also likely to be more stressed than those with partners. For both these reasons, they may be less able to provide for the physical or psychological needs of their infants and children. Children who are raised in female-headed households where women have adequate financial and social support obtain as much food as those in male-headed households (Onyango, Tucker, and Eisemon 1994) and do not appear to differ from other children in any important ways.

Divorce

Divorce is not new to African families. However, traditional life-styles probably meant that the impact of divorce on children of the marriage was less than it is in urban Africa today. Children remained in their own home, surrounded by a large number of relations, all of whom had been involved in caring for them prior to the parents' separation. These people continued to meet children's physical, social and psychological needs.

Divorce has always been higher in matrilineal cultures than in patrilineal cultures for a number of reasons. (In matrilineal cultures the husband usually moves to live with his wife in her village, whereas in patrilineal cultures the wife moves to live in her husband's village. There are also differences in female independence and inheritance, and in aspects of child-rearing.) Children in patrilineal cultures belong to the male line and traditionally remained with their father's family if the mother left the marriage (LeVine et al. 1996), whereas in matrilineal cultures they accompanied their mother back to her family of origin. A woman's control of financial resources also contributes to her ability to meet her children's needs, both during her marriage and if she divorces. In the matrilineal communities of West Africa women have long held a level of financial independence that is not possible in the patrilineal communities that are more typical in East Africa. For example, market women of West Africa have usually been able to retain control of at least some of their earnings, whereas in East Africa women are still expected to hand over any earnings to their husband. The situation in East Africa was worsened by the behaviours of colonists whose insistence on male ownership and inheritance of land removed the women's traditional sources of independence (Okeyo 1980). Finally, in the matrilineal cultures of West Africa, women's societies have also been a major source of psychological, social and financial support for women. Many belong to several societies. Women who divorced probably also obtained support from these societies in times past.

The relatively higher divorce rate in matrilineal cultures still exists today. In a study of 61 ethnic groups in seven countries (Senegal, Ivory Coast, Ghana, Benin, Cameroon, Kenya and Lesotho) Lesthaeghe and Eelens (1989) found that an average of 30% of women from the matrilineal societies of Ghana and Ivory Coast had been divorced and that this was markedly higher than in other groups. Differences in the socio-economic status of divorced and non-divorced women confounded the picture. Higher socio-economic status was associated with higher rates of divorce, except among the women from matrilineal societies, where higher status was associated with lower divorce. Divorce has also traditionally been high among Moslems in parts of Africa and remains so today (Ntiri 1993).

Higher rates of divorce in recent times reflect changes in the way marriage partners are selected. Onwuejeogwu (1975) discussed various ways in which Fulani adults choose a marital partner. He pointed out that where parents participate in the selection of their child's spouse, marriages are more stable and the likelihood of divorce is lowered. This is partly because parents are more involved, helping the young married couple to resolve disputes in a harmonious way. When the marriage is based on personal choice, parents' assistance may be neither requested nor accepted.

The impact of divorce on children varies according to the age of the child, his or her personality and gender. To date, studies of this problem have been done in northern hemisphere countries. These show that in the short-term many children of all ages are distressed by marital break-up. Young children, who cannot understand what is happening, may feel that they are guilty of driving away the parent who leaves the family home. They may become rather anxious and regress temporarily to behaviours from an earlier phase of development; for example, they may begin bed-wetting again after a period of control. Adolescents dealing with identity issues may also become difficult to manage, and some run away, becoming involved in early sexual relationships or delinquent behaviour.

The frequency with which children show a lot of distress is influenced by the quality of interaction between divorced parents. If the parents can find a way of negotiating about issues that arise from their new status, children are likely to make a better long-term adjustment than if parents keep arguing (Berk 2000). While there is a need for research into the effect of divorce on African children, they probably show much the same kinds of reactions as children elsewhere, unless they have really strong social supports. This may be the case in rural communities, but is less likely, perhaps, in the towns.

Absentee spouses

The pattern whereby men and, less frequently, women worked away from their family for extended periods was set during the colonial period. It has continued to the present because of the limited opportunities for employment in many countries. Even when men reliably send money home for their families, the income earned is split between the need to maintain themselves and the need to maintain their family. This creates an unstable situation and the probability of poverty for all. Because the African father is the symbol of authority, the wife and children may be deeply affected by his absence (Kayongo-Male and Onyango 1984). Women in this situation become more self-reliant, taking on tasks and authority that would not have been their responsibility otherwise.

When absentee fathers return home, they may impose their authority on previously independent wives and on children whom they do not know at all well. Arguments and anger may erupt with the usual harmful effects on all involved. Children may be afraid of the father they do not know well, or may be resentful, sad and confused about his temporary involvement in their lives (Reynolds 1990). Absentee fathers also quite often retire and return to the family home before all the children have grown up, imposing their new and unwelcome authority on teenage sons and daughters. This can contribute to problems in adolescent identity development. For the father, adjustment to life with the family can also bring problems. Kayongo-Male and Onyango (1984) say that, in their attempts to resettle in the rural environment, men who have worked away for long periods commonly spend their retirement money on marrying a new wife, abusing alcohol, or taking up new work or business activities that drain financial resources. Again, these behaviours can be detrimental to the physical and psychological wellbeing of the children in the family.

Socio-economic status

In northern hemisphere countries the socio-economic status (SES) of a family is usually calculated by measuring the father's level of education and ranking his occupation in comparison with other occupations. Some recognition of family income is also included. Individuals in high status occupations such as doctor and lawyer have typically had many years education, have high incomes and their occupations are seen as important in their community. This approach to measuring SES has not been found to be very useful in Africa, and other methods of assessing SES have not always been satisfactory. Researchers have found that they need to ask questions about characteristics of the home, including its water supply and toilet facilities and ownership of desirable items (e.g. a bicycle) in order to gain some idea of family income and modernity relative to others in the community (Cleland and van Ginneken 1998). People with more money and modern goods and those with high levels of education usually have better access to the limited resources available in poorer countries.

Differences in socio-economic status have been shown to be associated with differences in child-rearing practices in northern hemisphere countries. Kohn's (1969) study, mentioned earlier, showed that in the United States of America the child-rearing techniques used by middle-class parents encouraged children to act autonomously and make their own decisions. In contrast, the methods used by working-class parents produced children who conformed to the expectations of others. The situation in Africa, where social classes are still emerging, is less clear. Traditional obligations to members of the extended family, including obligations to help relations in need of financial support, reduce the differentials in personal wealth that are associated with differences in social class in the northern hemisphere. Similarly, the widespread perception in developing countries that education is a way into employment and access to resources may mean that parents in both high and low status occupations place a high value on education. Finally, the traditional expectations that children should be self-reliant from an early age may mean that children at all social levels are more autonomous (independent) than has been the case in the northern hemisphere.

Because schooling is frequently associated with both higher SES and modernity, unschooled women might be expected to be rather traditional in their ideas about children, but this is not always the case. Nsamenang (1992b), for example, investigated the beliefs of a large number of Nso men and women about childbirth and child-rearing. Sixty per cent of his sample had not had any schooling, with men and women equally likely to fall into this category. Women were less likely than men to believe that using traditional potions facilitated birth or to think it was important to dispose of the placenta according to customary practice. They were much more likely to prepare for the birth of their infant through using the modern health-care system. Sixty-five per cent of women and only 26% of men believed that modern drugs facilitate the birth of a child.

Women were less likely than their husbands to assume that characteristics of their children were innate and less likely to believe that physical punishment should be used. On the other hand, they were more likely to believe that boys and girls should be socialised differently. Thus, women in the sample were generally more modern than their husbands. This was possibly because the child-health clinics had provided good-quality up-to-date information about childbirth and child development. Within this sample, access to information overcame the lack of schooling and low SES of many respondents. It is possible that the relationship between SES and behaviours in Africa might also differ in other ways from the patterns found in northern hemisphere studies, but more research is needed.

Conclusion

Each of the many forms of family life in Africa has some advantages and some disadvantages for satisfactory child development. Advantages increase if there is marital harmony and if family income is sufficient for basic survival needs to be met. Where this is not possible, some children may be exposed to levels of family stress that limit development. Stress may arise because of shifts in culture, particularly shifts from traditional beliefs and practices towards modern ideas about family life and child-rearing.

Characteristics of the parents

The personality and values, experience, and history of the parents and other caregivers all influence the way they behave when raising their children. Some characteristics of African mothers have been studied quite intensively, although less is known about the influence of fathers.

The mother

Traditional and modern beliefs and behaviours of the mother, and the amount of schooling she has received contribute to differences in the duration of breast-feeding, and in the use of contraception or of post-partum sexual abstinence (not having sexual relations after the birth) to achieve socially desirable child spacing. The openness to new ideas that is one of the consequences of education is modified by some other characteristics of the mother. In a study of women from several regions in each of eight countries (Senegal, Ivory Coast, Ghana, Benin, Cameroon, Northern Sudan, Kenya and Lesotho) Lesthaeghe, Vanderhoeft, Gaisie and Delaine (1989) found that mothers who belonged to traditional African religions were more likely to breast-feed for long periods. Being a Moslem was associated with lower contraceptive use. Christianity was associated with higher levels of female education, lower use of post-partum sexual abstinence as a method of child spacing, and higher use of contraception.

Box 1 Women and education

When you educate a man, you educate an individual,
But if you educate a woman you educate a family.

Dr Kwegyir Aggrey, Ghanaian scholar and educationalist, 1875–1927.

(Cited in *Save the Children* 1990)

Research in the last 40 years has shown the importance of education in changing mothering behaviours in ways that enhance infant survival and child health. Infant mortality may be more than twice as high if the mother has *not* been to school than it is if she has had even a few years of schooling. Attending secondary school improves outcomes even further (Cleland and van Ginneken 1988; Palmer 1993). Where there are mother and child health clinics in the village or nearby, mothers who have been to school are more likely to attend regularly. They are also more likely to have their children vaccinated against a range of illnesses. (These results occur even where schooling is of low quality.) Schooled mothers may also be more likely to practise new techniques that they have been taught at the clinic. For example, Palmer (1993) describes an unschooled mother who could tell her all about oral rehydration therapy (ORT) as a treatment for diarrhoea, but had not used it, because she was afraid she would not make the mix exactly right. In contrast, mothers who had been to school confidently prepared and used the mixture.

The advantage to the children that comes from having an educated mother occurs even when her socio-economic status is not improved as a result of that education. Mother's education is more important than father's education in terms of promoting infant health. It seems that mothers who have been to school are more willing to use new facilities and approaches to caring for their children.

They are more alert to indications of ill health in their children, and are more likely to seek out help at a hospital or clinic than unschooled mothers. Most importantly, mothers who have been to school appear to have higher status and to be more autonomous within their extended family than unschooled mothers. Their comments about their child's illness are more closely attended to by the decision-makers (e.g. husband, father-in-law) within the family. These men might otherwise not have noticed the early indicators of child ill health (Palmer 1993).

The father

Interest in the role of the father and his impact on child development is relatively recent both in the northern hemisphere and in Africa. Fathers in traditional African cultures were the recognised authority figures (Kayongo-Male and Onyango 1984; Munroe and Munroe 1992), but their involvement with their children varied greatly among ethnic groups. This difference continues to influence fathering today. Kipsigis fathers, traditionally excluded from contact with their infants in the first few months, still have limited contact with their young children. This contrasts strongly with the Aka of the Central African Republic and nearby regions. Hewlett (1992:153) reported that 'Aka fathers provide more direct care and are near their infants more than fathers in any other human population that has been investigated'.

Hewlett (1992) suggests that the variations in fathers' involvement in the parenting of infants might arise because of differences in both biology and culture. Aka people travel between 5 and 15 kilometres a day when hunting. Infants are relatively heavy compared with adult weight, so neither mothers nor siblings can manage to carry infants throughout the day. As a result, fathers carry infants quite a lot of this time. In the camp they continue to hold their infant as the mother completes chores, especially when she leaves the camp for firewood or is doing the cooking. Thus, the relationship between an Aka husband and wife is one marked by reciprocity and mutual aid as they share tasks throughout the day. This is associated with a high level of paternal care for the child. This situation is quite unlike the one that prevails in more settled farming communities where tasks are gender-linked and men and women lead lives that are largely independent of each other.

Parenting style

Each parent has a generally preferred way of interacting with his or her children. Baumrind (1971) describes three different styles of parenting that are still being investigated today. These styles are authoritative, authoritarian and permissive (sometimes also called laissez-faire). Baumrind defined authoritative parents as people who are consistent in enforcing rules and who value obedience in their children. They expect mature behaviour, but recognise children's rights and are willing to reason with them. In contrast, authoritarian parents are highly controlling and do not encourage independence. They are unwilling to discuss rules with their children and expect them to do as they are told without debate. Finally, laissez-faire or permissive parents set few limits, do not require children to help with household chores, do not enforce rules, and rarely direct their children's behaviour. Northern hemisphere literature states repeatedly that the best outcomes for children from individualistic cultures are when they experience authoritative parenting (e.g. Fletcher, Darling, Steinberg and Sanford 1994; Steinberg et al. 1994).

Evidence about the preferred parenting styles in collectivist cultures is limited, and comes mainly from studies where families from collectivist cultures have migrated to the USA, one of the most individualist cultures in the world. In general, these studies show that parents in collectivist cultures are more controlling and authoritarian than parents in individualist cultures and that children are happy to be treated in this way. They see the rules imposed by parents as indications of parental concern about their development and wellbeing (e.g. Lin and Fu 1990; Rohner and Pettengill 1985). This may also be true of the collectivist cultures of Africa, although the situation in Africa remains unclear. A study of street children that was done by Matchinda (1999) in Cameroon suggests that modern urban African adolescents dislike the excessive demand for obedience to parental rules that is characteristic of authoritarian parenting. It is possible that this kind of parenting is less effective in cities today than it was in the rural communities of the past.

Other influences on social development

Specific members of the extended family, the broader clan and the community have had, and continue to have, rights and obligations with regard to children in their kinship group. Today, staff at child-care centres and schools also participate in the socialisation of children. These influences are outlined in the remainder of the chapter.

Members of the extended family

As elsewhere, African grandparents have an important role and are perceived as people who provide gifts and treats (Kilbride and Kilbride 1990). In one study reported in their 1990 book, the Kilbrides asked 62 Samia and 69 Nzoia adults in East Africa to describe the characteristics of good grandmothers and grandfathers. Adults in both groups were most likely to say that grandparents should ideally transmit culture through their skills as storytellers, teachers and advisers. Samia adults also emphasised the role of grandfathers in solving disputes, especially disputes about land. They expected grandmothers to take care of grandchildren and give them gifts. Nzoia grandparents were expected to love their grandchildren, to be peace-loving and helpful, sociable and friendly. Again, grandmothers were expected to take care of grandchildren.

At specific points in children's lives, certain members of the extended family traditionally provided young people with the information required for the subsequent phase of development. For example, Tswana informants told one of the authors that in the past grandparents taught young adolescents about menstruation, sexual, and marital relationships. There was a taboo against parents teaching their offspring about these matters. Among the Baganda, the father's sister played a similar role with regard to her nieces (Kilbride and Kilbride 1990). Changes in society mean that young people today may no longer obtain adequate information from these sources. As they seldom obtain good explanations from other sources, the loss of traditional practice is detrimental to development outcomes.

Foster parents, often members of the extended family, have also traditionally been involved in raising children in many parts of Africa. In West Africa, especially, fostering of older children served many goals (Page 1989). For some, placing a child with his or her grandparents enabled families to provide the grandparents with much-needed assistance. Doing this also showed that the younger parents recognised their own debt to this older generation. Other children have traditionally been placed with more powerful or more important members of the ethnic group with the long-term goal of improving the child's opportunities in life. (P. L. Kilbride and J. C. Kilbride (1990) also report this use of fostering among the Baganda of East Africa.)

Today, the advantage of fostering is often that it permits adolescent children to attend the better-resourced schools in the cities, thus improving their chances of entering tertiary education or finding a good job when they finish school. When children are old enough to understand the reasons for fostering, and when they are not entirely separated from their parents and home community, they may gain a great deal from the fostering arrangement. An unsatisfactory fostering arrangement with excessive demands for help with chores or excessive use of punishment has the potential to distress the adolescent, however. Unhappy children and adolescents are less likely than their more settled peers to be able to make good use of the apparent advantages of their placement. Their situation is worsened if cultural expectations about fostering make it difficult for parents to intervene.

Modern adaptations of this practice may be less conducive to the psychological wellbeing of the child, although physical needs may still be met. Bledsoe and Isiugo-Abanihe (1989) and Page (1989) have described a widespread practice whereby infants and very young children may be placed in foster-care with grandmothers and other kin. Page's data showed that in parts of Cameroon as many as 19.5% of children in the age range 0 to 4 years were fostered. However, the typical rate was much lower, usually less than 10% in many ethnic groups across Ghana, Cameroon and the Côte d'Ivoire. Early fostering has been made possible by the availability of alternatives to breast milk. When children have been fostered from such a young age, their strongest attachment is to the foster mother and others in her community. These foster parents, often grandmothers, may also 'spoil' the children, making fewer demands for compliance than parents would have done, and not insisting that children learn culturally required courtesy behaviours towards adults.

Problems may arise when children are up-lifted from an indulgent environment to live with their parents. Often this coincides with beginning school. The sudden loss of important attachment figures coupled with parental demands for compliance to requests and the pressures of beginning school can cause considerable unhappiness and anxiety, which may have long-term negative effects. Where fostering of children below the age of four or five years is necessary for traditional or modern cultural reasons, it would be better if children could return to their parents about a year before beginning school. This would give them time to adjust to life with their parents before they have to go to school.

Recently an abuse of the tradition of fostering children with wealthy relatives has been reported in some poorer parts of Central and West Africa. Slave traders are recruiting members of extended family groups and paying them to persuade relatives that their children's future can be improved if they can be taken to work in richer countries nearby. Children as young as four years may be sold for small sums by extremely poor parents. Children sold in this manner experience confusion and fear during the transition to their new employer, who does not always provide adequate food or show any concern for children's safety and who may beat them severely for minor misdemeanours (Astill 2001). These children suffer both physical and psychological harm that may be irreparable, even if they are found and returned to their families. In particular, abused children lose the capacity to trust others that is critical to the formation of strong relationships during childhood and later. If they have been punished excessively, they may be fearful of adults generally. Some may have nightmares and become depressed and withdrawn, while others will act out their anger in aggressive responses to minor provocation (Wright 1995).

Child care and school

A recent pattern in the care of preschool-age children involves placing them in a child-care centre while their mothers are at work in towns and cities. The quality of care provided varies, and there may be little stimulation for the children. But some recent work in the Republic of South Africa shows that paid caregivers may be keen to learn how best to help children develop social and cognitive skills. In one programme offered by the Gauteng Regional Department of Education in Johannesburg, women who were running informal crèches in their homes responded well to instruction in child development. One such caregiver openly acknowledged that prior to receiving training she had hit and yelled at children. Now she understood that they learned through experience. She was seen to use a totally different approach from her old one of yelling and hitting (UNICEF 2000a).

At school children learn a great deal that is not in the curriculum. The values, attitudes and behaviours of teachers and other children alter the way they themselves think and act. These influences are discussed in detail in chapter 5: The primary school years.

Conclusion

A large number of characteristics of the physical, personal and social environment influence child development. Because each child is different from all other children in some ways that are discussed in subsequent chapters, the impact of the broad environment varies among children. All children benefit from some aspects of their environment, and all have their development limited in some ways by it. Successful parents and teachers provide an environment that reduces the harmful aspects of the environment and takes advantage of its more positive features.

In your community (two)

Choose some of the following exercises to clarify your own ideas about child development:

1 If you are a parent, write a brief statement about the characteristics you would like your child or children to have by the time they are young adults. What values or attitudes would you like them to have? What kinds of behaviours would you like to see?

2 If you are not a parent, talk to your older siblings, cousins or others who are already parents and make some notes about what they want their children to be like when they are young adults.

3 Compare information obtained in exercise 1 or 2 with the information obtained by two or three other students in your class. How much similarity is there in goals for child development? Do parents want the same things for their daughters as for their sons?

4 Think about your own family of origin. What were its main characteristics (e.g. was it polygynous, monogamous, was your father at home? Away working? etc.). How do you think these characteristics of your family influenced your values, beliefs and behaviours?

5 Find one or two research articles describing some aspect of family life in the northern hemisphere. Compare your experiences as a child with those that are described in northern hemisphere research.

Chapter Four

Development in infancy and early childhood

Introduction

A large number of authors (e.g. Kayongo-Male and Onyango 1984; LeVine et al. 1996; Nsamenang 1992a) agree that children are greatly desired and highly valued across a wide range of ethnic groups in Africa. These authors agree that African child-rearing emphasises the social development of the child, but provide evidence showing that caregivers also are sensitive to issues in the realms of physical and cognitive development.

Box 2 The importance of names

Omonkaro	– A child comes first
Omonsigho	– A child is more valuable than money
Omonsefe	– A child is more valuable than wealth
Omonrotomwan	– A child is one's kin
Omonragbon	– A child is the world

Common names in Edo (Benin, Nigeria)

Source: C. O. Airhihenbuwa (1995:77)

Berry et al. (2002), Ogbu (1981) and others whose work was discussed in Chapter Two have pointed out that child development takes place within the physical and cultural environment of family and ethnic group. Values and attitudes that are generally held within the culture influence child-rearing practices, as do parental beliefs (Harkness and Super 1996). When considering child development, therefore, it is important also to consider the various beliefs about child development and parental responsibility for development outcomes that are held in different ethnic groups. There are a great number of ethnic groups in Africa, but relatively few researchers have reported on child-rearing practices amongst them. Most published studies come from research in only a handful of countries. This chapter presents some examples of the kinds of information that are available internationally, but teachers need to use these examples as cues to their own thinking about culture, rather than concluding that these are the only parenting beliefs and behaviours in Africa.

Some aspects of development appear to be universal, in the sense that they take place in all normally developing children. Thus, physical growth follows the same pattern in children everywhere, vision and hearing develop in the same way, and some social and cognitive skills develop in the same general sequence in African children as they do in children from other parts of the world (Werner 1988). This chapter gives a rather brief overview of these universal aspects of development. Students should read any one of the many texts that describe prenatal development, and physical and sensory development during the early years of childhood in more detail. Instead of emphasising universal features of development once again, the chapter focuses more on normally developing African children's relationships in the family and broader community and the ways in which children's cognitive and social skills develop in African communities. Difficulties and problems that might alter development outcomes are discussed in Chapters Six to Eight.

Some terminology

Researchers studying child development use a mix of medical and other terms to identify the age of the child to whom they are referring. The term *neonate,* which means 'newborn', is used to refer to infants in the first month of life. Thereafter, the term *infant* is used to refer to a child who is less than one year. Between the ages of about 1 and 2.5 years, children are often referred to as 'toddlers' and between the ages of 3 and 5 or 6 years, as preschoolers. These terms will be used in the present chapter.

Survival, growth and socialisation of body functions

The period around the birth of an infant, the perinatal period, has always been a time of quite specific danger for the majority of African mothers and infants. Even today many die at this time. The high risk has been recognised in the various practices, and rituals aimed at securing life during this period have long existed in many cultures (LeVine et al. 1996). The practices of referring to a child as 'it' during the first month or so and delaying naming until a few days or weeks after birth (e.g. Nsamenang 1992a; Zeitlin 1996) show that parents have long recognised the risk that the neonate might not survive. These practices are ways of delaying making an emotional commitment to the newborn at a time that his or her survival remains rather uncertain.

Traditional practices aimed at ensuring that birth was safe for both mother and infant are still used today by the Ganda and Luyia women who were interviewed in studies by the Kilbrides (1990). Following a traditional practice (now confirmed as helpful by modern medicine) all rural women in the group described how they maintain physical fitness and muscle strength through work and exercise during their pregnancy. A much smaller percentage (58%) of urban women did so. Massaging the stomach and abdominal regions is another traditional behaviour that continues to be practised by pregnant women in both these ethnic groups. Massage, too, is recommended in modern medical practice, although justifications for its use may differ from traditional explanations.

Practices that improved the chances of neonatal survival have also been part of the African tradition. For example, Nuer women in southern Sudan stayed in their own mother's compound, with the husband having visiting rights only, until the first child was born and weaned. Similarly, Fulani women returned to their own mother's home just before giving birth to their first child, also remaining there until they had weaned their infant. The grandmothers almost certainly provided guidance and advice at this critical time (Onwuejeogwu 1975). Some of the skills grandmothers taught may still be being used.

Traditional mothering behaviours which promote the physical development of the infant in the first few days of life have been reported by Brazelton and his colleagues (Brazelton, Koslowski and Tronick 1976), who assessed the health status of neonates in Lusaka, Zambia. These investigators reported that many of the infants had poor muscle tone and were relatively inactive in the first day of life. However, at ten days old they showed better than average muscle tone compared with infants in an American sample. They were also alert and interested. Brazelton et al. attributed this rapid gain in physical health to rehydration from breast-feeding, to the amount of vigorous physical stimulation of infants provided by each mother, and to the upright position in which infants were carried, wrapped in a long cloth that was tied around their mother's body.

Modern health practices that have improved neonatal survival rates begin prior to and around the time of birth. Programmes for village midwives in some countries teach about the hygiene procedures that reduce the risk of infection to mother and child. In Mali, for example, specialists in health care taught traditional midwives hygiene procedures that would reduce the risk of neonatal tetanus and the consequent death of the newborn. They also provided the midwives with some basic equipment that would help them to maintain mother and infant hygiene at this time (Gray, Baudouy, Martin, Bang and Cash 1990).

A similar programme in Cameroon was reported by Palmer (1993). This author also pointed out that each year traditional birth assistants in Cameroon attended a one-week refresher course to enhance their skills. Palmer cites, for example, a traditional birth assistant who had used her knowledge of possible risks associated with some births to enhance birth outcomes. This birth assistant routinely referred women to the maternity hospital if the pregnancy was their first one, if she suspected twins, if the mother had bled more than usual when giving birth on a previous occasion or had some other problems. Using approaches like this, it is possible to maintain the best of traditional culture and to permit village midwives to continue to earn their living, at the same time eliminating some potentially harmful aspects of their behaviour that have existed because of lack of knowledge.

Feeding practices

Naturally, survival and normal growth require adequate nutrition. Cultural factors that may influence growth include beliefs about feeding, whether or not the infant is breast-fed and if so, for how long and by whom. For example, in the first two or three days after birth the mother produces a thin yellowish fluid called 'colostrum', which is different from the milk she will produce later. Colostrum contains a great quantity of proteins and calories (kilojoules), antibodies that offer protection against disease, and lymphocytes that further assist in fighting disease (Thomas 1988). Neonates in some ethnic groups are not fed for the first few days because of traditional cultural beliefs about colostrum, so they miss out on this valuable food (Konner 1977). In the past, neonates and older infants in some ethnic groups were fed by various lactating women in the community (Tronick, Morelli and Winn 1987), a practice which is risky nowadays as the HIV/AIDS virus can be transmitted in breast milk.

In general, however, the best and safest form of food for infants is mother's breast milk, especially in homes where there is no electricity or gas for refrigerators, where water resources are limited, and water is of poor quality. Besides being safe, breast milk contains the antibodies that help protect infants against harmful viruses and bacteria. For these reasons a longer, rather than a shorter, period of breast-feeding is better for infant development in developing countries. Traditionally in Africa infants were demand fed throughout day and night. They were also likely to be offered the breast at any time that they showed distress of any kind (Berry et al. 1992; Konner 1977; Omolulu 1974). In ethnic groups where the child's sling was hung so the infant rested across the hip rather than on the back, older infants could often also reach for the breast themselves whenever they wanted food (Konner 1977).

In the past, African mothers breast-fed for two to three years, although larger infants might be weaned earlier and smaller ones later than average (LeVine 1977). Many (but not all) breast-feeding women are amenorrhoeaic (do not menstruate) and cannot become pregnant at this time. Extending breast-feeding, then, had a secondary role in assisting with spacing of births (LeVine et al. 1996; Palmer 1993; Shelley 1985). Thus, breast-feeding assisted in promoting the health of both mother and infant during the mother's childbearing years.

In modern times the period of breast-feeding may be shortened owing to the ready availability of substitute baby formula, the pressure on adolescent mothers to return to school, or on urban mothers to return to paid work (Bledsoe and Isiugo-Abanihe 1989). More educated and urban mothers are more likely to breast-feed for shorter periods than rural mothers and those with lower levels of education, although the relationship between education, residence, and breast-feeding is a complex one, and not well understood (Lesthaeghe, Page and Adegbola 1981). Mothers' attitudes towards breast-feeding may reflect broader attitudes to tradition and modernity. Women who reject tradition may choose not to breast-feed, associating bottle-feeding with modernity (Rabain-Jamin 1989). This change in practice may also be accompanied by a change in attitudes towards breast-feeding, with some women becoming self-conscious about feeding their infant in public places (Omolulu 1974).

The process of weaning a child can be gradual or more abrupt. This is one aspect of child-rearing where traditionally there was quite a lot of variation among ethnic groups and where this variability in practice continues. Among the Gusii and the nomadic Turkana, both of Kenya, the Nso of Cameroon and various tribes in Ethiopia, for example, weaning may be abrupt (LeVine et al. 1996; Palmer 1993; Ryback et al. 1980; Shelley 1985). Among the !Kung San of Botswana it is much more gradual. Boys may be breast-fed for slightly longer than girls (Konner 1977), a finding that is consistent with child-rearing in many developing countries where boys are valued more than girls (Werner 1988). African research on this topic is limited at present.

The degree of distress at weaning appears to vary from one group to another, irrespective of whether the process is gradual or abrupt. In Uganda, where the Baganda wean their infants gradually, Ainsworth (1977) found that the degree of distress expressed varied with the time at which weaning took place. Within the 8 to 12 month age range the mother's refusal to allow the child to suckle elicited significant distress reactions over a considerable period. But earlier or later weaning appeared to cause only very short-term upset.

Ainsworth believed that the differences in infants' reactions to weaning reflected other aspects of their development. In particular, she believed that weaning a child around the ages of 8 to 12 months was difficult because feeding and the formation of an emotional bond with the mother were closely interconnected at this time. For older children, whose attachment to their mother was well established, tantrum behaviour appeared to occur more because of their inability to access a source of satisfaction that had previously been freely available, rather than for any more serious psychological reasons. In contrast, Konner (1977) reported that !Kung San children became quite depressed around the time of weaning, and remained depressed for weeks or months, irrespective of when they were weaned.

The time at which solid foods are introduced in more traditional communities may also vary quite considerably. For optimum growth, solid foods should be introduced into the diet during the second half of the first year (MacGregor 2000). This has not been traditional practice in much of Africa and is still not widespread in rural communities. The delayed introduction of solid foods led Omolulu (1974:334) to conclude that, 'The average African child is . . . nutritionally famished from about the ninth month of life till he starts eating the adult diet, about the twenty-second to twenty-fourth month of life.'

Reasons for delaying the introduction of solids vary among groups. For example, Zeitlin (1996) found that Yoruba women, who introduced solid foods very late in the first year, had a preference for wiry active infants. They believed that fat infants were lazy and would walk late. Women who participated in Gray et al.'s (1990) study in Mali were reluctant to introduce solids at around six months for two other reasons. First, they recognised that the introduction of solid foods was often associated with the onset of diarrhoea. Naturally, they did not want to expose their infants to that risk. Second, their poverty was such that they feared the loss of income that would arise if they gave their infants food that they might otherwise be able to sell. In contrast, the Nso women of Cameroon who were studied by Palmer (1993) introduced additional foods into the infant's diet very early, some children receiving strained pap (maize porridge) as early as one to six months of age. Other foods, such as oranges, were also introduced to infants in the first year in this community.

In some ethnic groups children are not allowed the whole range of foods. In particular, Yoruba children, both urban and rural, may eat very little meat because their parents believe that too much meat is damaging to children's moral development (Zeitlin 1996). Whether or not children and parents eat together may also limit the amount and quality of food children obtain. Family eating patterns in educated middle-class families may enhance growth. In some of the Yoruba families who participated in the Zeitlin study the practice of having family meals, rather than feeding the men first, was associated with more equitable distribution of meat. Fathers who ate with their children were initially given the greater proportion of meat, but then shared it with others at the table. Fish, a food of less social importance, was generally distributed more evenly by mothers. This access to sources of protein that were traditionally denied to children is clearly likely to have health advantages for them.

Even when there is enough food for all, toddlers and preschoolers may miss out on food for some other reasons. In families and communities where members of the group eat from a common bowl, the young child has to compete with others for food. Times at which meals are served can also limit young children's access to food. Omolulu (1974) points out that in some rural Nigerian communities the first meal of the day may be in the late afternoon, with the evening meal also quite late, by which time children may be asleep. Unless there are leftovers from the previous day or these children can buy food from a local market or vendor, they are at risk of malnourishment.

Sleep and growth

Adequate growth also requires adequate sleep, because the greater part of growth occurs during sleep. Traditionally, African infants sleep with their mother until some time in their second year. Super and Harkness (1986), in their study of the Kipsigis of Kenya, have shown that as a result they develop a pattern of having several shorter periods of sleep in each 24 hours, compared with infants in the United States of America, who intersperse longer periods of sleep with longer wakefulness. The Kipsigis infants slept little and often. Their longest period of sleep was 4.5 hours, with a total of about 12 hours. The Efe infants studied by Tronick, Morelli and Ivey (1992) typically fell asleep while lying on their parent's lap. Toddlers in this community were often awake during the night, interacting with adults who were caring for the fire. They also frequently changed beds during the night, moving to share with preferred others. These differences in sleep patterns have no significance for physical development.

Modern sleep arrangements for infants may be changing. P. L. Kilbride and J. E. Kilbride (1974) observed, for example, that Ganda women were increasingly placing their infant in a basket, crib or pram next to their bed, rather than sharing their bed with him or her. The pattern of demand feeding at night is no longer so easy for mother or infant when this modern arrangement exists, but the risk of mother overlaying her infant while she is asleep is eliminated. In families following a modern lifestyle with parents sharing a bedroom, the infants in the Kilbrides' study were often placed in the father's bed in the morning for a period of play. Changes in developmental outcomes may be associated with these modern sleeping arrangements and with the increased paternal involvement with infants that occurs as a result.

Bladder and bowel control

The child's ability to control the urge to urinate or defecate is a result of development of the brain, nerves and muscles (MacGregor 2000) and generally occurs around the age of 2 to 3 years. (Parents in some cultures may state that their child develops control in the first few months. In fact, they have learnt to monitor signs that child needs to urinate and respond to these signs.) Toddlers gradually develop awareness of the need to urinate and of the social desirability of controlling the urge to do so until they can use the toilet or properly designated place. By about the age of 2 most can control the urge to urinate during the day, although they may still need immediate attention when they say they need to go to the toilet if they are to avoid accidents and remain 'dry'. Nighttime dryness is usually established by 3 years, but it may be much later. For example, around 15% of 7-year-olds are still not dry at night in northern hemisphere countries (MacGregor 2000). As with bladder control, physiological maturity is accompanied by increasing awareness of the need to void (empty the bowel) and by awareness of the social desirability of doing so in the designated place. Toddlers usually develop bowel control around the age of 2 to 2.5 years. Parents around the world, including those in Africa (Zeitlin 1996), generally recognise this timetable for control of these bodily functions.

Socialisation practices greatly influence the development of culturally acceptable toileting. Some infants are encouraged to develop personal control of bodily functions early. In other groups toileting may be of less concern, as among the Masai of Kenya and Tanzania (deVries and Sameroff 1984). Harsh punishments may be used during toilet training in some parts of Africa, making children anxious and upset about toileting. This harsh response to mistakes is reportedly quite common in Ethiopia. There 78% of young adults surveyed said that punishment was used during toilet training, 64% said shaming was used and 67% said parents expressed disgust at urine or faeces. However, 67% of respondents also said parents were patient and 82% said toilet training was a gradual process (Ryback, Sanders, Lorentz and Koestenblatt 1980). There does not appear to have been any research into the role of sibling caregivers in toilet training, although they might be expected to play a significant role in regard to this developmental task, since they often have a lot of involvement with children who are developing control of bodily functions.

Conclusion

Traditionally, African women have recognised that birth, the early days and the early months of life are times that the infant is very vulnerable. They have taken a range of actions to ensure child survival. But the need for older infants and toddlers to have access to the full range of solid foods has been less widely recognised. Access to modern knowledge and changes in family life have improved some young children's chances of attaining optimal physical development, but other changes, such as the reduction in the prevalence of breast-feeding, may be detrimental in communities where food and financial resources are limited.

Motor skills development

Besides rapid gains in length and weight, infants show rapid development of motor skills during their first year. Table 4 shows the average age at which northern hemisphere children acquire a number of motor skills without training, but some training practices in Africa promote the development of motor skills at an earlier age than the ages shown in the table.

Table 4 Some physical milestones in the first 15 months

Age	Physical milestone
At birth	When child lies on stomach, hips are held high, with knees under abdomen
6 weeks	Lying on stomach on couch/floor, readily lifts head up so face is at 45 degrees to the couch/floor
12 weeks	Holds rattle voluntarily. Pulls at own clothing
16 weeks	Holds rattle for prolonged periods. Reaches for objects but is inaccurate
20 weeks	Grasps objects deliberately. Plays with toys, splashes in bath
24 weeks	Rolls over. Holds bottle
28 weeks	Chews. Feeds self with biscuit/bread. Sits, head forward for support. Transfers objects from one hand to the other
9–10 months	Finger and thumb work in opposition (allows infant to pick up small objects). Creeps (crawls)
13 months	Stands alone for a moment
15 months	Constantly throwing objects away. Feeds self fully if given a chance, picking up a cup, drinking, putting it down without help. Walks without help

Source: Adapted from Illingworth (1991:144–150)

The practice of placing very young infants in a sitting position with support to help to keep them from falling has been widespread in Africa. Periods in a sitting position may be prolonged, as much as 60% of waking time among the Kipsigis for example (Super 1976). The Kilbrides (1975) found that the rural Ganda people of Uganda placed their infants in a sitting position from as early as the first few months. This occurred in association with a ritual at three months, for which children were required to sit while they were formally accepted into the clan. Samia infants, whose mothers were driven by the more practical need to be able to do farm work without carrying their young child, sit unsupported even earlier than Ganda infants (Kilbride 1980). Thus, the median age at which Samia infants sat unsupported with good co-ordination was 5.6 months, for Baganda it was 6.0 months and for a comparison group of American infants it was 6.9 months. These differences were all statistically significant. The early unsupported sitting that is very generally reported in the African literature is believed to occur because the child develops good muscle strength as a result of being regularly placed in a sitting position from an early age (Super 1976, 1981).

But not all motor skills develop early in all African ethnic groups. Crawling, correctly called creeping, may be relatively delayed, compared with the development of this skill in northern hemisphere infants. Again, this may be an outcome of practice. Northern hemisphere infants are regularly placed in a prone position (lying face down), a position that promotes the development of muscles needed for creeping. Placing infants in this position is less common in Africa (Super 1981), although it does happen in some ethnic groups (Super 1976). Some African mothers might deter infants from creeping in homes where there is a risk that they might crawl into the cooking fire. However, Yoruba mothers say they encourage early creeping by routinely placing objects the child wants just out of reach (Zeitlin 1996).

Walking may or may not begin early. In some cultures more traditional adults believe inaccurately that children will not learn to walk unless taught to do so (Konner 1977), so infants are regularly held in such a way as to allow them to make the stepping movements necessary for walking. Yoruba mothers in the Zeitlin (1996) study said they encouraged early walking, rewarding the child who attempted a few steps with singing and clapping. Similarly, Super (1976 1981) cites a number of his own studies, each of which showed evidence for early walking in East African ethnic groups. In contrast, LeVine et al. (1996) noted that early walking was not encouraged among the Gusii because of concerns that toddlers are prone to many accidents. DeVries and Sameroff (1984) reported that Kikuyu motor training was also later than in other ethnic groups.

Conclusion

The evidence for a common sequence of motor development across ethnic groups around the world is well established, and children in African ethnic groups follow the same sequence of development in this area. But socialisation practices, especially the amount of training given, influence the age at which motor skills are established. The advantage brought by practice can be quite large. The extent to which traditional practices continue to be used by well-educated and urban mothers is not known.

Social and emotional development

As with physical development, some psychological characteristics appear to have a genetic basis and each infant responds both consistently and in its own unique ways to environmental stimulation from the earliest days after birth. This tendency to respond consistently is referred to as the infant's temperament, and underpins later personality development. The formation of a close emotional relationship between the infant and a reliable caregiver is also important for later development. This is called forming an attachment with the caregiver. Because infant temperament and the quality of attachment both influence further development, they are discussed in some detail before socialisation practices are outlined.

Temperament

Temperament has been described as the behavioural style of the individual. Some infants are very adaptable and generally respond positively to new stimuli. Others need more time, or even respond negatively. Some have very stable moods, while the moods of others change quickly. Some have more intense moods, but others are less intense. Some are easily calmed down if they become upset, while others are not. These patterns were first described by Thomas, Chess and Birch in 1968. A large number of more recent studies of infant temperament in the USA, UK and Australia (e.g. Bornstein, Gaughran and Homel 1986; Pedlow, Sanson, Prior and Oberklaid 1993; Prior 1992) have shown that these characteristic ways of responding do not change much as children grow older. For this reason each child's temperament is regarded as forming the basis of his or her personality.

Infant temperament varies a great deal within an ethnic group. But, in addition, there may be more general differences in temperament among various ethnic groups. For example, Keefer, Tronick, Dixon and Brazelton (1982) reported some differences between 15 Gusii and 15 Anglo-American children. Gusii neonates were somewhat more capable of soothing themselves when they became distressed than American children. They calmed themselves by putting their hand to their mouth. They also showed a tendency to habituate (that is, to show decreasing reactivity to repeated stimulation of the same type) more rapidly to touch and other tactile stimulation, and to show fewer startle responses than American children. But they were more irritable than American children. This study suggests that ethnic group differences in temperament exist from birth, but at present not enough research of this kind has been done to allow any conclusions to be reached.

A study by deVries and Sameroff (1984) suggests that parents' perceptions of the characteristic temperaments of their children may also reflect cultural values. These investigators asked Kikuyu, Digo and Masai mothers in Kenya about the characteristics of their infants, using a standard interview schedule that has also been used in many other studies. Comparisons between the three groups showed that Kikuyu mothers rated their infants as most difficult, and Masai least, with the Digo responses in between. For example, Kikuyu infants were described as being more active, less adaptable, more intense and more negative in mood than infants in the other two groups.

Results also reflected differences in the extent to which families could be described as 'modern' (this measure included father's and mother's schooling, the quality of house, whether there was electricity, and some other measures). Compared with traditional mothers, modern Kikuyu and Digo mothers were more likely to describe their infants as active and intense. Modern mothers in all three ethnic groups thought their infants were more adaptable than did the traditional mothers in the same ethnic group. In the matrilineal Digo tribe, boys were perceived as much more difficult and negative, while the patrilineal Masai described girls in this way. The authors concluded that there were almost certainly cultural influences in the infants' behaviours and in the mothers' reports. Similar studies in other parts of the world have also shown that parental responses to questions about temperament are influenced by the parents' ideas about what children should be like (Hsu, Soon, Stigler, Hong and Liang 1981; Kyrios, Prior, Oberklaid and Demetriou 1989). When more objective trained observers assess infant temperament, the results are often quite different.

Parents' beliefs about 'normal' infant behaviour may make it difficult for them to raise a child who differs markedly from the cultural norm. De Vries (1994), for example, discusses what happens in various tribes in Kenya when the child's temperament results in behaviour that is not acceptable within his or her culture. De Vries' case notes describe a Digo mother's experiences in raising an energetic, lively, intelligent child in a culture in which parents and teachers expected children not to stand out from the group. In this instance the child initially developed patterns of withdrawal and shyness, which later developed into fear, anger and overactivity. In contrast, a fussy demanding Masai child whose behaviour was seen as assertive in a culture where assertiveness is valued was fed more often in response to his demands and survived a drought during which less demanding infants died.

Attachment

For successful social-emotional development to occur, the infant must first develop a close relationship with a caregiver who is reliably available to meet his or her needs. But in polygynous families a child may have multiple caregivers. A study of Hausa women living in walled compounds in north-western Nigeria, for example, showed that, although each mother of an infant aged 6 to 14 months had the major responsibility for feeding and bathing her infant and for other routine physical care, any one of four other women sometimes attended to the infant. These other women were especially likely to respond to infant crying. In fact, a person who was not the mother attended to the infant on 47% of the occasions when it cried (LeVine et al. 1996).

The consequences of multiple mothering for the development of an attachment figure are interesting. Northern hemisphere literature describes an increasingly intense reaction of the infant to separation from a single attachment figure, usually his or her mother. Around the ages of 8 to 12 months, with a peak at about 10 months, infants in northern hemisphere countries typically become very distressed if separated from the mother (Ainsworth and Wittig 1969; IJzendoorn (sic) and Kroonenberg 1988; Zach and Keller 1999).

The African situation may be different. Data from the studies of Gusii and Kikuyu infants and their mothers have shown that where more than one caregiver is reliably available, infants commonly show a strong attachment to their biological mother *and* to one other caregiver, although they may still show a preference for their mother if she is available. Some infants show attachment to more than one alternative caregiver besides their mother (LeVine et al. 1996; Reed and Leiderman 1981). It seems likely that such infants actually experience fewer episodes of distress during the period 8–12 months than many northern hemisphere infants. African infants whose primary caregiver is unavoidably absent may be content if their alternative caregiver is present. In monogamous marriages where the wife is well educated and in paid employment, the family maid is most likely to become an additional attachment figure. In the interests of the child, it is best if she remains with the family throughout this important period, if possible.

Infants continue to show distress when separated from their caregiver for some time after they have formed an attachment to that person. This may show as separation anxiety or fear of strangers if children are left with people whom they do not know well. The percentage of children showing this kind of distress between the ages of 1 and 3 years varies quite considerably from one ethnic group to another. For example, Super (1981) presents evidence that, at 15 months, about 90% of !Kung infants protested when their mother departed, and that 40% of them were still doing so at nearly 3 years. The duration and intensity of infants' response to mothers' departure may vary in relation to the number of caregivers with whom the infant has become attached, and to the frequency with which they are exposed to strangers (Ainsworth 1977).

Social development

Socialisation has been defined as the process 'through which children acquire the beliefs, values, and behavior considered appropriate for people in their society and culture' (Berndt 1992:429). As with other aspects of development, many aspects of early social and emotional development follow much the same sequence, irrespective of the learning situation (Werner 1988). Some of these aspects of development are shown in table 5. However, the age at which children show a number of social and emotional behaviours may vary according to the degree each behaviour is valued and practised. Thus, a study by the Kilbrides (1975) obtained data showing that at about six weeks of age Baganda infants smiled when someone talked to them and smiled at them, just as American infants do. Like American children, they began to vocalise in response to smiles and talk at about two months. The sequence in which they began to smile and vocalise when they saw their image in a mirror was also the same as that of American children, but it was considerably earlier. The researchers concluded that the earlier development of some smiling-related skills among the Baganda occurred because sociability is greatly valued in this ethnic group, and others with whom the infant interacts generally reinforce infant smiling.

Socialisation towards calmness, both motor quietness and emotional restraint, also begins in the first year. A number of early investigators in East Africa (e.g. Goldschmidt 1975; LeVine 1977) reported that mothers provided only physical care for their infants and that there was little emotional interaction between mothers and infants. But the Kilbrides (1983), who were aware of the sharp distinction between public and private expression of emotion in some African cultures, considered the question more closely in their study of the Baganda of Uganda. They arranged for a Muganda (woman of the tribe) assistant to do hour-long observations of mothers and their young infants in their own homes once or twice a week. In this setting, mothers showed a great deal of positive emotion towards their infants, stroking them, holding them in a face-to-face position and just looking at them, as well as hugging, kissing, and smiling at them. These results were confirmed in a study of the Gusii that was done by Richman, Miller and LeVine (1992). A difference between Gusii and American mothers in this latter study was that Gusii preferred to touch or hold their infant when it cried, while the American mothers looked at or talked to their child from an early age.

Table 5 Some social milestones in the first year

Age	Social milestone
4 - 6 weeks	Smiles at mother
12 weeks	Recognises mother. Squeals with pleasure
16 weeks	Laughs aloud
20 weeks	Smiles at mirror image
24 weeks	Smiles and vocalises to mirror image. Imitates adult who pokes tongue out. Laughs when head covered with towel and suddenly removed in 'peep-bo' games
28 weeks	Tries to attract attention by coughing
32 weeks	Responds to 'No'
40 weeks	Pulls mother's clothes to attract attention. Helps dress – holding arm out for shirt, transfers objects from one hand to the other in order to put hand in sleeve
44 weeks	Drops objects deliberately so someone will pick them up
48 weeks	Gives object to caregiver on request (e.g. ball). Repeats a performance that has been laughed at

Note: Norms for northern hemisphere infants. African infants may develop some of these skills earlier as a result of training.
Source: Adapted from Illingworth (1991:145–151)

Patterns of mother-infant play may also promote calmness. Dixon, Tronick, Keefer and Brazelton (1981) analysed videotaped material of mother-infant interactions. The data showed that although Gusii mothers' interactions with their infants followed the same sequence that had been obtained elsewhere, the amount of time they spent in each phase of the interaction was shorter. When infants became excited, 'talking' and playing, mothers were likely to avert their gaze, turn their head away, convey neutral to slightly negative emotion, and reduce body contact with their child. This and a more neutral response occurred on almost 45% of the occasions that the child became very stimulated. As a result, periods of play were extremely short, lasting less than 1.5 seconds on average, although Gusii mothers encouraged the return to play and 'talk' after this brief interruption. The abrupt withdrawal of attention when infants became too stimulated according to cultural norms promotes early control of emotional expression as infants seek to maintain the pleasure that occurs as they interact with their mothers.

Self-reliance and work

In northern hemisphere studies play has often been described as children's work (Millar 1968; Bornstein and O'Reilly 1993). However, work may involve skills in managing daily routines of dressing and washing oneself, and being able to do chores competently without close supervision. This is called self-reliance. In general, African parents traditionally believed that children should become self-reliant at an early age. As a result, there was an emphasis on teaching toddlers and preschoolers to run errands, to assist with water carrying, to watch that animals were kept out of vegetable plots and so on. Even today, young children in rural communities begin to learn these tasks in their second year, at first under maternal supervision, later sometimes assisting older siblings as they go about their chores. Mothers in some ethnic groups continue to believe that by around 4 years children are capable of running errands independently, and that by about 6 years they can be left alone for two hours. Between 6 and 7 years children are expected to care for younger siblings, and to help with farm work, trading and housework (LeVine et al. 1996; Nsamenang 1992a; Super and Harkness 1982; Zeitlin 1996).

Wenger (1989) reported that the amount of time spent working increases rapidly during the preschool years. Wenger made a series of observations of the activities of Giriama children in Kenya. She reported that 2- to 3-year-old children spent only 1% of their time working, by age 4 to 5 years, this had risen to 8% and by age 6 to 7 years children were working when 18% of observations were made.

Maternal employment outside the home may influence the age at which children show self-reliance. For example, Bloch and O'Rourke (1982), who studied the play of a small group of Senegalese preschoolers in a village not far from Dakar, observed that girls whose mothers were employed were more likely than other girls or boys to act out various roles in their play. These girls were also more responsible and showed more skills in the area of personal hygiene.

Play

Pellegrini and Smith (1998) state that the early play of infants consists of rhythmic stereotypes. Children repeat the same movements over and over (e.g. kicking their legs). Pellegrini and Smith believe that this kind of physical play assists in the development of the nervous system and is necessary before infants can play in more directed ways, such as manipulating toys. These same authors refer to the play of preschoolers as exercise play. This term refers to children in the preschool age range developing their muscle strength and endurance through long periods of physical activity.

Children's play also reflects their social development in other ways. In the countries of the northern hemisphere children aged around 2 years spend quite a lot of their time in solitary play. They play with toys that are different from those used by others around them, and ignore others' activities. Toward 3 years they begin to use the same toys, but still do not interact with others as part of the activity. This is called parallel play. Around 4 years there is an increase in associative play. Children use the same materials, sometimes sharing them, and talk to one another as they play. About a year later most play is co-operative, with children taking on various roles and sharing parts of the same activity.

In Africa, socialisation towards the group and children's work obligations might lead to different developments in social play. This is suggested in Wenger's (1989) study. The amount of time girls spent in social play increased only by 4% between the ages of 2 to 3 years and 6 to 7 years. In contrast, boys' social play increased markedly over this time. Wenger concludes that these differences occurred because girls' responsibilities for infant care meant they could not spend as much time with their peer group as boys did. Girls therefore had less opportunity for social play. Differences in play did not reflect differences in cognitive development. In Wenger's (1989) sample there was increasing separation of boys and girls from an early age, so that by the age of 4 to 5 years boys were already spending almost half their time working or playing only with other boys. In other communities the separation of boys and girls may have been traditionally later, reflecting differences in the economic activities of various ethnic groups. Herding and hunting economies probably resulted in earlier separation of boys and girls than was necessary in farming communities.

In the course of their play, toddlers and preschoolers begin to learn and practise the social skills they need if they are to function effectively in their peer group. One of these social skills is the capacity to deal with conflict. Many ethnic groups in Africa value avoidance of direct conflict, using intermediaries to solve problems when conflict arises, or seeking redress through the courts (Lowy 1974). Minor conflict may be dealt with through gossip or reference to witchcraft (Kilbride and Kilbride 1975). Preschoolers probably begin to learn about these strategies as a result of observing their use. For example, Jahoda (1982) notes that among the rather litigious Ngoni of Central Africa, boys aged 5 to 7 years frequently acted out the roles of people attending the law courts.

In communities where aggressive acts are tolerated or modelled, children learn to act aggressively. Traditionally some ethnic groups began to teach their children to fight at an early age. P. and I. Mayer (1970), for example, describe a practice whereby two Xhosa mothers would place their 2-year-old sons face-to-face. Each mother would then take her son's hand and hit the other child with it. Naturally, the boys became upset and began to fight more spontaneously. Their mothers and any other adults rewarded their efforts with attention and positive comments. Even where physical fighting among children is only tolerated, as has been reported in Ethiopia (Ryback et al. 1980), aggressive acts will be more frequent than where they are not socially acceptable at all.

Studies of children in collective cultures in other parts of the world suggest that a number of positive and helpful behaviours might occur more frequently in the collective cultures of Africa than they do in individualistic cultures such as those of the northern hemisphere. These studies have shown that children from collective cultures are more likely to share in general (Rao and Stewart 1999) and also to share rewards evenly, irrespective of the contribution made by individuals (Mann, Radford and Kanagawa 1985). They show awareness of others' feelings (empathy) at an early age (Borke 1973) and differ in their general social development from children in individualist cultures (Fang and Keats 1989). Research into the social-emotional development of young African children is needed to provide evidence about the ages at which African children in different ethnic groups show these behaviours, and the extent to which they do so.

Conclusion

Where there are many caregivers, most of whom are sensitive to the needs of infants and children and who help them as they tackle various developmental tasks, young children probably develop a strong sense of security and self-confidence. A strong emphasis on motor development, on the ability to get along with others and on contributing to the running of the household promotes the development of skills in these areas from an early age. Although there is less emphasis on the development of cognitive skills and speech, some investigations have been done. These are reported in the next section.

Cognitive development and language

The term *cognitive development* refers to an increasing capacity to make sense of the world, drawing on experience in manipulating objects, interacting with people and solving problems. The amount and quality of stimulation an infant receives contributes in important ways to cognitive growth. Obviously the cognitive skills that infants and young children in Africa develop reflect their experiences with objects and people. For children of this age, the mother and other reliable caregivers have a major role to play.

Assessing the cognitive development of infants is difficult, and relies on assessment of social and motor skills such as those listed in table 6. Measurement of the ability to solve problems cannot begin until children are about two years old. Cognitive development is similar to motor and social development in that the sequence of skills development appears to be universal, while there is some variation in the age of acquisition of a skill, according to how much it is valued and practised in different ethnic groups (Super 1981). For example, Konner (1977) found that !Kung infants showed early development of skills in visual tracking and visually guided reaching for objects. They also showed other signs of earlier cognitive development than American children of the same age. Konner concluded that the advanced visual development occurred because !Kung infants in a hip sling could to reach for and play with the beads that their mothers wore around their necks. Being carried in an upright position is associated with greater alertness so this may also have helped promote the early development of cognitive skills.

Table 6 Some cognitive developments in the first two years

Age	Indication of understanding
4 weeks	Watches mother intently as she speaks to him or her
6 weeks	Smiles when mother talks to him or her
8 weeks	Smiles and vocalises. Follows object with eyes if it is moved to and fro in front of his or her face
12 weeks	Smiles, vocalises and squeals with pleasure
16 weeks	Anticipates and excites when feed prepared. Shows interest in a strange room or environment. Laughs aloud. Turns head towards sound
24 weeks	When drops toy, looks to see where it has gone. Begins to imitate
28 weeks	Responds to name. Pats image of self in mirror
32 weeks	Reaches persistently for toys out of reach. Responds to 'No'
36 weeks	Compares objects by bringing them together
40 weeks	Waves bye-bye
48 weeks	Will give toy to caregiver if required. Shakes head for 'No'. Repeats performance laughed at
12 months	Responds to words, e.g. 'Where is daddy?' Uses two or three single words with meaning

Age	Indication of understanding
15 months	Asks for objects by pointing. Pats pictures, may kiss pictures of animals. Begins to tell caregiver about wetting
18 months	Copies domestic tasks. Names single objects. Points to pictures in picture book
21–24 months	Joins 2–3 words together spontaneously. Talks a great deal

Note: Northern hemisphere norms for development of the average child. Some of these skills may develop earlier if African parents value them and teach or reward them frequently.
Source: Adapted from Illingworth (1991:145–153)

Parental beliefs about learning influence the degree to which they become active teachers of their very young children. In traditional cultures parental teaching emphasised the acquisition of social knowledge and self-reliance. Children learned other skills primarily through observation (e.g. Nsamenang 1992a; Kayongo-Male and Onyango 1984). Today, mothers in some ethnic groups still do not believe that they need to use objects in play activities in order to teach their young children. One mother in a study by Rabain-Jamin (1989) made this clear. Rabain-Jamin asked French and West African mothers of 10- and 15-month-old children to play with their child in a pre-prepared room. The West African mothers came from Senegal, Mali and Mauritania, had not been to school, and had migrated to France as adults. One of these women said quite explicitly that one difference between French and West African mothers was that for French mothers play was an opportunity to teach children new skills, but that the African mothers thought children learned better when they were older.

Recent studies that have investigated the interactions between mother and child have attempted to discover which patterns of interaction are associated with more advanced cognitive development after the first year or so. In a Kenyan study of Embu children aged 15 to 30 months Sigman, Neumann, Carter et al. (1988) observed mothers interacting with their children in their homes. Each child was observed between six and eight times for a two-hour period. Records were kept of the amount of time the mothers spent caring for their child, holding or just touching it and talking to it. Late in the study a well-known test of early development was administered to assess the children's cognitive skills. This showed that the mothers who had talked to their child the most had children who obtained higher scores on the test of cognitive development. Other measures, such as how much the mother held her child or touched it, were not associated with higher scores on the test. Although they did not assess the contribution of older siblings to infant development, Sigman and her colleagues did point out that, because these children talk a lot to infants in the course of caring for them, they probably also make a real contribution to the infant's cognitive development.

Studies elsewhere have shown that the amount a mother talks to her child might reflect the amount of schooling she has had. Lloyd (1967, as cited in LeVine et al. 1996) reported that about 50% of the well-educated Yoruba women in her study said they talked to their infant. Only 20% of mothers with very little or no education said they did so. But Sigman, Neumann, Carter et al. assessed the relationship between mothers' literacy levels and the amount each one talked to her child. They found that mother's literacy level did not explain the results, and concluded that mothers who have had no schooling or only very little, but who talk a lot to their children, are capable of enhancing their child's cognitive development.

Another interesting finding obtained by Sigman, Neumann, Carter et al. (1988) was that mothers who had carried their child the most were more likely to have children with *lower* scores on the cognitive development test. The result is exactly the same as that obtained by Munroe and Munroe (1984) with a much smaller sample of children in Zambia. Sigman and her colleagues point out that there are two possible explanations for this result. The infant who is carried more frequently may be developing more slowly because of illness, slower physical maturity or some other reason. Alternatively, it is possible that being carried a lot after the first year restricts the child's opportunities to explore the environment, and this slows his or her cognitive development.

In a study by Dixon, LeVine, Richman and Brazelton (1984), Gusii mothers of 18 children aged 6 to 36 months were given some tasks from a test of infant development and asked to teach their child how to do these tasks (e.g. building a stack of two or three blocks; placing shapes in the correctly shaped hole on a board). This study assessed patterns of interaction between mother and child even more closely than Sigman and her colleagues were to do in 1988. The behaviours of Gusii mothers and American mothers, whose children were the same age, were also compared. Gusii mothers were more likely to instruct their children to do the task than American mothers. They were less likely than American mothers to offer either praise or encouragement or to scold their children, although if the child looked away from the task he or she might be scolded. They talked less to their children about the task, but helped by moving equipment, so that children could complete the task in the course of their general activity. They were more likely to use physical control, pushing or pulling their children towards task completion. Gusii children were more persistent than American children, trying more often with difficult tasks.

Dizon et al. thought that Gusii mothers had the goal of 'getting the job done, even if done accidentally by the child rather than staging a process of discovery for the child, or exploration of the limits of play' (1984:1260). They were teaching a new skill, rather than teaching their children how to learn. This kind of maternal behaviour is consistent with cultural beliefs that praise makes children proud and should therefore be avoided, and that learning consists of acquiring new facts. As Chapters Ten and Eleven point out, both these beliefs appear to be widespread in Africa.

Play and cognitive development

In addition to its importance for children's social development, play is important for cognitive development. It is a way in which children learn new skills, practise skills that have only recently been acquired, try out different roles, and use their imagination. Thus, cognitive skills (e.g. how to solve the problems involved in making a toy) develop during play as well as in more structured educational settings. Children who play games where they mimic adult behaviours (e.g. cooking like mother, pretending to go on a lion hunt) or pretend to be an animal, another child or fantasy creature are developing a range of imaginative and problem-solving skills that will benefit them in later learning.

Hughes (1995) reports that northern hemisphere middle-class children are more likely to show imaginative play than children in working-class families, probably as a result of greater parental acceptance and encouragement of exploratory and original play than is shown by working-class parents. In developing countries this freedom for middle-class children to play imaginatively may also reflect the greater ease of life in their families. More chores mean less time for play, despite children's capacity to incorporate play into everyday activities and work routines (Harkness and Super 1983, Wenger 1989). Legitimate fears of the harm that might arise in exploratory play may also lead some parents to restrict exploration. Mulder and Milton (1989), for example, reported that 56% of all injuries sustained by 11- to 15-month-old toddlers in one Kipsigis community were burns, and a further 42% were the result of falls. Parents would naturally want to prevent these.

Speech and language development

Infants communicate via sound from birth. In an early study Wolff (1969) found that even a very young infant's cry conveyed information to his or her mother about whether he or she was hungry, angry, or in pain, and mothers could tell the difference between these cries. More recent studies also show that infants communicate with their parents via the different sound of their cry (Worchel and Allen 1997; Zeskind and Marshall 1988). On average, infants vocalise at around 5 to 6 weeks, and 'talk' when spoken to by 12 weeks. By 28 weeks infants make four or more identifiable sounds, which are soon combined. At around 11 months infants use one word in a meaningful way, and by 12 months use two or three words meaningfully. Between 15 and 18 months they use a lot of 'jargon', sounds which follow the patterns of the language, but are not words in that language. Increasingly words replace the jargon, and by around 21 to 24 months toddlers are using two or three words in meaningful phrases (e.g. daddy home, drink milk). They repeat things that are said to them and use the words 'I', 'me' and 'you.' Between 2 and 3 years lisping and stuttering are common, but these correct over time in most instances. By 3 years most children's speech is normal by adult standards (Illingworth 1991). This sequence of speech development occurs only if the child hears well and is making the cognitive gains required for normal language use.

But there is evidence that patterns of interaction between mother and child may influence the use of verbal communication skills. Dixon et al. (1981) stated that Gusii mothers did not respond to their infants' vocalisations because they did not believe infants were capable of social interaction. This failure to respond would result in the gradual reduction in the frequency with which the infant vocalised – a process known as extinction in psychology. Similarly, Super and Harkness (1982) recorded that Kipsigis (Kenyan) mothers and their infants 'talked' only half as much as American mothers and children when children in the two ethnic groups were the same age. They reported that the Kipsigis mothers did not see themselves as having a major role in teaching their children to talk. They believed that this was a task for siblings and other children.

Dixon et al. (1984) found that when their children were about 2 to 3 years old Gusii mothers used labels for objects mainly when giving instructions (e.g. Give me the comb), but did not commonly just name objects that their child was playing with or looking at. Children were expected to respond to the instruction rather than talk to their mother about the object. This inequality in amount of speech, with younger members of the group speaking less than older members, is common in the hierarchical relationships that exist in many African ethnic groups. By complying with requests rather than talking about them, children are showing respect for adults in their community.

Zeitlin (1996) points out that when young children respond to verbal directions through action they learn a lot about prepositions (e.g. put the dish *on* the ground, go to the house *between* the trees, put the water *in* the cup). They also learn about sequences of events from listening to instruction about doing chores (e.g. take the dish to auntie's house and then go to the shop). Children in Zeitlin's study were encouraged to talk about whom they had met as they went about their errands, how they had greeted older persons, and what kinds of gestures others had used in their presence. The emphasis on functional language also encouraged children to be attentive to the language going on around them. Zeitlin observed that 3- to 5-year-old Yoruba children listened carefully to adult conversation about foods, market prices, the whereabouts of siblings and similar topics. Thus, speech interactions resulted in both increased cognitive skills and social understanding.

Modernity and early childhood

Although there has been some reference to the impact of modernity in the first few years, much of this chapter has focused on traditional beliefs and practices. This is because little is known about the extent to which modern living in Africa has altered the experiences and the social and psychological development of infants and young children. Changes may have negative or positive impact. For example, modern practices may result in reduced physical contact between mother and infant, perhaps decreasing the feeling of security that comes from constant touch.

The absence of older children when at school reduces the amount of care-giving they can provide, with an associated reduction in the amount of social, verbal and cognitive input from this source. This may alter the socialisation of young children in ways that are not well understood at present. Children who are living in a more traditional social environment and who have an important role as caregivers spend a lot of time helping and directing those who are younger than themselves (Whiting and Whiting 1975). Clearly, this is not possible when older children are at school during the day and still have chores to do when they return home. On the other hand, mothers who have been to school may talk to their preschool-age children more, promoting cognitive growth.

For urban children, reduced contact with extended family and others in the village from which the family originated may also alter children's experiences in ways that modify outcomes for development. But urban parents may have more time to spend with children, because they do not have to spend long periods getting water or weeding the vegetable patch, and this can bring advantages for the children. Family access to a greater range of activities, libraries, and other modern resources may also be beneficial, although parents' legitimate fears about permitting young children freedom in towns and cities may restrict children's independent exploration of the larger environment.

Conclusion

The period from birth to about age 5 is a time of rapid growth and development in all spheres. Even features of development that appear to be genetically timetabled may be influenced by the children's experiences within their particular ethnic group and culture. These and other experiences determine how infants and preschool-age children perceive themselves and their world, how they think about problems and about ways to solve them. In a time of rapid social change children whose families retain a more traditional lifestyle will have had markedly different experiences from those whose parents have received more education, and from those who live in bigger towns and cities. Variations in child-rearing practices across the continent will become even greater than previously as some members of each ethnic group retain traditional ways and others modify belief and practice as they learn more about how best to promote optimum child development. Teachers need to recognise that these differences in experience will influence the ways children respond to the demands of school life.

In your community (three)

Observing parents and children is the best way of examining development during infancy and early childhood. You can do this in a number of environments. Each period of observation needs to be a minimum of 10 minutes duration, but about 20 minutes will yield a lot more information.

Choose one or more of the following activities:

1. Find a public place and observe mothers of infants as they go about their tasks. Make notes of all the things the mother does (e.g. talks to another woman, rearranges clothing, feeds infant, chastises preschooler). What percentage of these actions involve interaction with the infant? Does the mother talk to her infant? Are all actions of a care-giving nature or are some more affectionate (e.g. gazes at infant, rubs his or her limbs).
2. Ask a mother that you know if you can observe her and her child at a time of rest or play. Make notes about the sorts of interactions that take place. Compare your findings with those of a colleague who has observed someone from a different ethnic group.
3. Observe several fathers and their children. How many fathers are involved with very young infants? How many are with boys? How many with girls? What does this tell you about what children are learning?
4. Observe some preschoolers in your extended family, street or community and, if possible, talk to their parents. What chores do they do? Do all of them have approximately the same number of chores? Do girls and boys do the same chores?
5. Compare your findings in any of the exercises listed above with information you have read in the present chapter. How closely do your observations match the information that has been provided? If it is quite different, discuss why this might be so with a colleague.

Chapter Five

The primary school years

Introduction

The early primary school years coincide with the period of development known as middle childhood. This period begins at about 5 to 6 years old and continues until the onset of puberty around the age of 11 to 13. The physical changes associated with puberty occur during the middle to late primary school years. At this time pupils enter the developmental period known as adolescence. Children's development during middle childhood and adolescence varies according to whether they attend school or not, but all children are expected to show increasing maturity and gains in social skills each year. As is usual in child development, the children are influenced by the behaviours of adults that reflect the adults' beliefs, values and attitudes.

The present chapter describes some of common beliefs held by African adults and the behaviours that are associated with them. This is followed by material on what is known about the social, emotional and cognitive development of children in Africa, both in and out of school. Physical development is not emphasised, as it follows the same pattern as that of children around the world. Detailed information about physical development during this period, especially the important physical development of adolescents, can be found in many general texts on child development.

Beliefs about child and adolescent development

In traditional times the period of middle childhood was one in which children developed the social and work-related skills needed for successful adulthood. This was followed by initiation rites at or around the beginning of the adolescent period. After initiation, young people were expected to gradually acquire the rights and responsibilities of adults. Parents in many rural communities still raise their children according to this age-old system that emphasises the development of different skills according to the child's gender. Thus, during middle childhood parents expect girls to become increasingly skilled in domestic tasks and crop-growing while boys, who are increasingly separated from the women in the village, learn skills such as fishing, raising cattle, and metal-working that are required for the survival of their future families.

Although parents may send both their sons and their daughters to school during middle childhood, those who hold traditional values commonly think that if their daughter becomes too educated or stays at school until she is older she will become unmarriageable. This belief is so widespread in traditional rural communities that girls themselves may tease older girls in their class. Younger girls in Ghana, for example, use the term 'skuul mama' to tease those older girls who have passed puberty and are still at primary school (Stephens 2000). Parents with limited financial resources may not see the point of educating their daughter, who, in the many patrilineal cultures of Africa, will marry into another family, taking the advantage of her expensive education with her. Parents with these kinds of traditional beliefs commonly withdraw their daughters from school at or around the age of puberty (11 to 13 years). These girls often marry and bear children within a year or two of leaving school (Stephens 2000).

Research in some African countries shows that parents, whether maintaining traditional lifestyles or living in a way that has been more influenced by modernity, frequently believe that boys are more intelligent than girls. This belief is maintained, although no studies anywhere in the world have ever shown any gender-related differences in overall intellectual abilities. Jean Davison and Martin Kanyuka (1992), for example, asked parents and children in Malawi whether boys or girls were more intelligent or whether they were equal in ability. In all, 70% of fathers and 69% of mothers said boys were more intelligent. About 20% of fathers, but only 8% of mothers, thought that girls were more intelligent than boys. Mothers were more likely than fathers to perceive children as having equal abilities. The 80 primary-school-age children (40 boys and 40 girls) who were asked the same question in this study were even more likely than their parents to think that boys were more intellectually capable than girls. Over 80% of both genders agreed that boys had higher abilities. Despite these beliefs, almost 100% of Malawian parents agreed that education was as important for girls as it was for boys.

Davison (1993) compared these finding with results she obtained in a parallel study in Kenya. Fewer Kenyan parents, around 85 %, thought education was as important for girls as it was for boys. A few mothers in both Malawi and Kenya thought it was more important for girls to be educated than boys, but no fathers thought this. The Kenyan mothers who favoured educating girls explained that girls who had been to school were more likely to help with the costs of sending younger children to school. They were also more likely than sons to retain links with their parents and help them in their old age.

As a group, Kenyan parents hoped that their children, boys and girls, would go to university, although 15% of fathers thought girls' schooling should be considered complete at the end of secondary school. However, Malawian fathers and mothers both accepted the idea that girls should have less education. Around half of them said that girls should finish at the end of secondary school. Malawian parents perhaps had more realistic aspirations for their sons, with about 27% stating that boys should complete their education at the end of secondary school, and the remainder wanting them to go to university.

Regional differences in ideas about the importance of education for girls are found in some countries. This may be associated with differences in religion or ethnic group. Thus, Cammish and Brock (1994) found that in Cameroon upper-primary-school-age children were *less likely* to agree that education was as important for girls as for boys if they lived in the rural north of the country than if they lived in less remote rural regions. In all, 52% of rural children in the north, 31% of those in less remote areas, and only 19% of those in urban area in the centre of the country thought education was more important for boys.

Besides valuing education, African parents value the contribution children make to household work. In general, parents describe children who are responsible workers in positive terms. Responsibility is seen as an indication of intelligence among the Kipsigis, who believe that this form of intelligent behaviour develops when children are about 6 years old (Super 1983). Occasional studies have also asked about who is responsible for various chores. Nxumalo (1979, as cited in Ferraro 1993) asked adults in rural Swaziland who had the most responsibility for various agricultural activities. Between 27% and 34% of parents said children had prime responsibility for tending goats, sheep and cattle, and taking animals to the dip. Between 8% and 11% said children also had prime responsibility for preparing the land for planting, ploughing, applying fertiliser and planting crops.

Conclusion

Parents' beliefs about development during middle childhood emphasise the differences between boys and girls both in terms of intelligence and in terms of the contribution they are expected to make towards maintaining the household. Ideas about the importance of schooling for girls vary from one ethnic or religious group to another. Not all parents believe girls and boys should have equal opportunities for education.

Development during middle childhood and early adolescence

The rapid gains in social, emotional, physical and cognitive skills that occur during the first five years do not continue at the same rate during middle childhood. Instead the rate of change, like the rate of growth, is slower. Socially, this is the period when children's play becomes more complex, and when the earlier preference for their own group can develop into the kinds of prejudice towards other groups (known as out-groups) that are called racism, tribalism and sexism.

This is also the period when differences in parental expectations and differences in children's behaviour based on gender become most apparent. Work is an important context for the development of children in more traditional environments and a great deal of social and cognitive development takes place in this context. Children who attend school learn to use cognitive skills more flexibly than those who do not go to school. This appears to be a direct consequence of the kinds of problems they are expected to solve during class lessons. There are only a few studies of this general period, and those studies that have been done have mostly assessed children's behaviour and learning in schools. These influences on development are outlined in detail in the rest of this chapter.

Social and emotional development

Very little is known about the social and emotional development of African children during middle childhood. For children living a fairly traditional life much social-emotional development is likely to occur in the process of interaction with other children. Children in many African communities, like children elsewhere, probably continue to develop the skills in controlling emotions and moderating expression of emotion in public that they began to learn at an earlier age (Altshuler and Ruble 1989; Rossman 1992). They almost certainly learn display rules (Davis 1995; Saarni 1988). These are the social rules that require facial expression of an emotion that is not necessarily the emotion being experienced on some occasions (e.g. not looking sad when receiving a bad mark for work in class). Children who learn these skills are probably also more popular than children who cannot manage their emotions in socially acceptable ways, as has been found elsewhere (Denham, McKinley, Couchoud and Holt 1990).

African children have been shown to respond in indirect but helpful ways to children who are distressed. Weisner (1989) studied the expression of social support for distressed children among the Abaluyia people of Kenya. He observed that Abaluyia children showed support for a distressed child by giving him or her a task to do, or asking the distressed child to help with some chore. They did this to distract the child from his or her upset. Teasing or aggression accompanied this social support, but it was still seen as support, perhaps because of the quiet emotional tone of the interactions. Empathy for the upset child was not necessarily openly expressed. The response to receiving social support was also quite indirect. The supported child frequently showed his or her appreciation for support by offering equivalent support for another child as soon as this was needed. Mothers began to train children both to tease and support others who were upset at an early age, and soon left much of the responsibility for solving problems in which children are distressed over small matters to older children. The mother remained more neutral and uninvolved. As a result, young children in a family were just as likely to seek reassurance from older siblings as they were to approach their mother.

Another study of social interaction among children was also done in Kenya (Whiting and Whiting 1975). Results showed that Gusii children aged 3 to 11 years offered help and reprimands to others, or made responsible suggestions for activities in 41% of their interactions with others. An additional 20% of time was spent in acting in generally sociable ways. These results contrast markedly with the behaviours observed among children in individualist American society. In America children spent a considerable amount of time demanding attention for themselves and were much less likely to help others. Casual observation suggests that northern hemisphere children are much more likely to reject reprimands from other children and more likely to seek help from their mothers if they are upset. Together these differences in social development reflect the differences in the values and styles of parenting between individualist and collectivist cultures.

Relationships between same gender members of the age band may change at adolescence as a result of traditional practices such as initiation into adulthood. For example, Barley (1986) discusses the relationship between Dowayo men who were circumcised together. After initiation, these men form a relationship based on jokes and insults and the use of each other's property. Thus, participation in initiation rites strengthens social and emotional bonds between members of the age band in ways that are important for the future wellbeing of each individual.

Today, however, initiation ceremonies may also mean that adolescents miss school, sometimes as much as a month, because of the seclusion that is part of the initiation into adulthood in many ethnic groups. Young adults of both genders may suffer ill health and pain as a long-term consequence of circumcision. This is especially likely for young women in those ethnic and cultural groups where extensive cutting of the labia (the fleshy area around the vagina) leaves scarring that restricts both the flow of menstrual fluids and the ability to urinate freely. In communities where cultural taboos prevent discussion of these kinds of problems young people's capacity to form mature sexual and social relationships may be limited.

Development of prejudice

Studies in various countries in the northern hemisphere have shown that children develop a sense of their own identity at an early age. Soon after this they develop a preference for others who are like them. Little girls prefer to play with other girls and may make unkind remarks about boys by the age of 3 or 4 years. Likewise, boys prefer to play with boys. This preference for one's own group, called the in-group, peaks at around 8 years. It then gradually decreases as children approach adolescence and develop the capacity to consider the personal characteristics of others before they decide whether to react favourably or unfavourably towards each individual (Aboud 1988; Brown 1995; Hirschfeld 1996).

The rejection of other groups, called out-groups, can become so extreme as to be called prejudice. Prejudice has been defined as an organised predisposition to respond in an unfavourable manner toward others because they are members of an identified group and not because of any unlikeable personal characteristics of an individual. Thus, for example, racial prejudice is evident when someone reacts unfavourably towards others because they belong to a different ethnic group (Aboud 1988).

The development of prejudice towards out-groups is not well understood, although northern hemisphere research shows that middle childhood is the period when it is most widespread. This northern hemisphere research has typically studied groups that are physically very different (e.g. majority white, others black, Asian or Native Indian in the USA). Hirschfeld (1996) questions whether children's prejudices are based on these physical differences. Even if they are, results from these studies may have only marginal relevance to African countries where physical differences between members of different tribes may be more subtle. However, children's preference for their own group and dislike of groups of outsiders probably follows the same sequence in Africa as elsewhere, since it appears to reflect social and cognitive development (Aboud 1988).

Characteristics of family life, especially some characteristics of the way parents behave, increase the likelihood that a child will continue to hold prejudicial attitudes beyond the age of about 12. Parents who are ethnocentric, that is, they value their own ethnic group above all others and respond unfavourably towards others on the basis of their ethnicity, are likely to raise children who are prejudiced against out-groups. This is especially likely if parents are also authoritarian. Authoritarian parents, as Chapter Three showed, expect instant obedience, have rigid rules for acceptable behaviour, and do not let children express anger towards them. Traditional patterns of parenting in much of sub-Saharan Africa have been authoritarian and, because of traditional enmities and fears of out-groups, parents have probably been ethnocentric.

Aspects of societal structure are important in determining whether the kind of prejudicial attitudes called racism are widely held and expressed. Northern hemisphere studies reveal that racial prejudice is more common in stratified societies, that is, those where one ethnic group is more powerful and has better access to resources than other ethnic groups. Adults at all levels in the society recognise the status of each ethnic group, and children develop this awareness around the age of 12 years. Conflict between groups strengthens adherence to the in-group and the sense of security people feel within their group. It also increases the probability that each group will know little about individual members of other groups. Members of these out-groups then become objects of fear (Aboud 1988). This kind of society is common in sub-Saharan Africa, and many children grow up with the fears and insecurities about out-groups that are common in their community. (More material on prejudice, discrimination, in- and out-groups is provided in Chapter Ten: 'Teachers and groups of children'.)

Work and play

African children generally do more real work from an early age than northern hemisphere children, but they still find ways of incorporating play into their daily lives. African children's play has not been studied, but it seems likely that some of the same sequences of development will occur as are found in children's play in other parts of the world. Some of the non-African research that has been outlined by Pellegrini and Smith (1998) shows that rough and tumble play such as wrestling, grappling, kicking and tumbling increases among boys during middle childhood. This kind of play reaches a peak at about 10 years before declining towards the onset of adolescence. When rough and tumble play does happen during early adolescence it is more likely to develop into real aggression, as adolescent youths attempt to establish socially dominant roles within the group. Play is also believed to assist in both social-emotional development and in learning. Children learn culturally appropriate ways of showing emotion in play contexts. They also learn to 'read' the feelings of others. In addition, play can give children a sense of mastery and provide a space or rest between tasks requiring more conscious cognitive skills. In this way it promotes the spaced or distributed practice on school tasks that is better for retention of new material than massed practice without breaks.

Gender differences in play have been widely reported in studies done outside Africa and are likely to be found in African communities. These differences in play preferences have been shown in the preschool years and become more evident as children enter middle childhood. Girls are less likely than boys to become involved in rough and tumble play. They prefer to use their more advanced verbal skills to solve problems that arise during play activities (Pellegrini and Smith 1998).

Work demands increase with age, but all children in the age range 5 to 11 years who live in rural communities across Africa are expected to contribute to household work and regularly do so (Ferraro 1993; Harkness and Super 1991; Wenger 1989). Work can occupy a significant part of the day. Wenger studied children's work and play among the Giriama of Kenya. She reported that children aged 6 to 7 were doing chores on 18% of occasions they were observed in her study. This increased to an average of 38% for children in the age range 8 to 11.

The average results for these older children hide a gender-based difference in amounts of work done by girls and boys. Girls in this age group were observed to be working on 51% of occasions, while boys were working on only 26% of occasions they were observed. Boys also performed a narrower range of tasks than girls, did not do any tasks that involved carrying (e.g. bringing water or firewood home) and did very little child-care. The great majority of their work time (62,8%) was spent doing errands. Girls' greater workload was more evenly divided between housework (33%), carrying (23,1%), child-care (15,4%), doing errands (16,5%) and gardening (10,9%). An exception to the general demand for girls to do more work than boys may occur in communities such as those in rural Botswana where families are financially supported by remittances from other family members who work in cities and towns. In these communities boys may still be expected to tend cattle or find a paid job. This may contribute to the higher academic success of girls in Botswana compared with boys (Fuller, Hua and Snyder 1994).

Cognitive development

All normal children begin to develop skills in coping with the enormous amount of information absorbed via their senses from the moment of birth. Bruner, Goodnow and Austin (1956), in work that is still often cited, stated that humans do this by developing concepts about classes of things. Each concept is an idea that describes a unique phenomenon, something that is different from other phenomena. For example, a child may see many objects, each of which is a similar shape, colour, length and so on, all of which are eaten and referred to by adults as 'bananas'. Through a gradual process, which takes place over time, the child develops a general idea or concept of a 'banana' and is then able to identify objects with most or all of the same characteristics as bananas. Having developed the concepts of banana, mango, and papaya the child later forms the more abstract concept of 'fruit'.

Bruner et al. (1956) state that the capacity to classify things reduces the need for constant learning (all objects with certain characteristics can be thought of as fruit, including new objects with characteristics common to fruit). Having many abstract concepts makes it easier for humans to cope in a complex environment and provides direction for actions (e.g. the concept of a knife includes the information that it has a sharp edge and can be used for cutting). More importantly, this capacity to classify encourages human beings to think about the order and relationship of classes of things in their environment.

Cognitive activity takes place when individuals use concepts to understand their world. Thinking, analysing, and remembering are examples of cognitive activity. Cognitive activity cannot be seen, but outcomes of this activity can be assessed in studies of behaviour. Some of these studies have been done in Africa. Various early studies of cognition in Africa, and those done under the apartheid regime in South Africa, appeared to demonstrate that Africans had difficulty with cognitive processing. But the studies may show more about the problems investigators have when assessing children from different ethnic groups or children with little or no schooling and need to be carefully evaluated.

Rogoff (1981) gives a good example of the kind of problem that exists with this early research. She cites the study done by an American researcher named Greenfield with unschooled Wolof children in Senegal. Greenfield used a test developed by Jean Piaget to measure conservation of liquids (Piaget and Inhelder 1966/1969). According to Piagetian theory a child understands about conservation of volume when he or she realises that a certain amount of water, poured from a short fat jug to a tall narrow one, remains the same, even although the water rises higher in the tall jug. A child who thinks the amount of water has changed has not developed advanced cognitive skills. Rogoff notes that the unschooled Wolof children in Greenfield's study often indicated they thought there was more water in the tall, narrow jug and this led Greenfield to conclude that if children did not go to school, they made no cognitive gains after the age of nine. Rogoff, however, suggests that perhaps the unschooled children were acting in a respectful manner to this strange adult who had come all the way from her own country to pour water back and forth. Would she have gone to all that trouble if she thought nothing was changing by her action? (Rogoff 1981:259–260).

Despite these sorts of problems, some of the studies of cognition done in the 1960s and 1970s do contribute to knowledge about African children's cognitive development. One important series of early studies that is still often referred to was reported by Cole, Gay, Glick and Sharp (1971). These investigators asked schooled and unschooled Kpelle children and adults in Liberia to recognise or recall verbal and non-verbal information (e.g. pictures on cards). They wanted to find out whether Kpelle classified information in the same ways as people in the northern hemisphere. To be quite certain that the data they were getting gave a true indication of the ways the Kpelle grouped or classified objects, the researchers chose foods, tools, utensils and clothes that were familiar in the local environment as the objects to be classified. Each study consisted of several parts, all of which aimed to obtain information about the same aspect of cognition. For comparison, the responses of Kpelle participants in the study were contrasted with those of Americans.

The studies showed clearly that Kpelle people, like people in non-African countries, grouped objects into classes, but also demonstrated that the ways they classified objects into groups varied according to the task. Sorting was sometimes done according the semantic relationships between objects (e.g. putting all the utensils in one group, all the foods in another), but on other occasions the Kpelle sorted according to the function of the item (e.g. putting knife and food in the same group because the knife cuts the food). All the groups tested, literate and non-literate children 10 to 14 years and non-literate adults, showed these various ways of sorting.

Schooled children showed more flexibility than unschooled children and illiterate adults in being able to use different bases for classification. For example, when given a task that involved sorting cards into different categories both young unschooled children and unschooled adults, and the 10- to 14-year-old schoolchildren all preferred to sort by number (two or five objects shown on the cards) or colour (red, white or black objects shown on the cards) rather than by form (objects were either triangles or squares). But when the researchers asked participants in the study to re-sort cards using a different basis for sorting from the one they had originally chosen, the schoolchildren were able to do so, while unschooled children and adults found the task extremely difficult.

Following this discovery, Cole et al. (1971) tried to discover the conditions under which members of the Kpelle community used different approaches to classifying. They did another series of studies assessing rates of learning, transfer of learning to new tasks, recognition and recall. Their results showed that both non-schooled and schooled children used mixed methods for learning. In some experiments they appeared to learn by rote. In other experiments they clearly learned the underlying concept required for successful transfer of knowledge to new but similar learning tasks. It was not clear to the researchers why children took one approach rather than another on different tasks.

Tasks involving memory showed that the children who had been to school were able to recall more information, but only when they were not given any cues. When culturally relevant cues (e.g. placing objects in a bucket during the teaching phase of the study) were provided for children and adults who had not been to school, their rate of recall matched that of the school children. It is interesting to note that cued recall among the non-schooled population varied according to the social situation in which cues were provided. This is interpreted as showing that people solve problems in ways that are well established in their daily lives. Because the daily lives of the schoolchildren included a demand that they recall information in the absence of any cues, they were more successful at this task.

Cole et al. (1971) also obtained data that showed increasing skills in solving logical verbal problems as children grew older. This is the general pattern of development among children around the world, and occurs whether or not they attend school. Cole et al. did find, though, that schoolchildren showed greater gains in this skill than others. The additional flexibility that accompanied schooling was again evident. Children who had attended school were more able to solve verbal problems that concerned hypothetical situations. People who had not attended school commonly indicated that they preferred only to discuss events they had personally experienced and people they actually knew. However, if given a hypothetical situation and its solution to discuss in a group, illiterate adults soon reached consensus as to whether the solution was correct and could explain why they had reached that conclusion. It is possible, therefore, that some of the results obtained by Cole et al. with regard to logical problems reflected the importance of the in-group as a social support in all kinds of contexts, rather than an individual inability to solve such problems. This was not addressed in the research.

The importance of Cole et al.'s (1971) research cannot be underestimated. These investigators demonstrated how important it was for researchers to be alert to the many possible factors that influence research findings in Africa. Their findings were confirmed by other investigators doing similar studies around the same time (e.g. Irwin and McLaughlin 1970; Nyiti 1976; Schmidt and Nzimande 1970). Carefully designed studies were more likely than less carefully designed ones to show no difference between northern hemisphere and African children or between schooled and unschooled African children in the development of cognitive skills (Rogoff 1981; Wagner 1981).

The facility for responding to school-like tasks that is shown by children who have been at school for varying periods may reflect other aspects of child development besides the impact of schooling. In communities where not all children go to school parents may decide to send only the children who seem most likely to benefit. Super (1977, as cited in Rogoff 1981), found that even before children began school, those who would attend later had advantages over children who would not. One of these advantages was that their parents were better educated. In addition, as Rogoff (1981:267) points out, parents who send their children to school 'may be wealthier, have more modern attitudes, or hold different aspirations for their children than parents who do not'.

Schooling itself prepares children for the kinds of tasks that are often used to assess cognitive skills. School children are familiar with tests, with written material and with the language used in assessment. They have experience with adults (teachers) who expect high levels of verbal interaction and who know the answers to questions, but ask them anyway. They have also learnt to work within time constraints. It is possible that classroom activities lead to the development of cognitive strategies that are also helpful in the research setting. For example, children at school are constantly expected to learn the general rule that underlies their actions (e.g. the sequence of numbers does not alter the sum when one is adding, but is important when subtracting). This may assist them as they seek efficient ways of solving the kinds of problems presented by researchers.

An interesting exception to the general advantage of children who have gone to school lies in the development of mathematical concepts in unschooled children, especially children whose work involves selling goods in the market. These children's mathematics concepts keep pace with those of children going to school up until about the age of 9 or 10 (Ginsburg 1997). In order to confirm the presence of these mathematics concepts, however, researchers have to find ways of assessing concepts that do not require the kinds of pencil and paper activities that can be used with schooled children.

Conclusion

Parents' beliefs and cultural practices continue to influence development during middle childhood and early adolescence, just as they influenced earlier development. During middle childhood children acquire many social and cognitive skills as they interact with peers and adults, but these have been studied only infrequently in an African context. Developmental changes at adolescence are rapid, and gains in cognition and moral development can be impressive, although, again, little study of these aspects of adolescent development has been undertaken in Africa.

Going to school

Today, children in sub-Saharan Africa may begin primary school between the ages of about 5 and 7 years, with some variation between countries in the age at which children are first admitted. Most do start attending school around the official age for entry, although a large minority may not begin until several years later. For a variety of reasons many children repeat one or more years of schooling (Robinson 1993; Swainson 2000). As a result, children in primary schools may be any aged from 5 to about 17 or 18 years of age (Lloyd, Mensch and Clark 2000).

Box 3 The UN Convention on the Rights of the Child: Education

The child has a right to education. The state shall make primary education free and compulsory and shall encourage the development of secondary and higher education, making education accessible to all and encouraging regular attendance at school.

Source: Save the Children (1990). *Prospects for Africa's Children*. London: Author. Appendix

Even if I could enrol in standard 1 for free, there would be no money for supplies.'

Piana 13, Lesotho.

'How can I continue education without having enough to eat?'

Street vendor 12, Ethiopia.

Source: UNICEF (2002:72)

In some countries (e.g. Belize, Benin, Rwanda, South Africa) enrolment in school is between 75% and 100%, and the majority of both boys and girls remain at school until the end of the primary school years. Other countries have high initial enrolments, but high dropout levels each year mean that fewer children receive a complete primary education. Still other countries (e.g. Mali,

Mozambique, Niger, Somalia, Yemen) have much lower rates of enrolment. This may be associated with poor retention (Stephens 2000; UNICEF 2000a).

Naturally, differences in national wealth influence the development of the education system. However, when Colclough, Rose and Tembon (1999) compared rates of enrolment in Guinea, a country with an income that is average for the sub-Saharan region, and Ethiopia, whose national wealth is much lower, they obtained some interesting results. Approximately the same percentages of girls, but not boys, were enrolled in primary school in these two countries, suggesting that other factors besides national wealth contribute to enrolment. Swainson's (2000) study of enrolments in Malawi, Tanzania and Zimbabwe cannot be easily explained on the basis of differences in national wealth either. Instead, the differences can be attributed to variations between countries in the amount of effort made at the political level to overcome discrepancies between female and male enrolments.

Regions within countries may also show considerable variation in the rate of enrolment and in the rate of retention of pupils. Again, poverty has been shown to contribute to lower rates of enrolment and retention in some regions, but socio-cultural factors are also extremely important in determining who goes to primary school, and who stays there long enough to complete the primary programme (Cammish and Brock 1994; Lloyd et al. 2000).

Socio-cultural factors in school attendance and achievement

Characteristics of the family and school environment both contribute to rates of enrolment and retention of pupils at African primary schools. In northern hemisphere countries children's eventual educational attainment is closely linked to characteristics of their family, especially family socio-economic status (SES). Children from middle and upper SES families do better academically than children from lower-status families overall (Kohn 1969). But in developing countries the quality of the school and of the teachers is more important. Good-quality school environments with good teachers have children who learn more than children who go to lower quality schools, with poorer-quality teachers (Heyneman and Loxley 1983).

Characteristics of the family

African children from poor families may not go to school because their parents cannot afford the costs associated with schooling, even if these costs are low. Davison and Kanyuka (1992), for example, report that both parents and their daughters mentioned lack of money for fees, books, and uniforms as a reason for girls' dropping out of school at all primary levels in Malawi. Cammish and Brock (1994) obtained similar information from parents in Cameroon. The time at which these costs occur may be a factor in some countries if the school year begins when money is generally scarce. Fees and costs involved in getting necessary documentation for enrolment (e.g. birth certificates) may be another factor in determining whether children even enrol (Colclough et al. 1999). Researchers in Malawi and Mozambique report that the hunger experienced by poor children may be a reason for their not attending school or for their learning little when in school (Davison and Kanyuka 1992; Johnston 1986, as cited in Robinson 1993).

For families practising subsistence farming, the loss of girls' work when they attend school may be a factor in determining continued attendance. Children who attend school have less time for work than those who do not, but may still be required to do quite a lot of work before and after school. This is especially likely to be a problem for girls. In one study girls spent about two thirds of out-of-school time on chores, while boys spent just over one third of their non-school time helping out at home. Thus, girls may have markedly less time for homework than boys (Davison and Kanyuka 1992). This is one of the pressures associated with membership of a low socio-economic group that reduces girls' learning, and increases the likelihood of failure and the risk that girls will drop out of school before completing their education.

Parental education levels form part of the measure for SES. Levels of parental education correlate with rates of repetition of classes and with school retention for their offspring in some developing countries. Cooksey (1981), for example, obtained data in Cameroon showing SES differentials in age at enrolment, attendance and success at primary school. SES was also associated with differences in success rates in the examination that would permit children to go on to secondary school. Younger pupils who came from higher status urban families were especially likely to do well enough to continue on to secondary school. In contrast, urban children from low socio-economic status families were more likely than any other group not to do well enough to go on to further education. High SES girls in Cooksey's study out-performed both boys and girls from all other SES groups. Cooksey concluded that many lower-class girls 'suffer both from being girls and from being lower class, which over-determines their educational failure' (1981, p.409).

A study of secondary school children in Maputo, Mozambique, suggests that social class does not completely explain all failure. In this study Robinson (1993) found that children who failed at least once were more likely than other children to have a father who had not gone beyond third grade in his schooling. But children whose mothers and fathers had each been to school for between four and six years were also at risk of failing. About one third of the latter group still failed at least some grades. These studies suggest that while socio-economic status is associated with different rates of success at school, some other factors also contribute to success and failure in African schools in ways that are not yet fully understood.

Characteristics of the school

Owono (1986), in an unpublished study cited by Cammish and Brock (1994), concluded that if the primary school is within easy distance of the child's home, he or she is more likely to enrol at an early age and complete primary school. (Interestingly, these children are also more likely to complete secondary school later on.) Children who have to walk long distances often enrol later and drop out earlier. This is especially an issue for girls once they reach puberty. Parents fear girls may be harassed or assaulted on the way to or from school and are more likely to withdraw daughters from school for this reason.

Many physical characteristics of schools, such as leaking roofs, and inadequate supplies of desks, blackboards and books, probably contribute to children's failure to complete the important primary school years. The teacher often cannot change these features of the environment, but some other features of school life may be more easily changed.

Matters relating to health are especially important, and some can quite easily be changed. Colclough et al. (2000) found that Ethiopian parents who were afraid that children might be exposed to disease were less likely to send their children to school. Health promotion activities might solve this problem. In Guinea, these same researchers noted that some schools did not have running water. Drinking water was brought in a bucket from the river and kept uncovered at the front of the classroom. All children drank from the same beaker. The likelihood that diarrhoeal disease would spread from pupil to pupil was therefore high. This practice can easily be modified.

Colclough et al. (1999) also reported that inadequate and dirty toilets can be a contributing factor to pupil dropout, especially for girls who have begun to menstruate. Some schools also have toilets that are shared by boys and girls, with the result that girls may not feel private as they change sanitary pads. Even where there are separate toilets for boys and girls, girls may be reluctant to use very dirty toilets when they are menstruating, and may stay at home for this reason.

General social environment

Schools may be unattractive to pupils, not just because of lack of resources, but also because of the general social environment. In some schools the level of punishment may be high. Lloyd et al. (2000), for example, describe a number of the schools visited in their study as being 'ruled by the cane'. In other schools, especially those where male teachers held traditional attitudes towards girls and women, physical and verbal harassment of girls by boys was tolerated. For the adolescent girls in this study, a high level of harassment by their male peers was associated with increased dropout rates.

Specific behaviours on the part of teachers and general teacher attitudes may also make the school unattractive to some pupils. Allocation of chores and selection of certain punishments can decrease learning time available to girls in particular. Teachers in some schools are more likely to give girls tasks such as sweeping the veranda or cleaning the toilets that remove them from the classroom during learning time. In areas where boys define certain tasks as 'girls' work' male teachers, who possibly agree with the boys, allocate these tasks to girls. In class, teacher behaviours also convey information about their attitudes towards boys and girls, their beliefs about abilities, and about the importance of education for male and female pupils. Many studies have investigated these aspects of schooling; these are discussed in detail in Chapter 10.

The impact of the socio-cultural environment on students' wellbeing

Much northern hemisphere research has shown that it is not just intellectual ability that determines academic success. More successful pupils are those who have a high self-concept, are highly motivated, are not too anxious and have a sense of self-efficacy, that is, a belief that their actions determine outcomes. These pupils are willing and able to take the risks that are associated with learning anything new. Little research anywhere in Africa has investigated how academic progress is influenced by these psychological characteristics, but anecdotal reports and the few studies that have been done tend to confirm northern hemisphere findings. These studies are discussed very briefly in the next few pages.

Self-concept

The self-concept is the set of attributes, abilities, attitudes, and values that individuals believe best describe themselves (Berk 2000). When asked about themselves, children may give their name and surname, gender or physical characteristics. They may say they are good at schoolwork, truthful, bad-tempered and so on. Children develop their self-concept before they come to school, but events at school can enhance it or have a detrimental effect. The self-concepts of both boys and girls are harmed when children are repeatedly criticised and punished, and enhanced when the teacher acknowledges their efforts and successes.

Girls in rural and traditional African communities learn from an early age to be submissive towards more socially powerful males, so their self-concept probably includes this dimension of submissiveness. It may be difficult for girls in classes with male teachers to practise some of the behaviours that lead to successful learning, such as challenging the ideas of their male peers or questioning the teacher. This kind of behaviour is inconsistent with culturally required submissiveness towards men. Difficulties caused by submissiveness are probably greater if male teachers adhere to traditional beliefs about female and male roles. Such teachers almost certainly convey their beliefs both directly through patterns of questioning and during verbal interaction, and more indirectly through patterns of body language or facial expressions of contempt or disgust when girls do not behave submissively.

Motivation

Motivation is the drive or urge that makes a person persist with an activity. In school, achievement motivation is the tendency to persist with challenging academic tasks (Berk 2000). Children who learn easily and who have a positive self-concept, especially as it relates to school learning, are generally highly motivated to do school tasks. On the other hand, pupils' motivation to achieve is decreased by constant failure, by excessive amounts of punishment, and by high levels of anxiety. Being required to repeat the same class as the previous year is extremely demotivating. Pupils' self-concepts as learners are adversely affected, and they begin to see themselves as incompetent failures. This, in turn, makes it more difficult for them to remain motivated and to take the risks involved in learning. If they already believe they cannot do a new task, they become less willing to try. Past experience has already shown that not being able to do some school learning task makes them feel bad, so motivation drops away.

Anxiety

A great deal of northern hemisphere research over long periods has shown that pupils learn best when they are only a little anxious about whether they can manage (Elliott, Kratochwill, Littlefield and Travers 1996). Pupils who have no concern about learning outcomes are unmotivated, and pupils who are experiencing high levels of anxiety cannot learn because feeling anxious disrupts attention to the learning task. Teachers who punish pupils excessively for minor misdemeanours or for mistakes in schoolwork have pupils who become too anxious to learn. Punishment can be physical (beating), verbal (sarcastic remarks) or even non-verbal (looks of disgust, sneers). Although it has not been possible to find published research into the relationship between anxiety and African pupils' learning, anecdotal reports from university students in Botswana confirm that some teachers induce very high levels of anxiety in their pupils. One student, for example, reported counting the weeks till the end of the year, when he would be able to escape from a classroom with a teacher in whose class he was 'too frightened to learn'. If pupils have come from homes where punishment is also common they will already be anxious and have a negative self-concept (e.g. I am stupid). The effect of teachers' responses on these children will be even greater than it is for other pupils.

Box 4 Fear

A year ago I was wondering how a child's fears might influence his strategies. This year's work has told me. The strategies of most of these kids have been consistently self-centred, self-protective, aimed above all else at avoiding trouble, embarrassment, punishment, disapproval or loss of status. This is particularly true of the ones who have had a tough time in school. When they get a problem, I can read their thoughts on their faces. I can almost hear them. 'Am I going to get this right? Probably not. What'll happen to me when I get it wrong? Will the teacher get mad? Will other kids laugh at me? Will my mother and father hear about it? Will they keep me back this year? Why am I so dumb?' And so on.

Source: John Holt (1982:91)

Action control beliefs

Action-control beliefs or attributions about success and failure can be considered from three different perspectives. Malmberg, Wanner, Sumra and Little (2001) have discussed these in their report of a study they did in Tanzania. They describe agency beliefs as the extent to which pupils believe they personally have some way (through their ability or effort, through having helpful teachers or through luck) of doing well at school. Control expectancy is more general and refers to the extent to which pupils think they can do well at school irrespective of the means they might use. Means-end beliefs are concerned with general causes of success for the group as a whole.

Malmberg et al. (2001) asked pupils what they thought contributed to their own school achievements. Pupils rated personal effort (e.g. I can really pay attention in class) as most important. Personal access to teachers who were willing to help them if they needed assistance was next most important. This access to teachers was more important than a feeling of personal control (e.g. If I want to do well, I can) and more important for success than personal ability or luck. When researchers asked what contributed to others' success, however, these Tanzanian pupils were more likely to say that the other person's ability was most important. Acknowledging others' ability, while not claiming high ability for oneself, reflects a Tanzanian cultural value. There, claiming personal ability is seen as arrogant, but ability is recognised at a community level as contributing to success in school. In contrast, a study in Kenya (Kivilu and Rogers 1998) found that older students, attending secondary school, were keen to attribute their success in mathematics to personal ability. They did not think that effort was important for maths success.

Some other important findings from the Malmberg et al. (2001) study were that boys and girls gave the same explanations for their success. There were also some differences between rural and urban children. Rural children more likely to attribute success to ability. In general, children were likely to believe that effort contributed to success in classes where they perceived their teachers as being generally fair and democratic. In these classrooms they also believed that they had good access to teachers who would help them if necessary. On the other hand, children in some classes were anxious, responding positively to statements such as 'I would rather not answer questions in class because I am afraid I'm wrong'. These pupils were much more likely to believe that neither effort nor ability contributed to success. Instead, they believed that success generally occurred because of luck.

This is an important study because it suggests that African children, probably not just those in Tanzania, can be encouraged to make the effort involved in learning if their teachers are fair and do not frighten them. African children respond to teachers in much the same way as children in other communities. In particular, they are like children in other communities where there are collective cultures, as Malmberg et al. (2001) point out quite specifically. Taken in conjunction with Kivilu and Rogers' (1998) study in Kenya, these results suggest that there will also be regional and perhaps even national differences in beliefs about the causes of success. Northern hemisphere studies have shown that pupils who attribute success to effort more than to ability generally do well academically (Elliott and Dweck 1988; Elliott, Kratochwill, Littlefield and Travers 1996). African teachers who encourage pupils to believe that effort matters are also likely to have more successful pupils in the longer term. But much more research in this area is needed in different parts of Africa before any more general conclusions can be reached.

Psychological responses to not completing primary school

It is important to remember that even when the reason for dropping out of school is beyond the control of pupils or their parents, each pupil will have some psychological reaction to that event. They may suffer lower self-esteem or sadness at not being able to complete their education or because they recognise that not completing it restricts their career options. For some children, however, more especially some boys, dropping out of school is associated with entering the work force and with increased financial independence. These boys may have a much more positive psychological reaction to leaving school, seeing it as leading to social acceptance as a mature adult member of their community.

Conclusion

A large number of factors in the general environment contribute to pupil success and failure in primary schools. These influences are beyond the control of the children themselves. Characteristics of schools that are beyond the child's control can also influence learning outcomes. They can have the effect of making children and young people feel good or bad about themselves. When children fail repeatedly, motivation decreases and anxiety increases. Both reduce children's capacity to stay in school and learn more. Failing children are at risk of dropping out of the system before they have acquired sufficient skills in literacy and numeracy to enable them to cope well in the modern world.

Children in school

A great deal has happened during infancy, toddlerhood and preschool development that is likely to influence the ways children will respond to being in school. If children are reasonably healthy and well, and have been so for most of their early years, they will have sufficient energy and skills to become enthusiastic learners during middle childhood. Teachers will see this enthusiasm and energy in the formal setting of the classroom. If parents have been reliable and caring, and have not been excessively punitive, children will also be psychologically healthy and eager for new experiences. However, if they have had insufficient food, have experienced extremes of poverty and ill health, if parents have been harsh or inconsistent, or have found their child difficult to raise, the children may make less satisfactory progress during middle childhood and may find academic tasks difficult.

Children come to school having already learnt many of their culture's 'rules' about teaching and learning, and about how a person should interact with others. They expect that these rules will also apply in school. In many traditional communities children have learnt by observation rather than direct teaching by adults (Nsamenang 1992a), although in some communities parents may give much more direct instruction, as Stephens (2000) found in his study in Ghana. During the preschool years children have learnt to co-operate with others who are both younger and older than themselves in their social group. In cattle-herding cultures they may have already been expected to function independently of adults, even in situations where they are potentially at some physical risk. In farming communities, they have begun to learn that doing things the same way as they were done in the past is best. They may have learnt that disobedience or discourtesy brings physical punishment, and that discourtesy includes questioning the statements of adults. If teachers want to interact with pupils differently, or if they expect children to behave differently in class, they need to introduce new expectations in a planned and careful way during the first few weeks and months young children are in school.

Teacher-pupil interaction and school learning

Being in school produces many changes in the child. Some of these are consciously valued, such as the achievement of literacy and numeracy. Some occur without conscious effort. The general culture and the specific culture of the school produce other changes. But relatively little is known about how these changes come about in African schools, because the literature to date has focused more on quality of schools and on gender issues than on what actually happens as teachers and pupils interact in the teaching-learning relationship. The few issues that have been discussed are outlined in this section.

Traditional ways and school learning

Cultural beliefs that appear to be unrelated to schooling may increase the difficulty in learning certain concepts and teachers need to be aware of where these conceptual differences exist. For example, core religious beliefs about the relationship of living people, recently deceased people, and ancestors who died long ago may be associated with concepts of time that differ from those usually taught in modern mathematics classes. Traditionally used number systems may also be different from the base 10 number systems of modern schooling. Pinxten (1997) has argued that teachers should not ignore these traditional forms of knowledge, but should use them to enhance conceptual development in their pupils. Teachers who are working with children from an ethnic group other than their own will also need to become familiar with the broad cultural beliefs of that ethnic group, especially where these cultural beliefs mean that children come to school with ideas about how the world works that are different from the teacher's.

Pinxten (1997) makes some quite specific suggestions about how to teach concepts where cultural beliefs differ from concepts presented in modern curricula and textbooks. He emphasises the need for children to explore concepts from their own culture fully before the concept from another culture is presented. Concepts being introduced from other cultures also need to be fully explored through activity and discussion. The teacher should make explicit comment about these concepts. He or she should give examples of how the local and introduced concepts can be integrated to form one complex elaborated concept, which acknowledges both perspectives. Only then will children link school learning to their own everyday lives.

This kind of integration of new and old concepts is unlikely to happen in many African classrooms just yet, largely because teaching methods do not encourage children to make links between ideas. Fuller and Snyder (1991) obtained observational data from ten minutes of teaching done by 127 primary schoolteachers in various parts of Botswana. In all, 54% of teachers spent this time lecturing pupils, and 43% listened to pupils reciting information as a group. Pupils in the remaining classes waited for the teacher to mark work and talked among themselves. Teachers rarely asked individual pupils to answer a question, and pupils were even less frequently heard asking teachers a question. The authors point out that their results over-estimate teacher talk and pupil listening times. They acknowledge that children also spent time in each lesson working silently on written exercises, but state that the pattern of not asking children to analyse and discuss has been reported in many parts of Africa. Fuller and Snyder cite unpublished work, also done in Botswana by Robert Prophet. Prophet reportedly observed that teachers asked factual questions requiring one-word answers. Answers were often chanted by the group. Even when they asked individual pupils for answers, teachers made no attempt to find out what kind of confusion led to incorrect answers, thereby depriving the child of a chance to learn.

Beginning to read

Because schooling involves such a lot of work with written and pictorial material, it can result in changes in the way children and adults respond to visually presented material. Some interesting work on visual illusions is relevant here. Visual illusions occur when what is seen can be interpreted in different ways. For example, the arrowheads on the lines in the Muller-Lyer illusion, as shown in figure 3, create the illusion that one line is longer than the other, but only for people who have been to school.

The Ponzo illusion, also shown in the figure, again has horizontal lines of the same length, but in this instance the background of converging lines creates an illusion that the top line is longer. Again, this only influences literate people. Non-literate people recognise that the lines are the same length, as has been shown in Uganda in studies by Leibowitz and Pick (1972) and by P. L. Kilbride and Leibowitz (1975). This is also true of various other visual illusions (Rogoff 1981). Children who go to school also learn to 'see' pictures in three dimensions, although pictures on paper exist only in two dimensions, top to bottom and left to right. Cues in pictures, which children learn to 'read,' give information about depth or distance – nearer or further away.

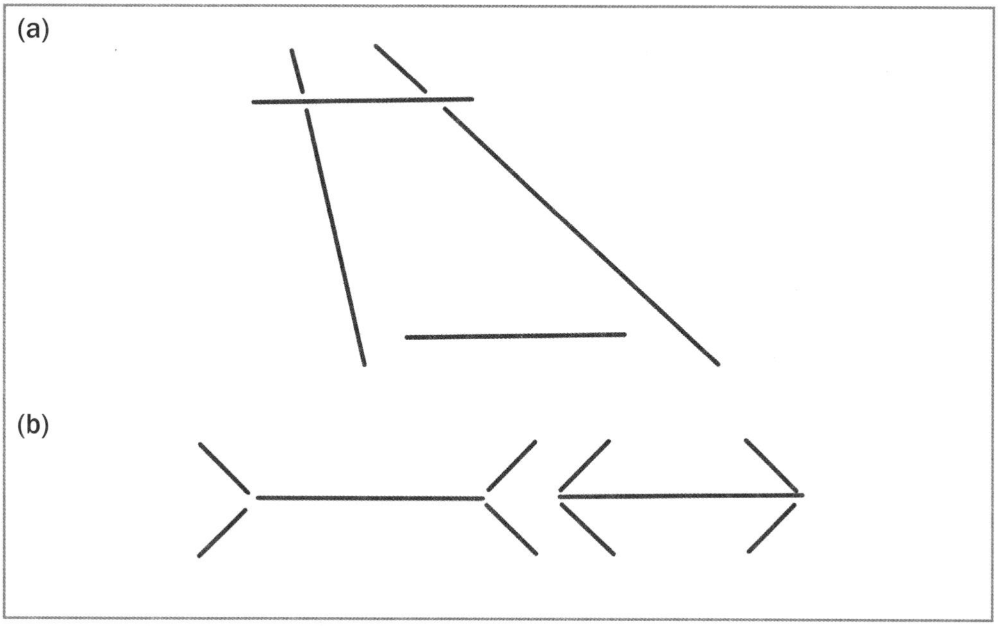

(a) modified form of the Ponzo illusion
(b) Muller-Lyer illusion as used by Segall, Campbell and Herskovits (1966). In each line drawing the horizontal lines are of equal length, but appear to be different lengths because of the surrounding lines.
Source: Berry, Poortinga, Segall and Dasen (1992:150)

Figure 3 Visual illusions

The lack of African research into how teaching influences the development of literacy is important in view of the over-riding impact of basic literacy skills on later school achievement. Even today, researchers who are unfamiliar with the patterns of interaction between teacher and pupil in sub-Saharan African schools may not do good research. A good example of this is the study done by Liddell (1997) in South Africa. This study of children's use of pictorial cues when learning to read is weakened by the way the question was posed. Liddell presented some evidence that beginner readers in schools in some remote parts of South Africa did not use picture cues to help them understand the story line. In her research they failed to develop a narrative about pictures they had selected from a set. Instead they labelled items in the picture right through the first three grades. In fact, Grade 3 children produced significantly fewer labels, made fewer statements linking two parts of the picture (e.g. the lady is behind the table) and offered less narrative than children in the first two grades.

Liddell concluded that the children's ways of responding to pictures remained very concrete, with little evidence of abstract thought. But another interpretation is possible. Liddell's research assistants asked pupils to 'Tell me what you see in the picture.' Such a question seems likely to elicit a list from children in teacher-centred classes where getting the one correct answer is emphasised. Teacher behaviour that might have contributed to children's continued use of concrete descriptors was not observed. A different question, such as 'Tell me about the picture', might have elicited a different range of responses.

Learning in a second language

Besides a lack of familiarity with pictures and books in communities where literacy is generally low, there is the additional difficulty of establishing literacy in a second language. Governments in many countries recognise that it is important to have a common language if there are many different regional languages in the country, and have imposed requirements that children learn a selected common language. Problems arise when children are required to use the second language, which they are still learning, while also learning new concepts in mathematics, science and other subjects. Cleghorn, Merritt and Abagi (1989), for example, investigated the use of English during science lessons with Standard 8 pupils in Kenyan primary schools. Although teachers were expected to be competent English speakers, only 6% of those who participated in the study were confident that they had no difficulties in expressing themselves in English. Most were unable to use English in flexible ways to enhance pupil understanding of new concepts.

Other problems arose if one language had two terms with subtly different meanings, while the other had only one word for both concepts. For example, Swahili does not discriminate between 'disease' and 'sickness'. Students studying intestinal parasites were confused when the teacher explained that the tapeworm did not bring any disease, but that people with tapeworms were sick. Teachers used a range of strategies, including use of an occasional first language word to clarify meanings, but both they and the pupils had additional difficulties with science because they were studying it in a language they did not know very well. Fuller and Clarke (1994) do note, however, that the English of Malawian teachers improved when they were provided with an adequate supply of texts to use in lesson preparation. This result suggests that with adequate resources and only a little regular practice the second language skills of teachers can be improved significantly.

Adolescents in primary schools

Teachers who have adolescent pupils in their primary school classes need to accommodate the changes in cognitive processing that occur during early and middle adolescence. Studies of adolescents in northern hemisphere countries show an increased ability to cope with abstract concepts and to solve complex problems (Berk 2000). Because African children's cognitive development has been shown to be just like that of children elsewhere (Cole et al. 1971) it can be assumed that adolescent Africans also develop cognitively in the same ways as other adolescents. It is important to recognise that cognitive development is not related to acquisition of literacy and numeracy. Adolescents will be able to reason in a relatively mature way, even if they have not been lucky enough to develop adequate literacy or numeracy. Asking these pupils to do the same tasks as much younger children increases the risk that they will lose motivation and drop out of school.

Social factors also have a marked influence on schooling, especially for adolescent girls who are less likely than their male peers to continue schooling once they reach puberty. Etori (1995), speaking from Ugandan experience, has pointed out that in the many rural areas where the majority of Africans live, cultural norms mistrust schooling for girls. Schools are believed to destroy customs; girls who go to school forgo learning the domestic tasks that prepare them for home-making and motherhood. But other factors limit girls' continued attendance at school once they reach adolescence. Many leave because they are pregnant. The rate of teenage pregnancy varies from country to country, according to how the culture and religion view it. In 1990, in Botswana, for example, a total of 2 047 pupils were reported to have dropped out of school. Three quarters of this number were female and two thirds of this group were pregnant (Ahmed 1990). Early pregnancy disadvantages young women permanently in terms of future choices and limits the contribution they can make to national development. Teachers who are unconcerned about these limiting factors are unlikely to behave in ways that encourage adolescent girls to continue with their education.

Conclusion

Changes during middle childhood are slow, but during this period children acquire many social and cognitive skills. These developments happen whether children go to school or not. For the child who reaches adolescence while still at primary school, there are more sudden physical changes that are accompanied by social and cognitive growth. However, despite the importance of the primary school years for African children's futures, little research has investigated the social, emotional, or cognitive development of children during this time. Moreover, research done by people who are unfamiliar with African cultures is not always helpful. Even today investigators from outside Africa may reach conclusions that are incorrect because they frame questions badly, or do not know enough about the culture of the people they are studying to consider alternative explanations for the results they have obtained.

Successful completion of primary school is important for the individual child, for his or her future children, and for national development. For the young people whose time at school ends with the completion of primary school, there are important decisions to be made about the future. Studies of this period of transition to the adult world also need to be done before the full implications of terminating education at the end of primary school can be understood. The effect of such early termination of education on the future social, psychological, and economic wellbeing of the young person may be quite different from the developmental consequences of later completion of education. As such, it is important that this transition, like other changes that are associated with primary school attendance, should be fully investigated and understood.

In your community (four)

A good primary school can modify the effects of family life and values, either improving the child's lot or, at times, making it worse. Choose one or two of the following activities to explore the impact of schooling in your community:

1 Discuss your ideas about the skills and development of primary-school-age students with some colleagues. Which ideas are based on tradition? To what extent are these ideas consistent with what modern research tells us?

2 Close your eyes and imagine you are back in the class with the unkindest teacher you had. Write about what this teacher did that was harmful. Think about what you need to do as a teacher to avoid harming children in these ways. Discuss ideas with two or three colleagues.

3 Close your eyes and imagine you are back in the class with the best teacher you had as a school student. Write about what this teacher did that makes you remember him or her as the best teacher.

4 Work with a group of colleagues. Decide which age group within the primary school age band you would like to talk to. Ask 5 or 6 students what 3 things they like best about their school and their teachers, and what three things they like least. Report back to others in your group.

5 Observe one experienced teacher in action for about 15 minutes. Make a list of all the positive and negative comments he or she makes. Do children get attention for doing good work and behaving well, or do they get it when they are misbehaving? Do boys or girls get more attention or are they treated in the same way? Present your findings to one or two others and compare results.

Chapter Six

Child health

Introduction

The child's potential for good health is partly determined by events that occur during its prenatal development. Thereafter, infants and children in Africa are vulnerable to poor health for a number of reasons. Parental knowledge about health and illness, dietary practices, and access to healers' support in times of sickness influence children's physical and psychological wellbeing. African parents may seek help from a traditional healer or may use medicines or medical techniques developed in the northern hemisphere and introduced to Africa.

The present chapter briefly describes traditional and introduced beliefs about management of ill health. It then outlines some health problems that are common in different parts of Africa, but does not generally reiterate information about problems that occur throughout the world. Despite the emphasis on the impact of inadequate food, on infection, and on the negative impact of these environmental factors on child development during pregnancy and later, teachers should remember that the great majority of pregnancies result in the birth of healthy children. Most of these children survive the dangers of infancy and early childhood and begin school healthy enough to acquire the cognitive and social skills required in their later years.

Traditional and modern understandings about health

Africans have traditionally understood illness in a different framework from that adopted in the northern hemisphere. Everyone is thought to be at some constant risk of illness and accident, and these misfortunes do not occur by chance. Therefore, an illness or accident at a specific moment must be due to some cause that can be found. Healers in Africa have asked, 'Why did this illness occur at this time?' and have often found the answer in some disturbance in social relations within the group. Thus, restoring social relations, or taking action to protect oneself from the harmful thoughts and actions of others can cure the illness. In contrast, northern hemisphere scientists and doctors have asked, 'How did this illness occur?' This has led to a search for the organism that causes the illness. Accidents are explained as occurring purely by chance (Airhihenbuwa 1995).

Some health practices that are now commonly used around the world were used in Africa well before they were accepted in the countries of the northern hemisphere. Airhihenbuwa (1995) presents evidence that the Baganda of Uganda almost certainly performed caesarean surgery on mothers who were unable to give birth naturally prior to European contact. They used techniques to prevent infection before the need for antiseptic conditions during surgery was known in Europe. Various kinds of medications have also been used for many generations. African healers use herbs and other plants to reduce fevers and may grow many healing herbs in their gardens (Palmer 1993). Mothers may actively teach daughters about these healing herbs (Shelley 1985). Just a few of the plants that have been used in traditional medical practice are those that have a tranquillising effect, some that act as laxatives, and others that provide insulin for people with diabetes (Airhihenbuwa 1995). The mechanisms by which these had effect have only recently been understood.

Other folk knowledge is not supported by modern medical research. For example, in Mali, Gray et al. (1990) found a widespread belief that the best way to treat a fever was to put additional coverings over the child, to 'bring the fever out'. Modern medicine has shown that the most important thing to do is to reduce the fever as much as possible by bathing the child in cool water. Similarly, rural Somali women listed several possible causes of diarrhoea, only one of which (the existence of worms in the stomach) is known to cause some gastro-intestinal problems. None of the traditional treatments that these women prescribed were useful (Ntiri 1993).

The African recognition of a relationship between disturbed social relations and ill health, whether physical or psychological, pre-dates northern hemisphere knowledge in this field by many centuries. Northern hemisphere researchers have only recently begun to understand that social and physical stress both affect the immune system, reducing the body's natural capacity to fight off infection (Plotnikoff, Murgo, Faith and Wybran 1991; Sapolsky 1998). Certain practices such as meditation and relaxation are now known to strengthen the immune system. Thus, the traditional African use of amulets, spells, and chants may promote healing, because they promote a sense of relaxation and control over events, and this has the effect of reducing physiological stress.

Clearly, then, Africans do not need to give up all the traditional practices with regard to health. Many still choose to approach traditional healers when suffering from certain health problems. They may seek help from pharmacists, nurses and doctors with training in introduced medical practice when other problems arise (Airhihenbuwa 1995). For educated urban Africans the choice is easily made. Most doctors live in the cities. However, about 80% of Africans, the rural people, are much more dependent on the local shaman because of the shortage of doctors in rural areas.

Box 5 The UN Convention on the Rights of the Child: Health

Every child has the right to enjoy the highest attainable standard of health and to facilities for the treatment of illness and rehabilitation to health. The State shall take steps to combat disease and malnutrition within the framework of primary health care, through the application of readily available technology and through the provision of adequate nutritious foods and clean drinking water. The State should also take steps to abolish traditional practices prejudicial to children's health.

Source: *Save the Children* (1990). Appendix

Optimally, parents need knowledge about, and access to, both systems in order to ensure the physical, psychological, and social wellbeing of their children. Parents and teachers are familiar with traditional practices, so the remainder of the chapter focuses on what can be learned from introduced knowledge, beginning with knowledge about prenatal and infant development.

Prenatal development and infancy

Much has been written about the nutritional needs of pregnant women (e.g. Stoppard 2001; Werner 1993). These texts emphasise the need for a range of foods that supply the carbohydrates, minerals and vitamins necessary for the development of a healthy foetus, and for the good health of the mother. If the pregnant woman's diet is inadequate, certain substances are drawn from whatever reserves exist in her body to feed the developing foetus. This leaves her even more depleted of substances essential for her own health. For example, if a woman does not have sufficient calcium in her diet, calcium from her teeth is used to promote bone growth in the infant. This leaves the mother with tooth cavities and may result in the eventual loss of some or all of her teeth.

Although most African women obtain enough carbohydrate in their diet to be able to perform daily tasks, they may not obtain enough for optimal health for either themselves or the foetus (Martorell 1980). In addition they may lack some micronutrients or trace elements, vitamins, and proteins essential for foetal development. An example of one of these is the B vitamin called folate or folic acid. Women who do not have enough folic acid in their diets are more likely to give birth to infants with spina bifida, a condition in which the spinal column does not close completely around the spinal cord during development in the womb. Drainage of fluid from the brain is also often affected, and when this occurs, the brain becomes progressively more damaged unless children have an operation to improve drainage of brain fluids. Children with spina bifida are also paralysed from the site at which the spinal cord has not developed normally. So, it is important that adequate levels of folate are established prior to the pregnancy and that pregnant women have sufficient folate from green leafy vegetables in their diets.

Almost half the pregnant women in sub-Saharan Africa are anaemic. The average rate of anaemia for this group across sub-Saharan Africa is 44%, with a range of between 7% and 74% (United Nations Development Programme (UNDP) 2000). Anaemia is a condition in which the body is unable to carry oxygen to the cells in the body efficiently because the red blood cells do not have enough haemoglobin. Haemoglobin is the part of the blood that transports oxygen. Anaemia occurs when people lack iron in their diet, are more generally malnourished, or have frequent illness, especially malaria. Besides being constantly tired and weak, an anaemic woman is more likely than one who is not anaemic to have a miscarriage (spontaneous abortion) some time during the pregnancy. Extremely anaemic women may also bleed heavily when giving birth, increasing the risk that they will die at this time (UNICEF 1999b; Werner 1993).

Illnesses such as malaria, which cause high fevers, may also adversely influence the developing foetus. Infants whose mothers have had malaria during their pregnancy are likely to be smaller than average at birth and are described as having low birth weight. Between 10% and 21% of infants born in all sub-Saharan Africa countries except Senegal and Ghana are of low birth weight, compared with 4% to 10% in the wealthy countries of the northern hemisphere (UNDP 2000). The malaria fever and the maternal anaemia that is often a consequence of the infection account for as much as 30% of preventable low birth weight infants in Africa. Malaria also contributes significantly to the rate of miscarriage, stillbirth and infant death, and is a major contributor to maternal death (UNICEF 1999b).

Knowledge about the cause of malaria remains low among people in developing countries. For example, half of the respondents who participated in a study in Ghana did not know that mosquitoes transmitted malaria (UNICEF 1999b). This ignorance of causes meant that pregnant women in the group could not take action to reduce the risk of infection during their pregnancies.

African foetuses are vulnerable to the same risks that are described in northern hemisphere texts about foetal development. The mother's general health, her use of both prescribed and illicit drugs, and whether or not she smokes cigarettes or drinks alcohol can influence the development of the foetus. A range of other infections besides malaria may also be harmful. The extent to which foetal development is influenced by any event may depend on the point in the pregnancy when the stressor comes into play. As elsewhere, the age of the mother may further influence the outcome of the pregnancy. Women over 40 are significantly more likely than younger women to have infants with some genetic disorders, such as Down's syndrome, a syndrome in which the child has a characteristic appearance, and is intellectually disabled to some extent. Older mothers, especially those who already have several children, also tend to have children who are smaller than earlier infants they have borne. In LeVine et al.'s (1996) study of the Gusii, these latter infants were more irritable, more active, and less easily consoled when they became upset. They did not respond as well as children of younger mothers to sounds when these were presented during assessment. Finally, they were less alert than infants of younger mothers and gained weight less rapidly.

Infant and maternal mortality

Some infant and maternal deaths are inevitable in the perinatal period (the few days around birth) in countries that cannot afford the expensive clinics and specialist doctors who are needed to save lives when there are complex problems. But the frequency of maternal death (maternal mortality) varies widely from one African country to another, as does infant mortality (see table 7). While some of the differences between countries reflect the social stability or wealth of each country, the relationship is not an exact one. Mortality rates are at least partly an outcome of government priorities and policies with regard to infant and maternal wellbeing.

Some of the maternal and infant deaths in Africa are a result of traditional practices. For example, studies in Botswana cited by Ball (1988) and Seboni (1993) show that women there reject the use of episiotomy. (This practice involves making a small cut in the wall of the vagina to reduce the risk of tearing. Tearing may result in a ragged wound that is difficult to stitch together.) Some still favour the practice of going off alone to deliver the infant in isolation. Thus, if there are any problems with the birth, they cannot obtain help. Another belief that may result in harm to the mother is the idea that post-partum bleeding is healthy because it helps the uterus and entire body system to heal after the birth. This is not correct.

Table 7 Rates of maternal and infant mortality in selected African countries

Country	Maternal mortality[a]	Infant mortality[b]
Sierra Leone	Not reported	182
Angola	Not reported	170
Rwanda	Not reported	105
Senegal	560	70
South Africa	Not reported	60
Ghana	210	67
Zimbabwe	400	59
Namibia	230	57
Botswana	330	38

a = Actual number of deaths from pregnancy related causes per 100 000 live births during the period 1990–1998.

b = Number of infant deaths (before age 1 year) per 1 000 live births in 1998

Source: Adapted from tables 1 and 7, UNICEF (2000a)

Similarly, the risk of neonatal tetany, which causes death from high fever and convulsions, is increased when mothers and their helpers do not know about the importance of good hygiene at the time of the birth. Neonatal tetany most often occurs when infection enters the neonate's body through the umbilical cord. This is most likely to occur when dirty instruments are used to cut the cord, or when the area around the umbilicus (tummy button) is smeared with oil or some other substance, as has been a traditional practice. Giving the mother a tetanus vaccination just before the birth reduces the risk of both maternal and infant tetany. This vaccination is not widely available in sub-Saharan Africa, however. Less than half the pregnant women are protected in this way in many countries (UNICEF 2000a).

Feeding practices and infant health

Health professionals state that breast milk is the best food in the first three to six months, with additional foods added in the second half of the first year (e.g.UNICEF 1999a; Werner 1993) The UNICEF report *Breastfeeding: Foundation for a Healthy Life* states that 'children who are breastfed . . . are less susceptible to pneumonia, asthma, allergies, childhood diabetes, gastro-intestinal illnesses and infections that can damage their hearing' (1999a:1) Breast-feeding also provides some protection against malaria (Werner 1993). However, the data from the UNICEF (2000a) report, presented in table 8, show that in many countries the tradition of prolonged breast-feeding that was widespread in Africa prior to European contact is not necessarily followed today.

Table 8 Percentage of infants who are breast-fed in some sub-Saharan African countries

Country	Exclusively breast-fed (at age 0–3 months)	Breast-fed, with additional foods (at age 6–9 months)	Still breast-feeding (at age 20–23 months)
Benin	15	97	65
Mali	13	33	60
Nigeria	2	52	43
Congo	43	95	27
Gambia	Not reported	8	58
Swaziland	37	51	20
Kenya	17	94	54
Chad	2	81	62
Malawi	5	61	93

Note: Data refer to the period 1990–1999, except for Congo where data do not cover the whole period.
Source: Adapted from table 2, UNICEF (2000a)

The small percentage of infants aged 0 to 3 months who are exclusively breast-fed is a cause for concern. Reasons for this are not known. It is possible that traditional feeding practices in some African communities required the early introduction of extremely watery porridge made from a staple food such as maize, millet or rice. Alternatively, the mother may not be able to produce sufficient breast milk because her diet is inadequate (Martorell 1980). A third possibility is that there may have been a widespread shift in recent times to include some milk substitutes in the diet from an early age. No food substitutes are as rich in nutrients as breast milk, nor do they contain the many protective antibodies of breast milk. Such substitute foods are extremely costly, and using them carries the risk that harmful bacteria will give the infant the gastro-intestinal infection that causes the diarrhoea. Use of milk substitutes is actively discouraged by governments in some countries (UNICEF 1999a). On the other hand, breast milk may not be the best in all instances. A serious problem faced by many African mothers is a consequence of AIDS. Information about infants and AIDS is presented in Chapter Eight: 'HIV/AIDS'.

Conclusion

African women and their infants have always been at risk of poor health and high mortality. Ignorance, poverty and poor health care mean that they are still at risk today. In fact, some changes in practice that are associated with modernity may actually increase the risk that infants will suffer poor health and that rates of infant mortality will remain high.

Foods for healthy development

Once infants have reached the age of about 6 months, they should gradually be introduced to a wider range of foods. In this way, children will continue to have good health and good rates of growth (Werner 1993). The new foods should be offered in addition to breast-feeding, which often continues until children are about 2 years old. As table 8 shows, however, parents in some ethnic groups delay the introduction of solids beyond this age. They may be concerned about the increased risk of diarrhoea for the child when solids are introduced, but the result is that some children do not obtain sufficient food for continued growth and health in the latter part of the first year (Gray et al. 1990).

Table 9 shows the range of foods necessary for good health. Werner (1993) refers to these as Main foods, Go foods, Grow foods and Glow foods. Werner's table for meeting food needs resembles the description of different food groups used by nutritionists, but shows more clearly how poor families may provide a healthy diet for their children. The emphasis is on giving as much of the main food as possible, with other foods, especially the 'Go' energy foods, included in the diet frequently. The table gives examples of each of these food groups. Some foods appear in more than one part of the table.

It is extremely important to note that cassava roots and leaves contain cyanide, a poison that can kill. Children in poor families in East Africa, whose diet includes a lot of cassava, are especially likely to be harmed by the poison if they eat a lot of this food and not much else. They may lose of sensation in their feet and hands, develop damage to the optic nerve in the eye, and have some degree of deafness. Worst of all are the stumbling gait and many falls when they try to walk. Eventually they may not be able to walk without help. This disability is called 'konzo' in Mozambique (Lee 2001) but is more correctly named tropical ataxic neuropathy (Cliff 2003).

Although the disability is less common in West Africa, it has been reported there. West Africans have always eaten cassava that contains high levels of cyanide, but they have developed ways of processing the roots and leaves to remove the poison. This involves mincing or slicing the cassava tubers very finely, then drying them, before cooking them slowly in an open pan. In this way the cyanide is released from the damaged cells into the air. (It means, too, that cassava is best cooked outdoors, so that the poison can disperse rapidly.)

Table 9 Foods required for optimal growth and health

Food group	What this food provides	Sources	Examples
Main foods	Cheap source of energy. Cereals also provide some low cost protein, iron and vitamins	Cereals and grains Starchy roots Starchy fruits	Wheat, maize, rice, millet, sorghum Cassava,[a] potatoes, taro Bananas, plantain, breadfruit
Go foods	Energy	Fats Foods rich in fats Nuts Oil seeds Sugars	Vegetable oils, butter, lard Coconut, olives, fatty meat Groundnuts (peanuts), almonds, walnuts, cashews Pumpkin, melon, sesame, sunflower Sugar, honey, molasses, sugar cane
Grow foods	Proteins and other body building helpers	Legumes Nuts Oil seeds Animal products	Beans, peas, lentils Groundnuts (peanuts), walnuts, cashews, almonds Sesame, sunflower Milk, eggs, cheese, yoghurt, fish, chicken, meat, small animals and insects
Glow foods	Vitamins and minerals and protective helpers	Vegetables Fruits	Dark green leafy plants, such as leaves of sweet potatoes, beans, peas, pumpkins, squash, young cassava leaves[a] Tomatoes, carrots, pumpkin, sweet potato, peppers Mangoes, oranges, papaya, etc.

a: Cassava may contain large quantities of cyanide poison unless processed correctly.
Source: Adapted from Werner (1993:111)

East Africans may be more at risk of konzo because many of them now grow modern hybrids of cassava that produce large quantities of food, but that come from the West African varieties of cassava. In East Africa the local variety of cassava had less cyanide than the West African variety. East Africans who used the local variety in the past were less likely to be poisoned even when they ate cassava in large quantities. Therefore they did not develop ways of getting rid of the poison before making cassava flour (H. Bradbury, personal communication, February 2001).

Cassava leaves carry more cyanide than roots, but they also contain about seven times as much protein and more vitamins than the roots, so they are a good source of cheap additional nutrients (Werner 1993).The cyanide can be removed from leaves fairly easily, by crushing them finely, preferably with a mortar and pestle, and leaving them in the air for up to 30 minutes. Again, the cyanide releases into the air from the plant cells that have been crushed and broken (H. Bradbury, personal communication 13 June 2001).

Deficiency diseases and malnutrition

Many children in Africa do not obtain the so-called Go, Grow and Glow foods in sufficient quantities for good health. A shortage of these foods results in the development of deficiency diseases or more general malnutrition, stunted growth and wasting (low weight for height). Common deficiency diseases in Africa are described in the following few pages. The information is from Werner (1993), but the same information can be found in nursing and other medical texts, and may also be found in some books on nutrition. Environmental factors and culturally based practices that contribute to these problems are also outlined.

Vitamin A deficiency

Vitamin A deficiency initially causes night blindness, a condition in which the individual cannot see well at night. If the person continues to have insufficient Vitamin A, his or her eyes become progressively more damaged. Eventually, the cornea (the surface of the eye) becomes dry and dull looking, then grows quickly and bursts. This results in infection, scarring or other damage.

Babies less than 6 months old who are breast-fed generally obtain sufficient Vitamin A from their mother's milk, unless the mother also lacks this substance in her diet. But when infants are breast-fed for longer periods, they will not obtain enough Vitamin A for healthy eyes unless dark green leafy vegetables (e.g. leaves of peas, beans, pumpkin, sweet potato, cassava) are added to their diet after 6 months. Vitamin A deficiency may also be managed through providing additional Vitamin A as a liquid or in a capsule from about the age of 6 months.

Countries in much of Africa provide supplementary Vitamin A, although the percentage of children who benefit from this treatment varies widely from one country to another. Thus, for example, in Benin all children aged 6 months to

5 years receive Vitamin A supplementation, while in Burundi only 15% do so (UNICEF 2000a). Besides protecting the eyes, adequate reserves of Vitamin A in the body can provide some protection against diarrhoea and measles (World Health Organization (WHO) 2000b). Vitamin A may be especially important if children are to avoid the eye damage that can occur when they have measles.

Anaemia

Pollitt (1990) states that the rate of anaemia among African children in the age range 5–12 years is high. He notes that some authors estimate that as many as 49% of children in this age band suffer from this deficiency disease. These anaemic children are 'irritable, apathetic, distractible and anorexic' (Parks and Wharton 1990:157). Parks and Wharton state that a large number of studies of severely anaemic children have also found anaemia to be associated with deficits in cognitive skills. These deficits appear to occur because the children lack interest in the environment, rather than because they lack ability. For example, iron deficient infants are more fearful, and show less visual and auditory attention to stimuli than children receiving enough iron to prevent anaemia. The long-term effects of this lack of interest can result in reduced school learning and possibly the increased likelihood of behaviour problems.

The iron needed to overcome this deficit is obtained from dark green leafy vegetables and in particular from red meat, especially liver. When mothers use iron pots for cooking, a tiny amount of iron from the pot reaches the food, and anyone who eats the food absorbs some iron. Thus, continued use of iron pots is an advantage for villagers who may not be able to obtain iron in other ways (Werner 1993).

Box 6 A French nun's view of health problems

'The big problem is still anaemia,' a French nun told me on the flight to Ouaga.* 'We still see Africans lying in the sun all day and think, what a great life, no worries. The fact is, most of them just haven't the energy to do anything else. I often think that instead of pouring all these millions into Africa in the form of aid, we should simply ensure that the Africans have iron to cure their anaemia, and let them solve their own problems . . .

'Well, why don't they do something about anaemia?' I asked the younger nun.

'I don't know. Too simple. Doesn't involve enough money. Not enough jobs for consultants. . .'

Source: Peter Biddlecombe (1993:54)

* = Ouagadougou

Iodine deficiency

Iodine deficiency occurs where there is insufficient iodine in the soil in which vegetables and fruits are grown. This commonly occurs in regions where there is high rainfall or where there have been floods. Mountain soils are especially likely to be lacking in iodine. Eating large amounts of cassava also causes iodine deficiency. The way the body processes cyanide reduces the availability of iodine, even when the diet contains sufficient amounts of this substance. Other less commonly eaten vegetables such as spinach, kohlrabi, cabbage, and turnip leaves may also reduce iodine availability but, because they are not staple foods, are less likely to be harmful overall (Draper 1977; Werner 1993).

Iodine deficiency affects development throughout life. Most importantly, foetal development is affected when a pregnant woman has not had enough iodine in her diet before and during the pregnancy. Even if she does not have a goitre, the growth in the throat that shows a marked lack of iodine, she is likely to give birth to an infant who will be intellectually disabled, learning only very slowly, and unable to become independent. The child may also be deaf. This condition is called cretinism.

Neonates, older infants and children all show delayed development when iodine deficiency continues after birth. Infants show slower brain development and reduced general growth. School-age children show impaired school performance (Hetzel 1990). Even children who do not show obvious signs of iodine deficiency may be affected. In particular, some studies have shown that very small (sub-clinical) deficits are associated with poor hearing. Increasing amounts of iodine in the diet to optimum levels can return hearing to normal levels in young children. Lack of iodine is also associated with lack of energy for daily activities. Deficits in visual-perceptual organisation, visual-motor co-ordination and possibly slower processing of information may also occur (Pollitt 1990). All of these problems reduce children's capacity to benefit from school learning.

The problem of how to get people to increase their intake of iodine is easily solved scientifically. A tiny amount of iodine is added to each bag of salt that is sold for daily use. In countries in the northern hemisphere where health-care systems are good, almost all salt in daily use (table salt) has iodine added to it. Salt with iodine added is also available in many parts of Africa, but sometimes salt without iodine is more readily available or costs slightly less. Consumers who do not know how important iodine is, who reject it because of tradition, or who cannot get it easily, may continue to buy salt that does not contain iodine. Thus, the percentage of people using iodised salt in different African countries varies greatly. Surveys show, for example, that iodised salt is used in only 10% of households in Angola, about 60% in Mozambique, Namibia and Niger and close to 80% in Zambia and Zimbabwe (UNICEF 2000b). It is possible that there is sufficient iodine in the soil in some parts of Africa for people to obtain enough of this substance from foods they eat, but people have no way of knowing whether this is true of their village. People who live in coastal areas may obtain sufficient iodine by eating fish and shellfish regularly. But in much of Africa provision of iodised salt is necessary. People's access to it may reflect government health priorities.

Kwashiorkor and marasmus

Kwashiorkor and marasmus are the names given to the diseases of general malnutrition. Kwashiorkor is also called protein energy malnutrition (PEM). It is subdivided into mild, moderate, and severe categories. All of these levels of malnutrition have some negative implications for future development. Kwashiorkor can develop in one of two ways. First, it may develop when children obtain sufficient calories for daily life, but get inadequate amounts of protein (found mainly in milk, milk products, eggs and meat). Additionally, they lack minerals and trace elements (e.g. zinc) that come from fruit and vegetables. Alternatively, children may not obtain sufficient carbohydrate to meet their energy needs, even when they obtain enough protein, minerals and other food elements. In this instance, the child's body attempts to gain the energy it needs by converting the protein and other substances into energy. As a result, growth and tissue repair are prevented. Children with this disease develop swollen abdomens, faces and legs. Their hair becomes brittle and falls out, and skin sores develop. Marasmus develops when a child lacks sufficient calories (kilojoules) and sufficient protein. Such children stop growing, their skin wrinkles and their tissues begin to waste away (Berndt 1992). This level of malnutrition also affects brain development, leaving children with a permanently reduced capacity for learning.

Kwashiorkor and marasmus are most common when there is prolonged drought, or when war disrupts food production, but less severe forms of malnourishment are common in developing countries. For example, Airhihenbuwa (1995) presented information showing that in the period 1988–1990 the great majority of people in sub-Saharan Africa were unable to obtain sufficient calories to meet daily needs. Most obtained less than 95% of daily requirements. Gray et al. (1990) report a number of studies in two regions of Mali where between 18% and 34% of school-age children were found to be mildly to moderately malnourished. Similar results have been obtained in studies in many sub-Saharan African countries (e.g. Palmer 1993; UNICEF 2000a). The great majority of these children are not malnourished in the first three months when they are breast-fed, but rapidly come to lag behind children elsewhere once they reach the age of 1 to 2 years.

Besides the immediately harmful effects of malnourishment on children's development generally, being malnourished is harmful in another important way. It reduces the body's resistance to infection. In particular, it makes the malnourished individual vulnerable to diseases that infect the mucous membranes of the respiratory and gastro-intestinal tracts. Thus, malnourished people are more likely to have both bacterial and viral respiratory tract infections, including tuberculosis. They will more often have diarrhoea, measles, herpes (cold sores) and whooping cough (pertussis), and will be vulnerable to cholera and leprosy. In addition, because of their weakened immune system, their bodies are less likely to be able to destroy parasites (e.g. gastro-intestinal worms, bilharzia) which further weaken their system once they become established (Ulijaszek 1990).

The body's capacity to develop immunity to some illnesses is reduced when children are malnourished and recovery is slow. Children whose diet is inadequate and who have been ill may take four to eight weeks to recover their pre-infection nutritional state. They lose weight because the initial loss of interest in food during illness is followed by a period when the body uses more than usual amounts of energy to fight off the infection (WHO 2000a). Studies also show that the BCG vaccination that protects children from tuberculosis is less effective when children are even mildly malnourished. Similarly, immune response to the measles, typhoid and poliomyelitis vaccinations is also reduced if a child is severely malnourished (Ulijaszek 1990).

Cultural practices as causes of malnourishment

Children may be malnourished for many reasons, not just because of a general shortage of food in the community. For example, a child from a large family might not be getting enough food because the parents cannot grow food in the quantities required for the family. Or the greater poverty of female-headed households may mean that an unsupported mother cannot buy food in the amounts required to feed her child satisfactorily (Panter-Brick 1998). However, there are some parental beliefs and practices that also increase the risk that their children will be malnourished.

Using milk substitutes when feeding infants

Problems arise when women believe that powdered milk or milk substitute (infant formula) is better for their infant than breast milk, or when they believe that using infant formula is somehow a more modern thing to do. Because of the high cost of these substitute foods, poor mothers may dilute the formula below the recommended quantities. Thus, the infant does not actually receive adequate amounts of food. In addition, poor women living without electricity and constant supplies of water cannot maintain feeding bottles in a sterile condition. In fact, there is some evidence that feeding even very young infants from a cup is safer than using bottles (UNICEF 1999a). Water added to make up the substitute formula may also contain harmful bacteria and other infective agents. As a result, infants are at increased risk of contracting gastro-intestinal disorders that cause diarrhoea. Because the child feels unwell, he or she also eats and drinks less for some time.

Food restriction

African children's access to various foods may be restricted for a number of reasons:

- **Beliefs about 'food' and 'sauce'**: In some ethnic groups people use the term food to refer only to their staple carbohydrate vegetable (e.g. rice, maize, millet). All other edible substances (meat, oils, green and yellow vegetables, fruits) are referred to as sauce or relish. This way of thinking about foods is sometimes associated with a mistaken belief that if children have eaten the staple food regularly and in sufficient quantities they cannot be malnourished (Cassidy 1980; Zeitlin 1996). Substances that are labelled 'sauce' are often only available in small quantities but, as table 9 shows, these 'sauce' foods provide the essential proteins, vitamins and trace elements necessary for satisfactory growth and health.
- **Access to prestige foods**: 'Sauce' foods often have prestige value and only certain members of the community may have access to them. In the rural Yoruba communities where Zeitlin (1996) worked, most of the meat and fish, both prestige foods, was allocated to the provider, usually a man. Sometimes the women in the household were providers and in these instances they obtained sufficient meat or fish.

  Children may gain access to prestige foods based on gender or age. Where boys' status is higher than that of girls, boys may receive more prestige foods, or just more food overall than girls. Sigman, Neumann, Jansen and Bwibo (1989) found, for example, that Kenyan boys in their sample obtained more calories per day on average than girls, although neither group received sufficient food to meet energy and growth needs. But Cassidy (1980) pointed out that the allocation of food among the Sotho people gave some advantage to women and girls.
- **Food and moral development**: Parents' beliefs about the relationship of food to development may also influence younger children's diet. Yoruba women in Zeitlin's (1996) study stated that children should only receive a tiny amount of meat because giving children more than that hindered children's moral development (66% of mothers said this), encouraged the child to steal

(31%), or spoilt the child (31%). As a result these mothers gave their children very little meat. An earlier study cited by Zeitlin showed a clear link between maternal beliefs about spoiling children through giving too much prestige food and the child's growth. Mothers of children who were small for their age had strong beliefs that giving prestige foods was spoiling the child. They had not given their children sufficient amounts of these foods to promote adequate growth. In this instance, their strong cultural belief about prestige foods and moral development suggests that education about children's need for protein would not be well accepted initially.

- **Eating and illness**: Mothers in many ethnic groups adhere to a traditional belief that infants and children who are sick should not be fed. The women who participated in Gray et al.'s (1990) study, for example, believed that the best way to treat a child who had diarrhoea caused by a gastro-intestinal infection was to withhold food and drinks. They also believed they should withhold food when children were ill with infectious diseases such as measles, even when the child had passed the initial period of not wanting to eat. By acting on this belief, mothers were actually increasing the risk that their child would not survive the infection, or that they would recover with some residual damage that would limit further development.
- **Eating from a communal pot**: Eating from a communal pot may mean that toddlers and preschoolers miss out on food. Slower and less controlled movements make it difficult for them to compete against older children and adults when all are hungrily reaching towards shared foods. Sharing from a communal container also increases the risk that gastro-intestinal worms and diarrhoeal diseases will be passed to these vulnerable young children, reducing the benefit they might otherwise receive from the food they have obtained.
- **Food deprivation as punishment**: Both Zeitlin (1996) and Nsamenang (1992a) point out that deprivation of food is one of the punishments commonly used by African parents. In communities where children's food intake is already small or excludes some of the high protein, high vitamin foods necessary for health, further food deprivation can only be harmful.

Conclusion

Although much is known about the range of foods needed for healthy development, many African children continue to suffer from deficiency diseases and from malnutrition. These children's development is adversely affected in ways that have long-term implications for health and education. Some parents cannot provide adequate food because of the extreme poverty of their family, but many others do not provide a range of foods because they do not understand the importance of different foods. Alternatively, they may have traditional or modern beliefs about food that prevent them from acting in their child's best interests.

Causes of infection and disease

When infants and young children become ill in Africa, the illness is often believed to be caused by the mother's carelessness or bad behaviour, or by the evil intent of others. For example, a difficult labour is believed to show that a woman has had an affair and is being punished for her sins (Gray et al. 1990). In some cultures a 'night bird' flying over an infant who has been deliberately taken outside by a co-wife after dark is believed to cause the convulsions of malaria or tetanus. Strangers may put the evil eye (bad eye) on the food or drink of infants and young children, contaminating it and causing illness (Shelley 1985). However, Gray et al. note that when mothers learn that they can take actions to soothe their child's symptoms and can nurse their children back to health with little risk of life-threatening complications, they become 'less preoccupied with witches' (1985, p.92) as causes of ill health.

Diseases that are easily prevented and, if infection occurs, easily managed, if medical systems are adequate, make large numbers of African children extremely ill. Many of them actually die from such infections. Between 10% and 30% of infant deaths per year are the result of tetanus infection. In addition, about 800 000 children die from diarrhoea, which often co-occurs with measles and poor nutrition. Pneumonia is one of the three most important killer diseases, with about 1.5 million children under 5 years dying from this disease each year. A further 1 million children, most of them also under 5 years, die from malaria and just over half a million die from measles. In all instances the children's vulnerability to these diseases is increased if they are malnourished (WHO 1996). This is not the full story, however, as a significant minority of Africans have the quality and length of their lives reduced through some disability that follows from childhood disease. For example, nearly 90% of African people are infected with hepatitis B at some time in their lives, often during childhood. This infection very frequently results in the development of liver cancer in adulthood. Adults who develop tumours generally die between the ages of 35 and 45 years (WHO 1996).

Common parasites, such as the gastro-intestinal parasites that inhabit the gut, result in loss of quality of life and some deaths. Like pneumonia, measles and diarrhoeal diseases, these worms are extremely contagious, spreading quickly from child to child unless parents and teachers insist that children follow basic rules for cleanliness. Careful hand-washing, preferably with soap (and hot water if possible), after going to the toilet and before handling food is especially important.

Parasites that require another host animal (e.g. water snail) or insect (e.g. anopheles mosquito) to transmit the parasite from one human to another cause other illnesses. These parasites may be more difficult to eradicate, but their effect on the health of children and adults in the community is such that special efforts to reduce their impact are extremely worthwhile. Features of the broad environment that permit and encourage the spread of infection are poor quality water, poor sanitation, and limited provision of, or poor response to, vaccination programmes. These are described in more detail in the following few pages.

Poor quality water

Overall, only 39% of rural Africans have safe water, while 77% of urban Africans do so (UNICEF 2000a). There is, however, considerable variation between countries in the percentage of residents who have access to safe water. For example, in the Central African Republic only 55% of urban dwellers had safe water in the last few years of the twentieth century, while in Senegal 96% of people in urban areas did. In both countries the percentage of rural people with safe water was much lower: 21% in the Central African Republic and 70% in Senegal. Because most people still live in rural communities, these percentages mean that the great majority of African people are using poor quality water. As a result, they are vulnerable to the many diseases of the gastro-intestinal tract that are carried in dirty water. For infants and young children this results in a range of illnesses. It is also associated with higher rates of malnutrition among preschoolers (Smith and Haddad 2000).

When river water is used for drinking, washing and recreational activities, children are likely to become infected with the tiny worms that cause schistosomiasis (bilharzia). Research across Africa has consistently shown that the small water snail carrying the worms is present in nearly all rivers and lakes. Farley (1991) states that the rate of infection can reach nearly 100% among children and adults who use river water daily. One form of this disease causes damage to the liver and intestines, while the second form found in Africa damages the kidneys and bladder. Both contribute to the high rates of anaemia among African children and have other long-term debilitating effects on the health of the sufferer.

The anopheles mosquito, which carries the malaria parasite, breeds in stagnant water, often water that accumulates in empty cans and jars, inside the rims of old tyres and in ruts left after logging or when heavy vehicles use unsealed roads during the wet season. Infants and primary-school-age children are more vulnerable to malarial infection than adults. Where cerebral malaria is prevalent, (as it is in all parts of Africa where malaria occurs) children may not survive the infection. Primary-school-age children in Africa average six bouts of malaria a year, and are too unwell to attend school for a week each time they have this illness. When they return to school they are likely to be anaemic, with recovery from anaemia slowed by poor diet (UNICEF 1999b). During this time they will be less able to take advantage of school lessons than their healthier peers, so the cumulative effect of even a few episodes of malaria can mean considerable loss of efficiency in learning.

Poor sanitation

Adequate sanitation can be provided in towns and cities where the sewage system takes waste water and body wastes to treatment centres for processing to make it safe. While African cities, like cities around the world, have sewage systems, these are often only partly developed, do not cater for the needs of people living in slum areas, and are poorly maintained. The result is that sewage seeps to the surface, where passers-by are exposed to any infective matter it carries. Alternatively, urban dwellers may prepare a concrete-lined septic tank in the ground to contain waste material, which is later collected and removed by truck for processing elsewhere. A well-made septic tank can be quite safe, but where waste matter leaks away through cracks in the concrete, people living nearby are at risk of infection. In rural areas, the safe disposal of body wastes depends on the placement of pit latrines, their distance from households and water supplies, their design and the depth of the pit. Where latrines are poorly placed, where children play in sewage-affected areas, and where village dogs search through wastes that have been poorly disposed of, the risk of infection in the community is high.

Overall, 70% of urban residents and 35% of rural residents in sub-Saharan Africa have access to adequate sanitation, about the same percentage as are receiving safe water. Again, as with water, there is considerable variability from one country to another with regard to the percentage of the population for whom sanitation is safe and adequate. In Tanzania, for example, 98% of people in urban areas and 83% of rural residents have adequate sanitation. This contrasts dramatically with the situation in Sierra Leone where sanitation is adequate for only 17% of urban residents and 8% of rural people (UNICEF 2000a).

For townspeople in most countries there is some relationship between access to safe water and access to adequate sanitation. This is not necessarily true of rural people, as the figures for the few years leading up to 2000 reveal. In Namibia, for example, 71% of rural people had safe water but only 20% had adequate sanitation. A similar discrepancy existed for rural people in Zimbabwe, Senegal and Niger, among other countries. The reverse was also true for some countries.

In Uganda and Zambia more rural people have adequate sanitation than have access to safe water (UNICEF 2000a). These differences between rural and urban areas obviously reflect government priorities with regard to provision of basic services to communities in their country. However, since clean water and safe disposal of waste water and body wastes contribute importantly to the health status of communities, both need to be provided in the interests of community wellbeing.

Poor sanitary conditions within home and community

Ignorance of simple sanitary procedures to follow when a child is ill may promote the spread of disease, as may some behaviours that arise from poverty or tradition. Keeping fingernails short, for example, reduces the spread of gastro-intestinal worms among children. In communities where children and adults wash their hands using soap after toileting and before meals, the rate of diarrhoea is significantly lowered. Using a rag for a handkerchief reduces the spread of the cold virus. On the other hand, clearing the nostrils or throat by blowing or spitting mucus onto the ground creates a pool of infected material to which others are exposed. Using the hands to eat when sharing food from a communal bowl increases the spread of gastroenteritis and gastro-intestinal worms. Changes in these behaviours must be made at the individual and family level. However, where adequate supplies of clean water for thorough hand-washing after using the latrine are not readily available, parents cannot easily teach children to wash hands often. This problem is beyond the control of individual families and needs to be dealt with at the relevant community or national level.

Lack of vaccinations

Today, vaccination programmes have been set up to protect African children from a wide range of diseases, but the overall rate of completed vaccination is still not high. An average of only about 50% of children have received all the vaccinations available by the age of 12 months in sub-Saharan African countries (UNICEF 2000a). There is considerable variation between countries in the numbers of children whose health is protected by vaccination. In some countries as many as 90% of children have been vaccinated against common infections, while in others as few as 30% are protected in this manner.

Most vaccinations can be given by staff at local mother and child health clinics. Vaccinations are usually given in the form of an injection, although in some instances the infant is given the treatment orally, a few drops of the substance required for protection being placed in the mouth. The number of vaccinations required and preferred timing for these vaccinations is shown in table 10.

Table 10 Vaccinations and recommended time of treatment

Vaccination	Protection against	Number of treatments and age of child at treatment
D P T	Diphtheria, whooping cough (pertussis) tetanus	3 injections. Usually at 2, 3, and 4 months
Polio*	Infantile paralysis (poliomyelitis)	Drops in mouth, at birth 1 2, and 3 months.
BCG	Tuberculosis	One injection, at birth or any time in life
Measles	Measles	One injection, between 9 and 15 months
Tetanus	Lockjaw (tetanus)	Children over 12 years and adults who have not previously been protected. One injection a month for 3 months, one a year later, and then one every 10 years.

Note: Recommended time of treatment may vary slightly from one country to another.
* Polio has almost been eliminated, so in future the vaccination will be necessary only in small areas in a few countries.
Source: Adapted from Werner (1993:147)

In some places vaccinations are given for yellow fever, typhus, mumps, and German measles (rubella). Some other vaccinations are given only at the time of disease outbreak. These are vaccinations against typhoid and cholera, life-threatening illnesses that become more common in times when life is disrupted by flood, famine, or war.

A problem for poor parents in some countries is that they may have to pay at least some of the cost of vaccinations. The demand for payment varies from one country to another. The costs are covered entirely by the government only in Botswana, Burkina Faso, Chad, Ghana, Mali, Namibia, Nigeria, Senegal, South Africa, Swaziland and Zimbabwe. More than 80% of the cost is covered by the government in a few other countries (Equatorial Guinea, Niger, Togo). Governments in the remaining countries mostly contribute less than 50% (UNICEF 2000a). Government priorities, which may have been influenced by the demands of loan agencies, such as the World Bank and the International Monetary Fund, determine the extent to which parents are required to cover basic vaccination costs.

Conclusion

African children experience considerable ill health, much of which is preventable. Parents may not be able to protect their children from ill health, however, unless they can access services and community education programmes. They need to know what they can do to prevent infection and to help their children make a rapid and complete recovery if they do happen to get sick. Efforts should also be made to ensure that all parents realise that providing a varied diet is a simple way in which they can improve their children's chances of living a healthy life, because a healthy body can fight off many common illnesses. Access to vaccinations is equally important, but at present only about half the children of Africa have this additional protection against a significant group of severe illnesses.

Health promotion activities

Parents naturally want to have healthy children and will take whatever action seems best in order to achieve this goal. To encourage parents to make informed decisions about best health practice, a large number of health promotion programmes have been set up by governments and aid agencies in Africa. To date, many of these programmes have been designed to encourage mothers to have their children vaccinated. These programmes need to continue into the future, as is evident from the low rate of vaccination achieved so far. A second focus has been on the use of oral rehydration therapy (ORT), which involves giving a predetermined mix of quantities of boiled water, salt and sugar to children (and adults) with diarrhoea. Today reports from sub-Saharan African countries suggest that, on average, between 30% and 50% of families use this mixture (UNICEF 2000a). Better-educated women are more confident that they can prepare the mixture correctly and therefore use it more than uneducated women (Palmer 1993). ORT use may also be restricted in areas where people believe that sugar is the cause of diarrhoea (Airhihenbuwa 1995). Airhihenbuwa is appropriately critical of the provision of packets of rehydration mix, which add to the cost and create a dependency on external suppliers, decreasing any sense of self-efficacy in the mother, who could easily learn the correct mix if well taught.

Like the ORT programme, other programmes designed to help parents enhance their children's health have to deal with long-held beliefs and practices. Changing parents' health beliefs and behaviours is a slow and complex procedure, especially where levels of education remain low, and funds are limited. Airhihenbuwa (1995) has criticised programmes for using inappropriate methods of communication. He notes that visual aids can confuse adults whose culturally preferred way of learning is through story telling. Similarly, Barley (1986) describes a malaria education programme in which film showed magnified pictures of mosquitoes. The village people concluded that such giant mosquitoes were certainly dangerous, but the small ones in their area were unlikely to cause harm.

Visual aids may be useful if well prepared. Gray et al. (1990) present guidelines on how to use line drawings when teaching about childbirth, for example. These authors used only black and white in the pictorial material, eliminated distance cues that had been shown to confuse uneducated women, and also always showed all of the woman's limbs in each drawing, even when this required some distortion of the picture. Airhihenbuwa (1995) has made some other suggestions for improving health education. He states that educators need to acknowledge the cultural beliefs that may limit change, and to seek out beliefs that might enhance prospects for change. Health educators can then encourage behaviours that flow from the helpful beliefs and provide culturally relevant information to decrease the impact of unhelpful beliefs. Airhihenbuwa emphasises the need to work not just at the individual level. Beliefs and practices of the extended family and broader neighbourhood need to be considered and programmes for change targeted at the appropriate level.

Teachers and children's health

Healthy children learn more because they have sufficient energy to listen carefully, to concentrate on their lessons, and to complete academic tasks. Teachers can promote child health in their school by taking a range of actions. Being among the best educated people in rural communities and also in some poor city communities, teachers can support the efforts of staff at the nearest health centre, clinic, or pharmacy, as they educate mothers about children's food requirements, and about infection and illness and how these can best be managed. Teachers cannot be expected to diagnose the various diseases and infections of children in their class, but they do need to be alert to indications that children are unwell. They can then take action to assist the child towards recovery, and help prevent the spread of infection to other children in the class and school. Some of the ways they can do this are described in the remainder of this chapter.

- **Asking about vaccinations:** When children enrol at school, school principals might ask which vaccinations the child has had. When vaccinations have not been completed, they may take the opportunity to encourage mothers to have these vaccinations done as soon as possible. Schoolchildren can be taught about the advantages of having vaccinations in those parts of the school curriculum that provide for health education. Where medical costs mean that poor parents cannot afford these treatments, teachers may also choose to work with others in the community, lobbying government for change in this vital health area.
- **Teaching about cleanliness:** Incidental teaching about cleanliness should become part of the daily routine, especially on the part of those teachers working with younger pupils. Reinforcing children's use of toilet paper, newspaper, handkerchiefs or clean rags to wipe their noses when they have colds, reminding pupils about thorough hand-washing (using soap and hot

water if possible) before meals and after going to the toilet (latrine) should be part of the daily routine. With older children, occasional use of reading material that describes advances in health as a result of medical discoveries or the development of public health systems might also be a useful basis for discussion about infection, disease, and health. These sorts of lessons are not solely the responsibility of the home economics teacher or the science teacher. The issue of health is a vital one for all in the community, and teachers need to model concern about health promotion to their pupils.

- **Observing children carefully:** Like a well-informed and caring parent, teachers need to be alert to indications of poor health, noting changes in appearance, activity, and behaviour that suggest the possibility of infection and illness. A teacher who suspects that a pupil is not well can then make sure that that child is well cared for and that other pupils are protected from infection. In particular, teachers should be alert to signs of fever, especially where cerebral malaria (plasmodium falciparum) occurs. Werner (1993) points out that where this form of malaria is common, any unexplained high fever should be treated as malaria. Urgent treatment is necessary if the individual is not to suffer brain damage or die from this illness, which is a major killer in most of Africa.

- **Promoting good eating habits:** Like other members of their community, teachers have certain beliefs about which foods are good and bad for them, about who should be given certain kinds of foods, about what foods should be eaten at different times of the year, and about food preparation and storage. These beliefs will influence their own food consumption and what they tell others, including their pupils, about food. Teachers need to explore their own preferences for and prejudices against certain foods, and learn more about the range of foods needed for good health and growth. Then they can help pupils understand the need to grow and eat a wider range of foods than has been traditional. Making use of their education and more advanced understanding about food values, teachers should challenge their own food prejudices and show others how to do so as well.

  Teaching children how to grow different food plants and growing a range of foods in the school garden can encourage children to experiment with foods that might not have been part of the traditional diet. Resistance to change may arise because families in many parts of Africa cannot take the risk of crop failure. If they make major changes to planting, they may risk starvation. Careful introduction of small crops of just one or two supplementary foods is probably necessary. Teachers are in an ideal position to encourage this, especially if the children do some gardening at school.

- **Temporarily modifying demands on pupils who are unwell, tired, or hungry:** Pupils who are physically unwell, tired, or hungry do not have the same amount of energy or motivation for academic tasks that they might have when they are well. Their concentration and capacity to solve academic problems are reduced when they are feverish, have sore eyes or earache, muscle or other pains. For teachers to expect high output from such children or to label them 'lazy' is unkind and may be harmful to the quality relationship that assists pupil learning.

Teachers need to be flexible in their approach to children showing signs of illness and exhaustion. The great majority of healthy children are keen to learn. A teacher who assumes that the reluctant child is just lazy may be ignoring evidence that there are many health reasons for his or her unwillingness and inability to participate in class.

Children who are unwell might learn better after they have had a short rest or sleep. Parents of chronically tired children who do not seem to be unwell might be asking their children to do an excessive amount of physical work at home, and teachers might want to discuss this problem with parents. Alternatively, they might let such children have a period of rest some time during the day.

In times of hunger children will have better concentration soon after a meal. Primary school teachers might be able to re-organise their timetable so that basic literacy and mathematics skills are taught at this time. Activities that make significant physical demand, such as sport and gardening, might be omitted from the programme for a few weeks or pupils might be asked to spend shorter periods of time on such activities.

- **Examining own health beliefs and practices:** Children learn a great deal by observing the behaviours of adults around them, and the teacher can be an important role model for good health practice. As educated people, teachers can be expected to follow simple practices for reducing the spread of infection, but those who want to check their own practice might like to consider the following basic questions:
    - If I use a rag or handkerchief when I have a cold or cough, do I keep it clean?
    - Do I blow my nose into a tissue or paper when I have a cold? Do I then dispose of the paper by burning or burying it?
    - Do I spit on the ground, leaving infected material around the school in this way?
    - Do I cover my mouth when sneezing or coughing?
    - Do I routinely, regularly and carefully wash my hands with soap after I have been to the toilet? After working in the garden? Before preparing or eating food?
    - Do I keep my fingernails clean and trimmed short?

Conclusion

African children's health is at risk from a wide range of sources. A relatively high percentage of children on the continent die because of exposure to contagious diseases, especially during their first five years. Despite this, the majority of children survive, although they are typically not very well a lot of the time. This will reduce their capacity to learn quickly and efficiently. Teachers need to be aware of possible health problems and take what action they can to ensure children do not spend their school years struggling with preventable disease.

In your community (five)

Most of the studies of African children's health have examined children during infancy and the preschool years. Choose one or more of the following exercises that focus on the health of children during their primary school years:

1. Visit a local school and discuss common health problems of the children there with one or more teachers. What are the commonest health problems that are reported? What percentage of these problems could be avoided if children were vaccinated against disease?
2. Talk to several children in the age band 6–10 years. Find out how much they know about the importance of washing their hands with soap as a method of preventing disease. Ask each one to tell you if he or she always washes his or her hands with soap after he or she has been to the toilet, sometimes does so, or never does so.
3. Talk to children aged 11–16 years about hand washing. Ask the same questions that are listed in exercise 2. Compare your findings with those of someone who has talked to younger children. Is there any evidence that hand washing with soap increases with age?
4. Go to your local council offices and find out which parts of the town have sewage pipes and piped water. Visit one of the areas and check for leaks or other evidence of broken pipes or leaking taps. Report back to your peer group.
5. Read about local development programmes and international aid programmes that are set in place in your country to ensure people have well-designed, hygienic toilets or a pump to raise water from village wells. Find out what percentage of people in your country or community have to walk long distances to obtain water for daily use. Report your findings to your peer group.

Chapter Seven

Children with special difficulties

Introduction

A small but significant number of children in many parts of Africa have special long-term physical and social problems beyond those dealt with in the previous chapter. Children with special physical difficulties include those who have sensory deficits, such as impaired vision and hearing, and those who cannot move around freely because of problems with co-ordination, poor motor skills, and arms and legs that have never functioned normally or whose function has been lost through injury.

Social difficulties may arise when children are coping with parental death or have experienced the horrors of war, either as villagers whose lives were disrupted by fighting or as child soldiers. Some of these children may have lived alone or in small groups as so-called street children. These children's difficulties mean that they need special care and teaching if they are to make satisfactory adjustment to their situation and experiences. The lives of these children are discussed in the present chapter. Some simple suggestions are made as to how teachers can help, but teachers who work with such children will need to ensure that they learn much more than can be dealt with in this introductory text.

African views of disability

African children who are born with some characteristic that makes them different from others may be perceived in different ways, depending on the characteristic itself. The Songye of Zaire, for example, traditionally divide these children into three categories, ceremonial children, bad children and faulty children. The birth of ceremonial children, such as twins, or a child born with the umbilical cord around the neck, is celebrated because they are believed to have special powers and the capacity for healing. In contrast, those with very severe impairments, such as albino or dwarf children, are labelled 'bad' and are described as 'born to die'. They are believed to have been in contact with the anti-world of sorcerers (Devlieger 1995). Many die at an early age.

The larger group of children who are born with some flaw (e.g. hare lip, malformed limbs) constitute the faulty group. These children's development is believed to have been affected by problems in the parents' behaviour and social relations. Often the problem is thought to arise because of the mother's behaviour during her pregnancy. In particular, a pregnant woman is often believed to have had sexual relations with her husband at a time that this is forbidden in her ethnic group. Parents therefore make a considerable effort to discover and correct the problems, and to re-establish a good relationship with their physical and social environment, with family members, and with ancestors. If all culturally required actions to restore the infant to health have been taken without effect the defect is attributed to the intervention of God and is accepted (Devlieger 1995). Similar explanations for physical deformity are common in a number of other ethnic groups (e.g. Helander 1995; Talle 1995).

Some problems, such as blindness that has been present since birth, may be labelled illnesses (Setumbwe 1995). Impairment that develops later in childhood is also generally labelled 'illness' or 'disease' in the first instance. Such illness may develop as a result of curses, sorcery, or even acts of God. Parents may spend many months, even years, trying to find a cure for these impairments. They may ask therapists from a wide range of disciplines for help. This includes local traditional healers, nurses at the local health clinic, and doctors or traditional healers in far-away places. Parents may spend a great deal of effort and money during this period of seeking a cure. After some time, however, the label applied to the problem slowly changes until a new label that recognises the permanence of the problem is eventually applied and further efforts to seek a cure come to a halt (Helander 1995).

Village Africans and those living a fairly traditional lifestyle are generally tolerant of those members of their community who have some limitation in their development and functioning. The limitation is considered to be important only when it restricts the child's capacity to interact in a sociable manner with the others in the group. Blindness is considered to be especially limiting in Uganda (Setumbwe 1995), while problems with motor development and walking are a special problem for children in nomadic ethnic groups (Talle 1995). Madness was not well tolerated among the Hubeer in Somalia who were studied by

Helander (1995). Epilepsy (the fainting illness) elicited fears of contagion in Whyte's (1995) study in Tanzania, although it is not contagious.

Although village people are generally extremely group oriented and supportive of one another, they may think that the actual care of a disabled child is the parents' responsibility (Talle 1995). As a result, they may not provide the kind of support needed when parents are exhausted by the additional demands of raising a child with significant impairment. Differences between ethnic groups in attitudes towards people with some defect or impairment of function may also reflect religious differences. The Somali, for example, may assist those with defects, because Islamic teaching requires them to show charity in this way (Helander 1995).

General terms for groups of people with limitations are not used, the term *disability* commonly being used only to refer to those with physical defects. Instead more specific terms that relate to each kind of limitation are employed. Thus, among the Maasai, for example, children are referred to in their presence as the deaf one, the blind one, and so on. Outsiders sometimes interpret this kind of labelling as indicating some degree of stigma, but the use of these terms needs to be considered in the broader context of community life. Healthy children and adults are also identified by some personal characteristic in Maasai compounds, so children with limitations are not being specifically stigmatised when these labels are used (Talle 1995). Helander (1995) reports equivalent labels for people with and without physical or sensory impairment among the Hubeer.

In much of sub-Saharan Africa no special effort is made to help the child develop as fully as possible despite the impairment. In modern times, however, some nomadic parents have realised that they can best help children with physical impairment if they place them in boarding school. There they can learn tasks permitting a more sedentary lifestyle rather than having to continue with a lifestyle that makes high demand on physical competence (Talle 1995). In general, village parents do not understand that changing the way in which they interact with their child can help the child develop many skills despite his or her physical or sensory impairment or very slow rate of learning.

Modern health and education systems could help parents to gain a clearer understanding of the nature of the child's problem and the ways in which they can help their child develop. But good rehabilitation and educational programmes are not commonly available. The necessary emphasis on keeping children in their community limits parental access to support, especially parents in rural villages. Parents may think that when a child does benefit from a rehabilitation programme or from special teaching, the improvement comes from a source of strength inside the child (Helander 1995). Parents may not know that modern treatments can ameliorate certain problems. For example, Whyte (1995) found that many Tanzanian parents of children who had epilepsy did not realise that with careful diagnosis and use of good medication their children need no longer have seizures. Health professionals may also need to help parents learn more about their child's condition. Whyte cites one parent who asked what was wrong with her child and was told it was not her business!

Disease, impairment and disability: northern hemisphere views

Traditional African ways of thinking about children with deformities or impaired function are different from those used by northern hemisphere researchers and teachers. The people from the northern hemisphere generally use the terms *disabled* and *disability* when referring to all persons whose activities are restricted because of physical, sensory, or neurological (brain or nerve) damage. A person is considered to have a disability if the impairment cannot be corrected through use of some kind of aid. For example, a shortsighted person who can see as well as others when wearing glasses is not described as having a visual disability or being visually impaired. These terms are used only when describing people whose problem cannot be corrected. Some texts also use the word *handicap* when referring to a disability. This is becoming less common in material written in English, but in French-speaking West Africa the word *handicappé* is widely used.

Another issue for students and teachers who want to learn about children with limitations is that northern hemisphere authors use different labels for children with certain problems according to the nationality of the authors themselves. American authors refer to 'mental retardation' when discussing children who learn extremely slowly because damage to the brain has altered the way it functions. Depending on the amount of delay in learning, children are further subdivided into groups described as educable mentally retarded or trainable mentally retarded. The terms mildly, moderately, severely, or profoundly retarded may also be used. British authors use the term 'learning disabled' and Australians use the term 'intellectually disabled'. Like Americans, British and Australian authors sub-divide the category, using the terms mild, moderate, severe and profound.

Sensory and physical disabilities

Sensory and physical disabilities can have a profound impact on the way children develop, how much they can learn in school, and how well they can fit in with others in their community. The impact of a disability depends on its severity, the time in the child's life that the disability became evident and on others' reactions to that disability. Children who are born with defective vision or hearing, or the cerebral palsy that causes them to walk with unsteady steps have never had another kind of life. Their experiences and the issues they have to deal with are different from those of children who have had a period of normal development that has then been disrupted so that further development takes a different path. Children who develop disabilities as a consequence of ill health or accident often go through a period of confusion and mourning for the permanent loss of health. They may become angry or depressed, losing interest in activities that they previously enjoyed and finding it difficult to make the adjustments to their new, more restricted range of abilities.

Visual impairment

Children may have visual problems for a variety of reasons. Some problems arise because of the way the eyes have developed, as shown for example in children who are described as cross-eyed, having a 'wandery' eye or a squint. This problem arises because of the way the muscles that control eye movement have developed. Children who are cross-eyed usually cannot see well out of the eye that turns in or out unless the problem is treated before the child is about four years old. Other children may not see well because past injury to the eye has caused scarring.

A common chronic eye infection of African schoolchildren is trachoma. This infection is transmitted to humans by flies, or when infected material is passed from one person to another, either directly by hand contact or indirectly via towels, handkerchiefs, or other shared materials. When a person has a trachoma infection, one or both eyes initially look red and watery. Later small lumps appear inside the upper eyelid. After some months these lumps disappear, leaving whitish scars. In later adulthood many people who have this scarring will become blind because the shape of the eyelid means that the eye cannot be closed properly, or the eyelashes brush against the surface of the eye, causing scarring to develop on the surface of the eye itself (Werner 1993).

Trachoma is the world's leading cause of preventable blindness. It is a disease of poverty and is widespread across Africa. Where it is common, the rate of infection among children is often greater than 50% and may be as high as 90% (Bejiga and Alemayehu 2001; Mabey and Fraser-Hurt 2001). Within any one country rates of infection may vary considerably. For example, in Gambia Dolin et al. (1998) found that only 1.2% of children were infected in some areas, while up to 11.5% were infected elsewhere in the country.

Teachers and visual impairment

Teachers cannot be expected to diagnose the visual problems of children in their class but, as with poor physical health, they need to contribute to the reduction of preventable disease where possible. They can be alert to evidence that children are having problems seeing and reading written material and can take some actions to reduce the impact of such problems.

Clues that a child is having visual difficulties are listed in table 11. When teachers note these difficulties, they should refer children to the local health clinic as soon as possible for detailed assessment and treatment. This is especially important if the child shows several of the symptoms and these persist over time.

Table 11 Signs of possible eye trouble

Appearance

- Crossed eyes, wandery eye
- Red-rimmed, encrusted or swollen eyelids
- One eye higher in relation to other
- Eyes do not move smoothly in all directions of gaze
- Inflamed or watery eyes
- Recurring styes (infection at the base of an eyelash)

Behaviours

- Rubs eyes excessively
- Shuts or covers one eye, tilts head or thrusts head forward
- Face contorts when attempting to focus
- Has difficulty reading or doing other work requiring close use of eyes, or avoids close work
- Blinks more than usual or is irritable when doing close work
- Unable to see distant things clearly
- Squints eyelids together or frowns when looking at objects
- Loses place frequently when reading or holds book very close
- Makes many errors when copying from the blackboard, or approaches the blackboard to check what has been written there
- Avoids visual tasks, shows poor attention to visual detail
- Moves head excessively when reading

Complaints

- Eyes itch, burn, feel scratchy or sore
- Dizziness, headaches, nausea or fatigue following close work
- Blurred or double vision
- Eyes hurt in bright light, sensitive to glare
- Print moves when reading

Source: Adapted from Cartwright, Cartwright and Ward (1995:90), Kirk and Gallagher (1983:186) and Howell and Peachey (1990:244-245).

Children who are having difficulty seeing the blackboard should be encouraged to sit in the position where they see best. While this is usually near the front of the group, some long-sighted children will be better placed further back. Others will find that they can see better when sitting at the side of the group rather than directly in front of the blackboard, and they may see well from one side of the room but not from the other. Children who are albinos are extremely sensitive to bright light and should not be placed near a window. Finding the best spot for each visually impaired child may take a little while, but will gradually become obvious as the child's work will be better from the position where he or she sees best.

Teachers can contribute to the reduction of trachoma-induced blindness in their community in some simple ways. Research shows that daily face washing results in reduced prevalence of the disease in the community. The fly that transmits the disease from one person to another breeds most successfully in human faeces (shit) so building and using pit latrines (privies or toilets) also reduces disease prevalence. Reductions of up to 80% over no more than ten years have been reported (Emerson, Bailey, Walraven and Lindsay 2001; Mabey and Fraser-Hurt 2001; O'Connor, Lynch, Vitale and West 1999; Solomon et al. 2001). Teachers can ensure that children learn about and use these two methods for reducing trachoma.

Children with very severe defects of vision and hearing generally do not attend school in sub-Saharan Africa. In most countries, a very small number of such children who live in major cities attend special schools or classes where specialist teachers help them to learn in spite of their disabilities.

Box 7 Blind and bitter

Martin, a thirty-year-old partially blind informant . . . remarked with bitterness: 'Most people are not aware of the fact that given the chance, blind people can do almost anything. They see a blind person as useless; as one who is a loss to his family and society . . . The worst thing is that in most cases, persons with the preferred handicaps are treated no better than the blind are.'

Source: Setumbwe (1995:161)

Hearing impairment

Studies of hearing impairment in Africa are difficult to compare, because various researchers have assessed hearing in different ways, with different amounts of background noise, variable age groups, and different definitions of normal hearing and hearing loss (e.g. Bastos, Mallya, Ingvarsson, Reimer, and Andreasson 1995; Hatcher et al. 1995; Minja and Machemba 1996; Swart, Lemmer, Parbhoo and Prescott 1995). Overall, though, these studies show that there is a high rate of preventable deafness among African children.

Difficulties in hearing may have a number of causes, the extent of hearing loss varying according to which part of the ear is affected and how badly. The ear is divided into three parts, known as the outer, middle, and inner ear, and problems can arise in any one of these parts. Inner ear problems are generally referred to as sensorineural problems, because it is here that sound is transmitted to the brain for interpretation and understanding. Sensorineural problems can occur if the mother has rubella during the first three months of her pregnancy; as a result of meningitis (inflammation of the covering of the brain); if the child has had severe cerebral malaria; and after a few other illnesses. Thus, the rate of sensorineural hearing loss can be as high as 14% in some rural parts of Africa, although it appears generally to be markedly lower in major towns and cities (e.g. Minja and Machemba 1996). Sensorineural deafness is often severe and children need specialist education if they are to overcome the difficulties this imposes. Few African children have access to the special schools and specially trained teachers that are needed and so they cannot go to school at all.

Most mild to moderate hearing loss occurs because of a build up of wax in the part of the outer ear that is called the ear canal or as a result of middle-ear infection (correctly called otitis media). Most children who have impaired hearing have one or both of these problems. Between about 5% and 20% of the African children who have been assessed in the studies listed earlier have a build up of wax in the ear canal; this varies considerably within and between countries. Between 6% and 10% of children with this build up of wax have some hearing loss because of it. The hearing loss is usually fairly mild, but may be sufficient to make it difficult for pupils to hear clearly in the general noise environment of a school. Brandes and Ehinger (1981), for example, report that children with only mild hearing loss in one ear are more likely to show reduced language skills compared with their peers and to require more individual help if they are to progress satisfactorily through school.

A great number of children have episodes of otitis media (commonly called earache) during infancy and the preschool years, up until the age of about six or seven years. Early identification and treatment of these infections can ensure they clear up rapidly, but lack of treatment can mean that the infection becomes chronic, with 'weepy' ears where fluid drains from the ear at a slow but constant rate. Minja and Machenda (1996) reported that 9.4% of a rural sample and 1.3% of urban children showed evidence of chronic otitis media, although rates do vary considerably when different national and ethnic groups are studied. Also, the rural-urban differences are not always obtained, as shown by Bastos et al. (1995).

In a study by Hatcher et al. (1995) two out of every three children with chronic otitis media had sufficient hearing loss to interfere with understanding of oral communication and school learning. Children whose infections have been severe, but have cleared up later, may also have longer-term damage to the ear drum that prevents sound being conducted into the inner ear. Swart et al. (1995), for example, found that 2.3% of children in their sample had perforations (holes) in the eardrum. They report other studies where 6% of children had such perforations. All perforations interfere with hearing. Scarring of ear membranes, a sign of earlier infection, is also widespread.

Teachers and hearing impairment

Teachers need to be aware of the indicators of ear infection and hearing loss listed in table 12. When they suspect hearing loss from any cause, they should try to get parents to refer the child to the local health clinic for assessment and treatment as soon as possible. As with vision, this is especially important if the child shows several symptoms and these symptoms persist over time.

When the teacher suspects that a child does not hear well, he or she should attempt to find out where in the class the child hears best. Usually this is near the front of the class, in direct line of sight. This enables the child to make good use of visual clues as to what is being said through lip-reading skills. Teachers should also routinely check that pupils with hearing loss have understood oral instructions by having the child repeat what he or she has to do. Asking 'Do you understand?' is not useful because most children will automatically answer 'Yes'.

Table 12 Signs of possible ear trouble

Physical signs
• Ear discharge ('wet', 'weepy' or running ears)
• Breathing through the mouth (even when sitting, not because the child has been exercising)
• Frequent use of cotton wool in ears
• Tired, strained expression early in the day (but not otherwise ill, or exhausted from physical work)
Behavioural indicators
• Does not attend to speech or sound
• Turns head or ear towards speaker, puts hand behind ear when listening
• Fails to follow spoken instructions, especially in group settings
• Requests repetition of spoken words, particularly questions
• Speech problems, does not speak clearly, speaks unusually loudly or shouts
• Reluctant to volunteer answers in class or group discussion
• Withdrawn behaviour
• Unusual concentration on speaker's face or mouth
• Inconsistent or inappropriate responses to speech
• Better work in small group or one to one
• Uses a lot of gestures
• Relies on classmates for directions and assignments
Complaints
• Earache
• Ringing or buzzing in ears, discomfort in ears
• Noises in head
• Stuffy feeling in ears
• Sores in ears
• Frequent colds, sore throats that are often quite severe and last several days

Source: Adapted from Cartwright, Cartwright and Ward (1995:130) and Kirk and Gallagher (1983:233)

Physical disabilities

Children may come to school with any of a number of physical disabilities. The commonest of these is probably some form of cerebral palsy. Pupils with this condition do not have the capacity for smooth muscle movements of their limbs. They make sudden uncontrolled movements of the head, arms and legs. They may also have tremors or unsteady gait and walk with legs widespread. The condition is caused by damage to the part of the brain that controls smooth movements of muscles. The damage can occur before or during birth, especially if the infant lacks oxygen during a difficult or prolonged birth. It may also occur as a result of extremely high fever or because some illness or accident has harmed the brain. Other physical disabilities include malformation of limbs or loss of limbs from exploding landmines in former war zones.

Box 8 Poverty and poor health

As we turned into one village* and stopped in the market square, a young boy with one arm and no legs was propelling himself along on a primitive skateboard. Roughly 10% of the country's population were mentally or physically disabled, the nun told me. Around 25 per cent were affected by disabilities directly or indirectly, by having to look after somebody disabled. Yet, she said, nearly half the disabilities could have been prevented. 'Forty per cent of cases of cerebral palsy can be prevented. Eighty per cent of blind people can be cured,' she said. 'Guinea worm – from 60 per cent incidence it can be cut to zero in two seasons.'
'But why aren't they?'
'Money. It doesn't cost much, compared to how much is spent on other things. A piece of nylon cloth, that's all you need to reduce the transmission of guinea worm. But the money is not there, so we have to cope with the consequences.'

* = in Burkina Faso
Source: Peter Biddlecombe (1993:88)

Note: Treating guinea worm infection and teaching people to filter their drinking water through a tightly woven cloth have now greatly reduced its prevalence in much of Africa.

Children who learn slowly

The brain is a sensitive organ that can be damaged before or during birth owing to lack of oxygen. Later damage may be the result of very high fever or infection (e.g. meningitis, cerebral malaria). Damage may also be caused by an accident such as falling from a tree or being bumped hard on the head and losing consciousness for more than a few moments. Children with more serious limits to their ability to learn, that is, those who are described as having moderate, severe, or profound intellectual disability, generally cannot go to school in Africa as only a few schools for such children exist in major cities. Staff at such schools may be untrained and poorly paid, and schools may lack the basic resources needed to teach children with significant problems in learning (M.-C. Oudot, personal communication, April 2001).

A group of children who learn somewhat more slowly than most others, however, do sometimes attend school and can benefit from schooling if teachers recognise that they need to make special efforts with them. These children have a smaller vocabulary than others of their age, even in their mother tongue. They have difficulty coping with abstract ideas, and prefer to play with children who are younger than themselves. Their motor skills may also be less developed than others of their own age. In school, they learn best if tasks are broken into simple steps, with each step taught separately. Teachers need to use simple, concrete language when explaining new material and check frequently for understanding. These children experience a lot of failure and are at risk of developing low self-esteem, so it is important for teachers to acknowledge their efforts and to find ways of making them feel they are important members of the class.

Teaching children with disabilities

Although there are almost certainly pupils with some disability in most classes in African schools, teachers' attitudes towards and management of these pupils has not been widely assessed. In one study, Barnartt and Kabzems (1992) asked nearly 200 teachers whether children with a range of disabilities should be in regular classrooms in general, and whether they should be in that specific teacher's class. Overall, teachers were more willing to agree that they should have children with disabilities in their own class than they were to suggest that such children should generally be in regular classrooms. They were personally more likely to accept children with physical disabilities (79%) than to accept children with visual impairment (33%), hearing impairment (21%) or intellectual disabilities (14%). Nearly 17% of teachers said they were unwilling to accept children with any of the four types of disability in their classroom, and an additional 41% said they would accept only children with one kind of disability (the actual disability was not specified in the report).

Most teachers who were willing to accept children with physical disabilities in their classrooms said they would ignore the disability and not change their teaching in any way (40%). Others said they would do their best to help (20%) without specifying what they would do, that they would try to ensure that they encouraged and motivated the child (20%), and would encourage peer support and acceptance of the disabled child (10%). In contrast, the few teachers who accepted that children with visual, hearing, and intellectual impairments should be in their class commented on the need for changed teaching methods, use of more teaching aids, more individual attention and sometimes different academic tasks. Teachers were aware that they needed to change the seating arrangements for children with visual and hearing impairments and that they could seek help from other teachers and from specialists.

It is evident that some of these teachers were willing to make special efforts to help children with disabilities. But difficulties remain. For example, African school students with sensory impairments complain that teachers and others tend to generalise from their single area of disability to other aspects of their development. Most importantly, they state that they are often treated as if they are intellectually impaired as well as having a sensory impairment. This is referred to as 'spread' (Brook 2002; Setumbwe 1995) and reveals the teacher's ignorance about the various conditions. Children who have visual, hearing, or motor impairments have the same range of intellectual abilities as other children. Some learn more slowly, some at the same rate, and some more rapidly than others if they are taught in such a way as to optimise their chances of learning. Despite good abilities, however, some may find that trying to learn in spite of their impaired hearing or vision is extremely tiring and time-consuming. They may learn more slowly for this reason alone. Teachers need to be aware of these reasons for slowed learning and not treat children with normal abilities as if they lacked the capacity to learn.

It is most important for teachers to recognise that children with sensory and physical disabilities have some additional psychological issues to deal with. Children who have eye and ear infections may have fever and pain, and may generally tire easily as their body is using energy to try to fight the infection. Children with physical disabilities use more energy than other children, as they struggle to move about, and they are often tired by the struggle. Even doing schoolwork may be a struggle because of poor motor control. Children with disabilities are often neglected as playmates. They have to learn to cope with the self-esteem issues that arise as a result of social isolation and from their inability to participate in playground activities. For disabled students entering adolescence there are identity issues, concerns about future employability and poorer prospects for marriage.

Children with disabilities, especially sensory impairments, sometimes behave in ways that are culturally unacceptable. A young student in Swaziland who became deaf after having meningitis, had to watch his teacher's face very carefully in class in order to gain visual clues as to what the teacher was saying. In his culture, children are expected to show respect to elders by not looking directly at them, so his behaviour was perceived as rudeness rather than being seen as a sensible reaction on his part to the need for more visual information now that he was deaf (Save the Children 1990). Teachers in this situation must carefully consider whether the child is showing disrespect. If not, they need to work towards overcoming their personal discomfort at being looked at directly.

Conclusion

Whether they realise it or not, most African teachers have children with some degree of disability in their class. In particular, there are likely to be children in most classes who have some degree of loss of vision or hearing, or both. Teachers can improve these children's chances of making good progress by being alert to indicators of impairment. They need to encourage parents to have their child's sensory and physical health checked if it seems there are possible problems that could be corrected. In class, teachers can take some simple steps to ensure children with sensory, physical, and intellectual limitations learn as much as they can. In this sense teachers are acting as good parents themselves, caring for the total development of their pupils, not simply for academic achievements. In some rural villages they may be the only people in the community who have enough knowledge of these kinds of problems to be able to help parents ensure their children develop well.

Disruption of children's social world

Children in Africa live in an environment that is often quite unstable. The physical environment is characterised by problems with drought and, sometimes, floods. As elsewhere, some parts of Africa are vulnerable to earthquakes and volcanic action. More commonly, the social environment is also unstable, with civil war occurring in many countries. Some national leaders, who care more for power than for the wellbeing of their people, encourage violent expression of tribal, religious, or other differences of opinion. Disruptions to physical and social security are generally associated with the spread of disease and with high levels of psychological distress. Each of these disruptive influences alters the physical, social-emotional and cognitive development of children in ways that are generally detrimental to their wellbeing. Teachers need to understand the effects of these influences and realise that they can help children recover from harmful events in their lives. The remainder of this chapter discusses these issues.

Losses for children in difficult circumstances

Children in difficult physical and social circumstances experience a number of losses. First, they lose physical safety. In times of drought and flood, parents cannot always supply good food and clean water. Children are more likely than usual to fall ill with gastro-intestinal disease and may not be able to obtain satisfactory treatment. Epidemics of typhoid and cholera occur. In times of war, vaccination rates decrease significantly, and children often live in crowded refugee camps, with a consequent increase in outbreaks of preventable diseases such as measles (Cliff and Noormahomed 1992; Dodge 1990).

Children are often unable to obtain adequate food because planting or harvesting is disrupted, or family plots have been overrun and destroyed by soldiers. They may lose their homes as soldiers raid villages and set fires. Bombs are dropped, destroying homes and farmland. Children are at risk of becoming physically disabled, losing limbs, hearing or vision as result of bombing or from treading on landmines. They may be tortured or suffer deliberate mutilation of their bodies. In many instances these events happen at times that children are separated from the parents and caregivers who might otherwise have helped them to meet their needs for safety and health. Destabilising events in the physical environment, such as earthquake and volcanic eruption, also cause some, but not all, of these losses.

Kilbourn (1995a) points out that children also lose the conditions that promote satisfactory psychological development. They lose contact with important attachment figures, including parents, siblings, and friends when they become separated from them, or when these important people are killed. They lose a sense of security and can no longer trust parents or other adults to keep them safe. Their developing sense of themselves as autonomous beings who can control what happens is lost. Moral development may be hampered, as they see adults around them behaving in ways that are self-seeking and harmful to others.

Box 9 A child's right to safety: The UN Convention on the Rights of the Child

The child must be protected from all forms of violence, injury, abuse, neglect and exploitation . . .

No child under 15 should take direct part in armed conflict or be recruited into the armed forces, and priority in recruitment should be given to older children. The State must ensure the protection and care of children affected by armed conflict.

Source: Save the Children (1990). Appendix

Children who are forced to become soldiers, killing others in order to survive, or who are tortured, raped, or threatened with death are particularly likely to feel that the world is generally unsafe. Many develop psychological and social responses such as lack of trust, low self-esteem, and antisocial behaviour that may limit their future development. Kilbourn refers to the 'loss of childhood' that occurs when children are required to cope with events that are normally dealt with by older members of the community. Children miss out on the opportunity to play, to go to school and to learn social skills within their peer group, because they have to take on the responsibilities of adulthood, finding food, clothing, and shelter for themselves and sometimes for younger siblings.

Children's psychological response to loss and social disruption

A number of authors (e.g. Goodyer, 1990; Wright, 1995; Shaw and Harris, 1994) point out that children's responses to the kinds of losses outlined above are influenced by a range of factors. These are summarised below.

- **The child's age and developmental level:** Younger children have had a shorter period of development in which to establish their sense of themselves as worthy, autonomous beings. They are more dependent on others to meet attachment needs, and are still developing the trust in others that is essential for satisfactory psychological development. Very young children do not yet have enough language to be able to describe their reactions to events. In particular, they do not yet have the range of words needed to describe their emotional reactions to the events that have been so distressing. Primary-school-age children may have angry fantasies about their role in the events and show these in aggressive play. Adolescents may become distressed because of their newly developed sense of themselves in the world, an awareness that they, too, might have died and will do so some day.
- **The child's personality:** Children who are temperamentally more anxious may respond with anxiety to situations that elicit an angry response from other children. Children who have good social relations with others may be able to draw some support and strength from these relationships. They may be more able to cope with distress than others who do not have such good relationships with members of their group.
- **The child's understanding of the situation:** Children's understanding of the complexities of situations develops as they grow up. A very young child may perceive only that part of the event that has immediate relevance to his or her needs. Primary-school-age children gradually develop a broader understanding but, because they are still quite young, they may not be able to understand the relevance of the broad political factors or weather conditions that have produced the traumatising events. Older adolescents have the capacity to understand the full picture, but may not have enough information to do so. The way in which they think about events may continue to be based on inadequate information, myth, gossip and fear.
- **The child's ways of coping:** Children develop patterns of coping with stressful situations that they tend to use in all situations of stress. Thus, one child may withdraw and become very quiet and thoughtful, while another may become overactive in order to avoid thinking about horrid events. A third may use his or her intellectual capacities to try to understand what has happened, and a fourth may become emotional and dependent, clinging to others for psychological support.
- **The response of the family:** Children from families that are generally coping have a better response to traumatic events than children whose family was not functioning well before the disruptive events. In coping families, older family members can help the child deal with trauma. In less adequate families, the parents may themselves be overwhelmed and become psychologically unavailable to their children. These parents model excessive

fear and anxiety, disorganisation, and lack of problem-solving skills. Children learn to behave in the same way.

Individual psychological responses

Traumatic happenings produce confusion at a cognitive level as children struggle to understand the deeply troubling events they have experienced. Children also have emotional reactions to these events. When the events are extremely confusing and quite terrifying, children may show reactions that are beyond their control. Common and less common reactions to trauma are outlined in the present section of the chapter.

Emotional reactions

Normal emotional reactions to traumatic events include fear and anxiety, guilt, anger, and shame. Behaviours indicating these emotions are common. Fearful and anxious children often regress to behaviour patterns from an earlier phase of development. Pre-schoolers may whine and cling to their caregiver, weeping readily if faced with any new situation or challenge. They may start wetting the bed at night after a period of nighttime dryness or resist playing outside because they feel unsafe.

Primary-school-age children often feel guilty that they did not do more to protect others from harm, even although the reality of the situation was often such that they could not help – they were too small, or too young, to understand or they were paralysed by their fear for their own lives. They may feel angry that adults hurt them or that their parents did not protect them. They may feel ashamed of being afraid and of showing fear, or of stealing food from others to survive. Adolescents who have participated in sexual activity to obtain food may feel dirty and unworthy of respect. Because of this, they may indulge in behaviours that are risky and self-harming, such as excessive alcohol use, sexual excess and drug use.

The pattern of response may reflect general values within the culture. Members of collective cultures are generally described as experiencing shame when others see them failing to live up to group expectations for behaviour (Triandis, 1995b). Like other collective cultures, African cultures are probably shame based. The strong impact of Christianity, however, may mean that many Africans also experience the internalised feeling of guilt that is usually more widely associated with individualist cultures. In ethnic groups where moderation of emotional expression is valued, high levels of anger or deep sadness may be especially difficult for others to cope with. Children who are thought to be showing excessive anger may find themselves rejected by their group. Group rejection is psychologically extremely powerful in collective cultures and is especially likely to be additionally harmful to African children who have already lost important attachment figures in some traumatic event. Finally, in ethnic groups where boys are expected to be more dominant than girls, and where boys' control of emotions such as fear is expected to be well established from an early age, boys may have more difficulties in dealing with some emotions than girls in the same group.

Grief

Only a limited amount of research into parental death and children's grief at such deaths has been done in the northern hemisphere and it has not been possible to find studies done in Africa. But it seems likely that the grief process follows the same general sequence in all cultures, as people everywhere experience sadness and loss when someone important to them has died. Death is characterised by three features: it is inevitable, universal and irreversible. Children learn this as they develop cognitively. As with other cognitive development, early exposure leads to earlier understanding of the features of death, but children generally do not fully understand its characteristics until they approach their teens (Berlinsky and Biller 1982; Kastenbaum 1992).

Many African children experience the death of a parent or sibling at some time during their childhood. The way they understand death influences their reactions to the news of parental death. Surviving adults need to help them cope with this distressing event. Infants and toddlers respond to the death of a parent in the same way as they respond to other separations. They become upset and spend time searching for the missing person. When the person does not return, they may become apathetic and refuse to eat. These vulnerable children need special care and attention. African children who have formed a psychological attachment to more than one caregiver, as has been shown in some studies reported in Chapter Four, have the advantage that they may still have one important person available to them at this time. Pre-schoolers, aged up to about five years, do not realise that death is final, and may show concern for the dead person's continued wellbeing (e.g. Where will Mummy go to get water? Who will feed my little sister?). They may think that unrelated events, such as their own thoughts or actions, caused the death. Children of this age need clear explanations of the facts in simple language. Saying the dead person is asleep or has gone on a long journey can add to confusion and fear.

Children in the age range 5–10 years may still hold some immature beliefs about the cause of death, but are more able to express their thoughts and to empathise with others' grief. About this time, gender differences in expression of grief begin to appear. Boys in many ethnic groups find it more difficult to talk about their emotional reactions to the death of a loved adult or sibling than girls. After the age of about 10 years, children and adolescents understand about death, but still need help to cope with expressing their emotions, and their thoughts about it. These young people sometimes feel pressured to control their emotions and to behave in a mature way in order to help the surviving parent (Dyregrov 1991; Silverman and Worden 1993; Worden 1996)

The few northern hemisphere studies show that initial reactions to being told of the death of a loved one may include shock and denial. Like adults, children may not be able to accept the news immediately. Children in shock and denial may react as if they have not heard the news, perhaps asking if they can go on with earlier activities (Dyregrov 1991). But once they have fully realised that a death has occurred, children mourn their loss, although they may show their grief in ways that are easily misinterpreted by adults. Dyregrov lists the following indicators of childhood grief:

- **Anxiety:** The child has fears about his or her own death, the death of siblings or of the surviving parent. This may show in phobic responses to certain activities or places if the child has witnessed a violent death.
- **Vivid memories:** Fantasy or real recall of the death scene, especially if the death was violent.
- **Sleep difficulties:** Fear of sleeping alone, difficulty falling asleep or staying asleep, bad dreams.
- **Sadness and longing:** Crying with varying frequency and for varying periods, withdrawal and isolation in order to hide sadness from others, searching for the lost person, clinging to the dead person's clothes or objects belonging to him or her.
- **Anger and acting out:** Anger against him- or herself, health professionals, surviving parent, other adults, death (as personified) or God for causing the death or for not preventing it.
- **Guilt, self-reproach and shame:** For their actions, thoughts or wishes, for unkind things they said to the deceased just before that person's death. Shame at expressing emotions or for feeling relieved when a person who has been very sick finally dies.
- **School problems:** Difficulties with attention and concentration, slowed thinking, lack of energy and initiative.
- **Physical complaints:** Aches and pains in the stomach, head or limbs.

Some of these indicators of grief gradually decline over the first year after the death, but others decline more slowly. Silverman and Worden (1993) reported that 23.7% of an American sample still cried several times a week four months after their parent's death and 11% still cried frequently at one year. One fifth of the children reported frequent headaches during the first year. Nearly 15% were finding it difficult to concentrate in school four months after the death of a parent, and 12% still had problems concentrating one year after the death. Children who are mourning the loss of a parent may also feel that the surviving parent is not available to provide the support they need. This is because the parent is immersed in his or her own grief.

Children everywhere benefit from being involved in the rituals surrounding death (Young and Papadatou 1997). In African families where people still believe that all events have a cause, and that ill health and death can be caused by magic, curses or the ill wishes of others, children's involvement in rituals can be especially beneficial in helping them grieve in a healthy way. Where people believe that ghosts and spirits abound and may be harmful if proper rituals are not undertaken, these rituals are especially important, because children who are grieving often report feeling that the dead person is near. This can be a frightening feeling unless spirits are harmless or, better still, protective.

Parental death during troubled times bring additional issues for grieving survivors. If parents have died during war, and rituals have not been able to be completed at the time, the completion of these rituals as soon as peace or safety is restored can help children to finish grieving. Those children who witnessed the violent death of their parent may have difficulty thinking about how the parent looked and acted before the violence. They may need help to focus on happier memories. Children also grieve for parents and siblings from whom they have been separated in conditions where it is likely that the persons who disappeared may have died. It may be difficult for them to resolve their thoughts and feelings without seeing the body or participating in burial rites. These children often find it difficult to complete the mourning process satisfactorily.

Many children of school age, especially boys, hide their grief, isolating themselves when they feel overwhelmed by the need to cry. Little children experience grief in short, intense bursts that sometimes occur during play and are often not witnessed by adults. They resume their interrupted activity after a few minutes. Adolescents may avoid talking about their dead parent because they do not think their peers will respond well to such talk. They may also be reluctant to talk about the deceased to the surviving parent because they do not want to remind him or her of their loss. For these reasons, adults sometimes assume that children have completed their grieving before they actually have.

Post-traumatic stress reactions

Post-traumatic stress is the name given to a cluster of psychological and physiological reactions and behaviours that occur when people have had experiences that are far beyond those of normal life and that would be markedly distressing to almost anyone (Wright 1995). People may have symptoms of post-traumatic stress or, if the symptoms are extreme and prevent the person from doing normal things, they may be diagnosed by specialists as having post-traumatic stress disorder (PTSD). PTSD is characterised by the features of experience and behaviour that are shown in table 13, on page 162.

Children show these symptoms in age-appropriate ways. Primary-school-age children may find it difficult to interact with peers, withdrawing to spend time alone. Because they are easily angered, some get into many fights. Others find it difficult to concentrate in class and forget newly learned material, even when it is fairly easy. They may come to school exhausted after disrupted sleep and terrifying nightmares. Older children and adolescents may show their distress in additional ways, indulging in risky behaviours such as drug taking or sexual activity as they try to avoid thinking about the past. Children of all ages may show signs of depression and anxiety.

Shaw and Harris (1994) and Naslund (1997) briefly review studies that show PTSD occurs in a large number of children and adolescents who have been exposed to traumatic events. These studies show that between about 30% and 50% of children exposed to war show enough of the symptoms listed above to be diagnosed as having PTSD. Many children continue to show these symptoms for as long as three years after the war has ended.

Because there have been a number of civil wars in Africa in recent times, some of these studies assessed African children, reporting very similar patterns of distress to those reported elsewhere (Boothby 1996; McCallin 1996). But there may be some gender and ethnic group differences in presentation of PTSD. Naslund (1997), for example, presents data showing gender differences in the PTSD symptoms of adolescents and young adults from the Horn of Africa (Somalia, Eritrea, Ethiopia) and Zambia. These differences may reflect differences in the kinds of traumatic events they had experienced and the extent to which these traumatising events co-occurred. Thus, for males, rape and sexual assault commonly occurred in the context of severe beatings. Females were less likely to report the combination of rape and beating. For these young Africans PTSD was associated with grief rather than with the symptoms of anxiety and depression that have been reported in studies from other parts of the world.

Table 13 Post-traumatic stress syndrome

Re-experiencing • Recurring and distressing memories of the event in situations unrelated to the original event • Recurring and distressing dreams of the event • Suddenly acting or feeling as if the event was happening currently, at the present moment • Distress when exposed to events symbolic of earlier experience, e.g. anniversaries of event
Avoidance • Trying to avoid thoughts or feelings associated with the trauma • Avoiding activities or situations that remind of trauma • 'Forgetting' an important aspect of the trauma • Loss of interest in previously important activities • Feelings of detachment and separation from others • Less emotional responsiveness. For example, loss of pleasure in play, emotional flatness • Belief that their future has been cut short, inability to imagine a future for themselves
Increased arousal • Difficulty falling asleep or staying asleep • Easily angered, annoyed or made irritable • Difficulty concentrating or remembering important information • Constantly alert, looking out for danger • Very tense, jumpy, startle easily in an exaggerated way if unexpected events occur (e.g. a loud bang) • Signs of physical tension. For example, stiff muscles, fast pulse, breathing quickly, sweaty skin.

Source: Adapted from Wright (1995:34–35)

Although about half of all children with PTSD recover when provided with a safe, caring environment, some do not. PTSD of more than about one year's duration is important because children who have these symptoms cannot participate fully in daily life and cannot learn the skills and ways of behaving that are appropriate for their age. For example, preschool-age children who are constantly alert to danger cannot play freely with others and schoolchildren who have difficulty concentrating lag further and further behind in their studies, so future prospects are limited. Adolescents, trapped by their past, cannot undertake the tasks required as indicators of maturity in their community. These children need specialised additional help to overcome their problems.

Childhood depression

Little is known about childhood depression, but northern hemisphere research suggests that children and adolescents whose grief for the death of a loved person has gone on for more than about 18–24 months may be depressed (Barker 1995). Children who have been traumatised by war, sexual abuse or other trauma, or by living in a highly stressful situation for a long period may also be seriously (clinically) depressed (Wright 1995). These young people lose interest in life and schoolwork, refuse to eat, become slow and lethargic, lose concentration, and often complain of aches and pains for which there is no physical basis. They may complain often of being criticised, picked on or blamed when this is not apparent to others. If asked, they may admit to sleeping poorly, eating less or more than usual, feeling sad for long periods of time, feeling worthless or guilty, and having no sense that things will get better. Some young people who have this illness, especially adolescents, attempt suicide and a few are successful in their attempt (Barker 1995; Epanchin 1987).

This kind of depression is different from the sad, low mood that is sometimes called depression, but which lasts only a few hours or so after some unpleasant event. Clinical depression can last for months or even years. Teachers who fear that a child in their class is seriously depressed can try to make sure that he or she is supported and encouraged to interact with others. They should help the child to make choices and gain feelings of control over events as much as possible, but they should also seek help from other professionals such as doctors or social workers, if possible.

The development of conduct disorders

Some child soldiers and children who are homeless are at great risk of developing in ways that are harmful to themselves and to society. Child soldiers are generally severely traumatised by what they have seen and what they themselves have been forced to do. If they have been soldiers for more than a few months, they may begin to see themselves only as killers, losing the urge to escape from the violence, and adapting to the lives demanded of them (Boothby 1996; Shaw and Harris 1994). Children who live as so-called street kids may also have been traumatised, either by the events (e.g. physical or sexual abuse) that forced them to leave home or by experience of rape, prostitution, hunger, and fear as they have attempted to survive without a home to return to. They are at risk of malnutrition, general ill health, and sexually transmitted diseases. Often they develop addiction to drugs and alcohol as they try to avoid feelings of intense psychological distress.

A very small number of these children lose, or never develop, the capacity to form an attachment to others. They see people as objects to be used as they struggle to survive. Because they have no real relationships with others, they do not develop the moral codes that children in better circumstances are taught. These children are unlikely to attend school regularly unless they have had considerable psychological and social rehabilitation. If enrolled at school without having had such help, they steal from others, become verbally abusive, and may get into vicious fights. They do not abide by school rules and show little concern about them, or about the effect of their actions on others. Occasionally a teacher with special attributes can help them to trust enough to try to work through some of these issues, but generally these children do not stay around long enough to be helped. They are the ones whose lives have been truly destroyed by their experiences.

Promoting psychological recovery

Although extremely disturbed children need professional help, the very resilience of children means that many of them recover from their psychological distress if certain basic conditions are met by teachers and caregivers. Various authors (e.g. Kilbourn 1995b; McCallin and Jareg 1996; Jareg 1996; Shaw and Harris 1994) suggest ways that adults can help these children sort out their feelings, thoughts and reactions to their experiences. Some of these are listed below, but teachers who are working with numbers of children with significant psychological problems need to seek more detailed information about how they can increase their effectiveness with this group.

When dealing with children's emotions teachers need to:

- **Recognise that young children often do not have the language to discuss their emotions:** These children need opportunities to draw and act out their emotions, with teachers providing brief comments on what they think is being shown. Comments such as 'You must have been really scared', 'You seem to be angry about . . .' 'Do you feel ashamed about . . .' can help children recognise how they feel.
- **Accept children's emotions:** Saying 'Well, nothing bad happened, did it?' or 'Just forget it' is not helpful. Children need time and talk to deal with their reactions and will sort out what they think about what happened in their own way.
- **Find time to talk to older children and adolescents about their thoughts, beliefs, and feelings about what has happened:** Like younger children, adolescents may need help in labelling their reactions. Sometimes they benefit from having more information about the political events that underlay the war, or that contributed to the famine that uprooted their family.

- **Accept the reality of children's grief about deaths they have witnessed or learnt about:** Although children sometimes grieve in a different way from adults, they do not 'just forget' in a few days or weeks. Adolescents in particular may feel very vulnerable when someone close to them has died, because their recent cognitive development gives them an adult-level understanding of death.

More generally, teachers should:

- **Provide security through having a well-structured programme with good routines:** Anxious children need the security of knowing what will happen next, of knowing what the teacher's expectations are with regard to behaviour, what the class rules are, and so on. They need to know that reading and mathematics lessons are at certain times or that sport is scheduled for a particular afternoon. When times have to be changed, these children need as much advance warning as possible, with clear explanation about why things are different.
- **Act in a trustworthy manner:** Trustworthy teachers help children to become emotionally attached, and to regain self-respect. Such teachers provide an environment in which children can learn to feel safe, and make good choices about how they will behave and what they will do. Teachers who are trying to be extra trustworthy need to be consistent in the way they respond to pupils; they need to avoid emotional upsets, unnecessary shouting and punishments. They need to show loving concern for pupils' wellbeing, not merely concern for academic progress. They should encourage children to make decisions so that they sense they have some control over events. These decisions can be about minor or major issues (e.g. Do you want to use the red or blue crayon? Do you want to study woodwork or extra biology?). Culturally appropriate reward for effort should be offered, as outlined in Chapter Eleven.
- **Help children re-establish self control:** Angry children often act out their anger, having verbal disputes with the teacher and with other children, or getting into physical fights, throwing books or chairs across the room. Teachers can help children to learn alternative ways of expressing anger, such as talking about their emotions, breathing slowly when beginning to feel upset, briefly leaving the room to sit on a bench outside and relax. Teachers need to remember that some children who constantly express anger are hiding their fears. If they suspect that this is true, teachers can help by acknowledging the fear (e.g. saying 'Not knowing how to solve this maths problem can make you afraid others will laugh, as well as making you feel frustrated and angry'). Clear rules about what happens if children threaten

or harm others are important. Equally importantly, these rules should be consistently applied.

- **Help children relax:** Teaching children simple exercises to slow their breathing is easy and all children enjoy the experience of being relaxed. A good exercise is to ask pupils to close their eyes and breathe in and out as the teacher repeats slowly 'In . . . Out . . . In . . . Out' or provides a slow count for breaths. Some traumatised children will not want to close their eyes. These children can be asked to focus their attention on a plant or tree outside the classroom, or some immoveable object across the room. Children can then be taught a cue word or phrase that the teacher will use to remind them to relax a bit. Asking children to put their heads down on their arms, while the teacher reads a non-violent story, or plays some relaxing music can also be helpful.
- **Help children re-establish a positive sense of their identity:** Children who can no longer live with their parents may feel that they do not belong anywhere. But they remain the 'son of . . . and . . .' or the 'daughter of . . . and . . .' even when their parents are dead or missing. They are also 'the friend of . . .' and the niece or nephew, grandson or granddaughter of other important people. Class lessons on relationships can help here. A few children who have been traumatised may have developed the feeling that they are always going to be victims. Class lessons in which pupils list skills, strengths and resources can help them see that they are survivors, with potential to develop in positive ways. Traditional stories, dance and song can also help children to re-establish their identity.
- **Avoid loading extra humiliation onto children who are already upset:** Jareg (1996), for example, describes the situation in which a child who had seen her father shot and killed was punished in front of the whole class for not wearing a school uniform that her mother could not afford to provide. Punishing children who have gaps in their knowledge because of disrupted schooling also adds to their anger and humiliation.
- **Help children re-establish relationships with others:** Children who have been traumatised may be afraid of going out into the playground or may lack skills in some of the games played there because they have been too busy surviving to learn these games. Teachers can help children to interact with others, at first with just a selected or caring one or two, later a larger group.

Conclusion

Teaching classes that include children who are disabled or disturbed and difficult makes heavy demands on teachers, especially in education systems where class sizes are large and schools have few resources. Teachers are not therapists and cannot be expected to work intensively with one troublesome child at the expense of all others. On the other hand, teachers do have an obligation to act in a caring fashion and a concern for developing young people has often been one of the motivations for entering a teaching career in the first instance. Thus, teachers need to make some special efforts to help the pupils who are suffering as a result of sensory, physical, or intellectual limitations or because their lives have been disrupted by the instability of the personal and physical environment.

Sometimes a small amount of extra thought can make a difference. This was the experience of one of the present authors early in her career. A disturbed little girl joined the class part way through the year and began acting in ways that disrupted the learning of others. This child had lived in several foster homes and had gone to five different schools in the first two years of her school life. She was obviously feeling very insecure and responded well to being asked to place her desk right up close to the teacher's desk, not as a punishment, but so that she could experience the physical and psychological security of knowing that a caring adult was right near by. Although she needed careful monitoring, this was easy from her position close to the front of the class, and problems with her behaviour rapidly decreased. African teachers are just as capable of making these kinds of adjustments to classroom life as any others, and many probably already do so. These teachers are likely to be very effective in helping *all* pupils to develop as fully as possible.

In your community (six)

Teachers need to be alert to indications of disability and distress on the part of the children they teach. Some of the following exercises offer an opportunity to develop this awareness. Choose one or more.

1 Go to a school playground or other place where there are many children and observe them carefully for 10 to 20 minutes. Try to decide whether you are seeing any indications that one or more children are having difficulty hearing others' speech.
2 Visit the local health clinic and talk to the clinic nurse about the commonest disabilities in your area. What are they? How severe is the disability? What is the commonest cause of this disability?
3 Ask a teacher if you can visit his or her classroom and observe children while he or she is teaching a lesson. Try to discover whether any children are having difficulty seeing or hearing. Talk to the teacher afterwards and discover if he or she has identified any children with these problems.
4 Visit a group for parents of children with one or other disability. Ask them about the ways in which having a disabled child affects life in their family.
5 Choose one disability. Read any material from your country's Ministry of Health or other similar agency, on the subject of this disability in the country. Report your findings to your colleagues.

Chapter Eight

HIV/AIDS

Introduction

Almost everyone in Africa knows about AIDS, the fatal disease referred to as 'slim' in many countries. But there is still confusion about how it is transmitted, whether it can be cured, and what other illnesses are associated with it. The enormous amount of research into this disease, by African researchers and others from many parts of the world, means that scientific knowledge about it is expanding rapidly. Material in this chapter presents facts that were established at the time of writing, but new facts about the transmission of the disease and the care of those who have it will soon add to what can be presented here.

The presence of HIV/AIDS in the community can influence child development in several ways. Infants may be born with the infection, or acquire it during the early months or years of their lives. This is called paediatric AIDS. Children who are not infected themselves may suffer from seeing one or both parents die slowly from the disease or from diseases such as tuberculosis that frequently co-occur with AIDS. They may find their lives further disrupted by changes in where they live and who cares for them after their parents' death, even while they grieve for their parents. Adolescents may find that they are expected to take on parenting roles after the death of one or both parents. They are also at risk of becoming infected with HIV because this is the time that young people become sexually active.

HIV and AIDS: What do these terms refer to?

Like the common cold, AIDS is caused by a virus. The abbreviation HIV refers to the virus that infects people and is the cause of AIDS. HIV means 'human immunodeficiency virus'. People who have this virus in their bodies are sometimes referred to as being HIV positive (HIV+) and those who are not infected are HIV negative (HIV–). These terms come from medical test procedures. The term HIV refers to the fact that this virus causes illness by attacking the human immune system. The immune system provides the body's natural resistance to all kinds of infection.

When the immune system is weakened by HIV, people start to get sick with a cluster of apparently unrelated infections. Once a person has many of the infections that are typical of the disease called AIDS and very few of the cells in the blood that would normally fight infection, he or she is diagnosed as having this disease. The term *AIDS* means 'Acquired immunodeficiency syndrome'. People can be infected with HIV for weeks, months, or even years before they develop AIDS. Currently, some people in Africa believe that it is possible to tell whether others are sick with the virus just by looking at them. A person who looks healthy is not considered a risk. However, because people do not get sick with AIDS immediately they are infected, many people who are HIV positive look well and continue with daily life just like others who are not infected.

Transmission of HIV

As many teachers probably already know, the human immunodeficiency virus is passed from one person to another in male sperm, female vaginal fluids and the blood of males and females. The commonest mechanism of transmission is unprotected penetrative sex. This occurs when the male ejaculates his sperm into the vagina, mouth or anus (bottom) of his partner. These kinds of sexual activity are referred to as vaginal, oral and anal sex respectively. As elsewhere in the world, all of these kinds of sexual activity take place in Africa, despite strong taboos against anal sex in particular in many communities.

Although women in Africa are often blamed for the spread of HIV/AIDS, it is much more difficult for a woman to infect a healthy man with the disease than it is for a man to infect a woman. This is because male fluids always enter the female body when the male ejaculates into her vagina, mouth or anus, but her bodily fluids enter the male body during sexual intercourse only if he has an open injury site on his penis. Halperin and Bailey (1999) state that female to male transmission may be 'as rare as one per 9 000 acts of unprotected vaginal intercourse *in the absence of facilitating risk factors*' (1999, p.1814, italics added). Risk factors that contribute to the transmission of the virus are discussed later in the chapter.

The non-sexual transmission of HIV occurs when blood from an infected person enters the body of another person, usually during a blood transfusion with blood that has not been screened for HIV. An injection given with a used hypodermic syringe (needle) may also transmit the virus. The hypodermic syringe may have a residue of HIV+ blood in it, which is then injected into the next person who is treated. This kind of transmission is common when hypodermic syringes are reused in hospitals, or among intravenous drug users who inject illegal drugs and often share needles. As elsewhere, intravenous drug users can be found in Africa, although this method of using illegal drugs is not widespread.

Paediatric HIV/AIDS

Infants who are born to HIV positive mothers are at some risk of being born with the infection, which has been passed to them either in utero (in the womb) or, less commonly, during the process of birth. This may account for around 15% of paediatric infection. But in Africa the picture is confounded by the high rate of breast-feeding, because breast-feeding also permits the transmission of the virus to the infant, via mothers' milk. LeCoeur and Lallemant (1996), in a close analysis of several studies, concluded that about 14% of infants are infected through breast-feeding. These figures are consistent with findings suggesting that around 25% of infants born to HIV infected mothers are themselves infected by the time they are 12 to 18 months old (approximately 15% at birth plus up to 14% as a result of breast-feeding). LeCoeur and Lallemant note, however, that paediatric infection rates as high as 44% have been reported in some studies.

Box 10 A child speaks

'We are normal human beings, we can walk and talk.'

Nkosi Johnson (now deceased), 12, South Africa

Source: UNICEF (2002:40)

High rates of paediatric infection are more common in Africa than in northern hemisphere countries. The UNAIDS (1998) report for example states that paediatric HIV infection rates of 30% to 40% are common in the region. Women who are not HIV positive at the time they give birth, but who become infected during the period that they are breast-feeding, are more likely to infect their infants than those who were HIV positive before becoming pregnant. Thus, some mothers can provide protection for their infants by ensuring that they use safe sex practices while they are breast-feeding. Higher rates of infection also appear to occur if the child is still being breast-fed at 18 months (LeCoeur and Lallemant 1996), although the reason for this is currently not known.

The figures raise the question of whether HIV positive women should breast-feed their infants. At present UNAIDS (the specialist United Nations agency dealing with the AIDS epidemic) still recommends breast-feeding because of the risk that infants will die from diarrhoea if they are fed infant formula in conditions where the cleanliness of the water and of bottles cannot be guaranteed (UNAIDS 1998). Feeding practices are unlikely to change in rural communities where knowledge about HIV/AIDS is low. Kunii and Shibuya's (1995) study of rural mothers in Côte d'Ivoire showed that although almost all of them had heard about AIDS, only about half knew it was fatal. Not one knew HIV infection could be transmitted via breast-milk. These authors point out that early weaning would probably be associated with increased risk of malnutrition and diarrhoeal disease because rural women in the region usually wean children to water or juice. In addition they do not provide sufficient food to meet the infants' calorie (kilojoule) requirements in the period immediately after weaning.

Besides breast-feeding, infants and young children are most likely to become infected if they need a blood transfusion and receive blood that has not been screened for HIV. In some parts of Africa children who are extremely anaemic as a result of malaria may receive a blood transfusion. This practice is possibly less likely today than it was once. For example, in 1988 Greenberg et al. assessed this source of HIV infection in Kinshasa in what is now the Democratic Republic of Congo. At that time 87% of paediatric transfusions were given to anaemic children, a rate of blood use that was expected to lead to high rates of new HIV infection. A less risky treatment can be used today. Unless a child is nearly dying from the effects of anaemia, he or she can be treated with iron supplements given in the form of drops or tablets. Recovery will be slower but children are spared the risk of HIV/AIDS.

Not all infants who are infected with HIV immediately develop AIDS (European Collaborative Study 1991) but those who do have a much higher mortality rate than children who are not infected with this virus. Taha et al. (1995) for example reported that 36% of Malawian infants who were infected by HIV positive mothers had died by the age of 36 months, compared with only 12% of children whose mothers were HIV negative. Many of the infected children die in their first year, probably because AIDS develops very rapidly in infants once the virus is present in the body (Preble 1990).

An additional health problem that arises when there is AIDS in the community relates to parents' beliefs about treating other common childhood infections. Preble (1990) notes that because diarrhoea is an early indicator of AIDS, and because oral rehydration therapy (ORT) is not likely to be effective in this instance, parents might come to believe that ORT is not useful with any diarrhoea. If they give up using ORT, many children will die unnecessarily from diarrhoea that has another cause. The European Collaborative Study (1991) expresses similar concerns, stating for example that common infections of the middle ear that are unrelated to AIDS may remain untreated if parents believe they are a result of AIDS.

Conclusion

Most infants and young children who have HIV/AIDS have been infected by their mothers. The infection is most likely to have been transmitted during breast-feeding. But African village women have little choice about whether to breast-feed or not, because not breast-feeding carries a high risk that the infant will develop another life-threatening illness, the most common one being diarrhoea.

AIDS orphans

The life experiences of children whose parents die from AIDS are different from and much more adverse than those of children whose parents do not contract the disease. These children are referred to in the literature as 'orphans'. The term includes children whose mother *or* father has died, as well as children whose parents have both died.

Poverty increases during the period that a parent is ill with AIDS, as the immediate family and the extended family spend considerable amounts trying to find a cure for the illness. (There is no cure.) Household goods are sold off to meet daily living costs, young children's enrolment at school is delayed, and older children are removed from school to care for the dying parent and their young siblings or to earn money through paid work (World Bank 1999). Later, funeral costs may be high. Research in Tanzania and Uganda reported by the World Bank showed that in the period immediately after a parent died, families spent less on bought food. Although this shortage of bought food was partially compensated for by increased home production of food, the total food intake of orphan children dropped on average by 15%. In poor communities where children are already suffering chronic low levels of malnutrition, this further reduction in food intake has harmful effects on developing intellectual and physical capacities that will last throughout the children's lives.

The decision about what will happen to children who are orphaned by AIDS depends on a variety of factors. If the father dies from AIDS, the children generally stay with their mother, although sometimes his family unfairly blame her for the infection, and drive her and the children away. If the mother dies, children generally go to relatives, although some will be unwilling to take them because of their own poverty. If both parents die, the father's family usually decide on the placement of the children. In some ethnic groups, where the children are believed to be members of the father's family, a mother may leave her children with her dead husband's family and go off to seek another husband (Hunter 1990). This culturally acceptable practice may be less common today than in the past as cultures change in response to the presence of HIV/AIDS in the community.

Box 11 A young adult speaks about his family

'They (our relatives) want to split us up. They want us to be their servants. No one has suggested a way to keep us together and help us. They have picked who they want to take – to make us work for them – not to help us. And we are not willing to be separated. We want to stay together. We would rather eat nothing but beans, as long as we are together.'

Yemisrach, 21, Ethiopia, whose parents died of AIDS

Source: UNICEF (2002:40)

Outcomes for orphaned children can be excellent if they can find satisfactory substitute care after the death of one or both of their parents, but may vary according to the age and gender of the child. Very young infants and children make high dependency demands on the substitute family, and may be seen as an additional burden that cannot be managed. In contrast, older children, especially girls, may be more readily accepted into substitute families because they can do more work. Poor outcomes can result in economic and sexual exploitation, especially of girls. Children of both genders generally lose rights to family property if placed with another family, so may be faced with long-term poverty and hunger as adults (Levine, Michaels and Back 1996).

Generally, African governments and local community members believe that children should remain in their home town or village after they are orphaned. Adoption by strangers is not common and orphanages in Africa are often of poor quality. It also costs ten times as much to keep each child in an orphanage as it does to support that child if he or she remains with a family (World Bank 1999). In contrast, keeping children in their own community is both cost effective for governments and ensures that children remain integrated into their ethnic group, developing the values, skills, and behaviours required for acceptance by the group (Banda 1995; Levine, Michaels and Back 1996; Preble 1990).

Members of the extended family usually take these children into their homes, although their own poverty and the total numbers of orphans in the community may make this extremely difficult for them. For example, Shuey, Begarukayo, Senkusu and Ryan (1996) found that some families in Uganda were coping with as many as 17 orphans in the household. Interestingly, Webb (1997) obtained data showing that people in extremely poor communities were more likely to accept the idea of keeping AIDS orphans in their midst than those in slightly wealthier communities. Webb attributed this to the social value placed on helping others when times are bad, which he thought was stronger in poor communities because of their recurrent experience of difficult times.

After the parents have died, many households are kept together by older siblings or by the introduction of an unmarried adult relative to the house to care for young children living there. Banda (1995) states that these adolescent and young adult caregivers may need material and emotional support as they try to cope with a role that requires considerable maturity. Some governments provide limited financial assistance with the costs of schooling, clothing, food and bedding for families who have taken in orphans. A final option suggested by Banda is that more boarding schools should be provided. While more expensive than most other options, boarding schools permit children to gain an education and to return to their home village during school holidays, retaining links to their home community. These kinds of arrangements all increase the chance that children will be able to retain hereditary rights to their family property (Banda 1995; World Bank 1999).

Orphan children's health and education may be adversely affected as a result of their status. In poor communities orphan children are even more stunted (shorter in height) than other children of the same age. They remain stunted even when cared for by substitute adults who take over the role of caretaker, or when they are fostered with relatives. The reason for this continued problem is not known. It may be that the orphan children's own health has been harmed by exposure to the tuberculosis that very often co-occurs with HIV/AIDS (World Bank 1999). If substitute families are poor themselves, they may not be able to provide adequate food for additional children. Finally, some families may discriminate between their own children and those they are fostering through a sense of obligation, allowing orphans less food in times of scarcity.

School enrolment of orphans is lower than that of children whose parents are living. Data presented in the World Bank report (1999) suggest that this effect is greater in countries where enrolment is already low. In Côte d'Ivoire and the Central African Republic for example enrolment rates of about 56% and 64% respectively for children with both parents living dropped to approximately 38% and 45% for children whose parents were both dead. Thus, orphan status is a significant additional factor in determining who goes to school in these countries, and being an orphan condemns many additional children to lives of restricted choice and knowledge. In contrast, in countries such as Zimbabwe, where enrolment is generally high, the reduction in school enrolment of orphans is very small. Over 80% of all primary-school-age children in Zimbabwe were enrolled at school in 1994, irrespective of whether they had one, none, or both parents living.

A problem for some children is the stigma attached to AIDS sufferers and sometimes to the children of parents with AIDS. Webb (1997) points out that some of the increasing numbers of street children in Kenyan cities have been driven out of their communities because their parents died from AIDS. Teachers, too, have been shown to interact less with children whose parents have AIDS than they do with other children in the class. Children in some countries have also been thrown out of school, 'not for being HIV positive but because their parents have AIDS' (McGreal 2001, p.22).

Conclusion

The few studies of what happens when one or both parents die show an increase in child poverty and reduction in food intake. School enrolment may fall off for a number of reasons. These problems arise at the very time that children are additionally vulnerable because they are dealing with their own psychological responses to having cared for a dying parent, observing his or her great pain and distress. Children's grief can be intense and prolonged. This may contribute to their reduced food intake and poor school attendance.

Adolescents, sexuality and HIV/AIDS

In modern psychology, adolescence is considered a time of transition during which young people renegotiate their relationships and patterns of interaction with parents, peers and the wider world in preparation for adult roles (Bloom 1990; Jackson and Rodiguez-Tomé 1993). Bloom emphasises the development of the competencies needed for adult life, pointing out that the behaviours of others in the community can help or hinder adolescents as they try to establish these competencies. Important developments during adolescence lead to competence in the chosen occupation and in the development of culturally acceptable general values, goals and social behaviours. One necessary additional competence stands out as a major issue in the context of the HIV/AIDS epidemic in Africa. This is the safe expression of adolescent sexuality.

The physical changes that culminate in sexual maturity on the part of African adolescents generally follow the same sequence as the changes of adolescents in other parts of the world, although the onset of puberty may be a little later in communities where there are food shortages. In many parts of Africa large numbers of adolescents are still at primary school, and many of these will not continue on to secondary school. As noted elsewhere, adolescent girls are generally less likely to proceed to secondary school than boys (UNICEF 2000a).

To date, the studies of African adolescents' knowledge about and attitudes towards sexual activity have often only measured the knowledge and attitudes of those who are attending secondary school. In many countries these are the children with relatively richer, better-educated parents. Urban secondary school pupils are even more likely than those in rural areas to have more privileged and modern family backgrounds. Studies of adolescents at primary school (e.g. Leshabari, Pounds, and Celentano 1988) and the few community-based studies such as that of Magnani et al. (2002) therefore provide important information about adolescents who are less well educated or less advantaged.

Sexuality: traditional and modern beliefs and practices

Modern African beliefs and knowledge about sexuality continue to reflect tradition. Some traditional practices were established to enhance the sexual satisfaction of the two partners. These practices come in different forms and vary from ethnic group to ethnic group. In Botswana traditional doctors still give charms to individual adolescent women to enhance their enjoyment of sexual intercourse. In other cases girls are instructed to pull the labia majora (the outer fleshy part of the female genitals) to make 'ditlopi'. The practice lengthens the labia majora and tightens the vagina, thus enhancing sexual gratification. Women in the parts of Botswana where this practice is followed believe that any adult female who does not have 'ditlopi' is not a proper woman because she would be an unsatisfactory sexual partner. In fact, the absence of 'ditlopi' in a girl has often resulted in the termination of an affair or engagement (Seboni et al. 1999).

Boys are also taught ways of enhancing sexual skills. After their first wet dream boys in Botswana are instructed to pull their penis to make it longer (Seboni et al. 1999). The findings of Seboni et al. confirm the durability and spread of culturally valued practices aimed at enhancing sexual pleasure. These authors note that their 1998 findings are very similar to results obtained by Ammar in 1954 in Egypt and by Oduntam and Onadeko in Nigeria in the same year.

In contrast, some traditional beliefs and practices in the area of sexuality were harmful to one or both partners in a sexual relationship. These may also continue to be followed today. Female genital mutilation, which can result in painful menstruation, painful intercourse and additional pain and risk during birth, is still practised and may even be spreading (Lightfoot-Klein 1989). The traditionally low status of African women has also contributed to some harmful beliefs about sexuality. Sexually transmitted diseases (STDs) are frequently perceived as 'women's diseases', amenable only to magical cures. In some instances men wrongly believe that their sexually transmitted disease can be cured only by having sexual intercourse with a virgin. Likewise, pregnancy and birth are characterised by some harmful beliefs and practices, ranging from food taboos to mismanagement of labour and phobias about operative delivery or other hospital procedures. Because these beliefs are prevalent in many communities, they are passed from adults to children and adolescents during the early lives of young people.

Techniques such as aggressive sex, an emphasis on full vaginal intercourse during which the semen is ejaculated into the vagina, and an aversion to handling one's own or one's partner's genitals pose problems for condom use and safe sex. Similarly, there are other practices that are geared to enhancing libido or sexuality, such as drug stimulants and insertion of herbs into the vagina, which can damage the reproductive system. Traditions that sanction sex outside monogamous relationships as part of the rituals of puberty, inheritance, twin birth, or widowhood ceremonies also contribute to the spread of sexually transmitted diseases, including HIV/AIDS.

Religion, too, influences sexual behaviour and beliefs. Moslems and Christians explicitly forbid some sexual practices. These faiths both place an emphasis on female virginity. In Moslem communities the honour of the family may depend entirely on female virginity at marriage and her sexual fidelity to her husband afterwards. This value has resulted in the pattern of early marriage of Moslem girls in many parts of the world. Christianity, while not protecting young women to the same degree, still holds that women should be chaste and virginal until marriage.

There are problems about adolescent sexuality in both faiths. Thomas and Carver (1990) for example state that even in the modern world, committed Christians define adolescent sexual activity as socially deviant. Thus, they are more likely to oppose easy access to condoms, which they believe encourage adolescents to become sexually active. Mathews, Everett, Binedell and Steinberg's (1995) study in South Africa revealed that Muslim teachers there had the same difficulty in coping with the reality of adolescent sexuality that Thomas and Carver had reported for Christians. Matthews et al. point out, however, that it is also possible to perceive condom use as a sign of social competence. People with this view may think that sexually active adolescents who want to use condoms to prevent early pregnancy or the spread of a range of sexually transmitted diseases are acting in a socially responsible and mature manner. These people are more likely to think that condoms should be readily available to adolescents in order to promote competence in this area of development.

In the past, pre-marital sexual relations were forbidden and subject to social sanction in many ethnic groups except on the designated ritual occasions listed above. Despite this, sexual activity on the part of young people was often tolerated as long as they were discreet. Sanctions were applied only when taboos were broken in a very overt way, often when the young woman became pregnant. In some communities, however, premarital pregnancy was valued as a sign of the young woman's fertility. Sexual experimentation was more readily accepted in these ethnic groups (Caldwell, Caldwell and Quiggin 1994). Boys were universally expected to indulge in sexual experimentation.

Today, early sexual experimentation on the part of both boys and girls is widespread in some countries. Adolescents in Botswana and Nigeria for example no longer consider that it is necessary or desirable to be a virgin at the time of marriage (IPPF 1994; Omoegun 1997; Owuamanam 1982). As a result, teenage pregnancy has become a major problem in Africa. Botswana tops other countries in its rate of adolescent pregnancy with 23.5% of all adolescent females becoming pregnant. Teenage pregnancy rates are also high in countries such as Zimbabwe (16%), Ghana (19%), and Kenya and Togo (21%) (Network 1993). The stigma attached to this status varies from one country to another country, depending on how culture and religion view it. In addition, many African governments do not support abortion and therefore do not have provision for safe abortions. Together, these factors have resulted in high rates of single parenthood in some countries with some very young mothers who are too immature for parenthood. Thus, teenage pregnancy may result in psychological problems for the teenager and her family. It certainly limits her choices about further education and career training. In this way, teenage pregnancy has a negative economic effect on any given nation.

Some, but not all, teenage pregnancies are unwanted. In Botswana, the high rate of teenage pregnancy, which contributes 30–35% of total fertility in the country, is a reflection of a combination of factors, including sexual harassment, cultural norms, lack of knowledge, and lack of access to contraceptives. Seboni et al. (1999) found in their study in Botswana that some girls used pregnancy to trap boys into marrying them or to obtain damages from them. The study further revealed that adolescent girls also became pregnant because some men deceived them by pretending to possess herbs that prevent pregnancy when in fact they do not and the girls still became pregnant. Alternatively older men enticed young women into sexual relationships with money. Finally, some girls became pregnant when condoms split, allowing semen into the vagina.

Personal and social factors influencing HIV/AIDS risk

Disagreement among adults about adolescent sexuality does not alter the fact that many adolescents are having sexual relationships by the time they reach their mid-teens. Consequently they are potentially at risk of becoming infected with HIV. But the risk to each individual varies according to a number of his or her personal and social characteristics. These include traditional and modern cultural practices and beliefs, and the extent of education and knowledge about reproduction. These risk factors are discussed in the present section.

Knowledge about and attitudes to sexuality, and sexual behaviours

Bloom (1990) notes that social taboos against discussing matters relating to sexuality and parental inadequacies such as not knowing the facts about reproduction, not being able to communicate facts, or refusing to accept children as sexual beings are strong inhibitors of adolescent sexual competence. For traditional and modern cultural reasons these taboos remain powerful. They prevent the 'acceptance of one's sexuality [that] is viewed by many as a protector against threats of indiscriminate and unplanned sexual activity' (1990:22). Bloom's comments were made about taboos in the United States, but Courtois, Mullet and Malvy (2001a) have described similar problems arising from African taboos. They point out that African parents may not give information about reproduction and reproductive health for two reasons. The first reason is the long-standing cultural taboo against discussing sexuality even within intimate relationships and within the family. Second, parents may not know some of the necessary facts themselves.

Only relatively few adolescents obtain information about sexual matters from parents (Adjahoto, Hodonou, De Souza, Tété and Baeta 2000; Courtois et al. 2001a; Leshabari et al. 1988). Some studies show that maternal aunts and cousins may be culturally identified as sources of sex education for young people (Ball 1988; Seboni 1993), although very few adolescents today say they have obtained information from adults in positions of authority, from health professionals, teachers, or church leaders. Adolescents in a number of African countries report that they learned about sexuality via the radio or television, with some learning from newspapers, or school biology lessons (Asuzu 1994; Ndlovu and Sihlangu 1992). Some discuss aspects of reproductive health with their close friends (Magnani et al. 2002). However, because they are not able to talk about these matters with informed adults, they do not have any opportunity to ask questions and clarify confusions. Information from the adolescent peer group is very likely to be inaccurate.

Failure on the part of parents or other adult authority figures in the community to provide adequate information about reproduction reduces the likelihood that adolescents can protect themselves from unwanted pregnancies and sexually transmitted diseases. In the first instance, lack of information means that young people are ignorant about their bodies. For example, Leshabari et al. (1988) in Tanzania reported that only 10% of the adolescents in their sample knew that a woman is most fertile about mid-cycle (approximately two weeks after she last began to menstruate, that is, after her last period began), even although many of them were sexually active. Half of the sample did not know that it was only possible for a woman to become pregnant once she had reached puberty.

Similarly, the majority of adolescents in a large study in Botswana (n = 600) did not know that a young woman could become pregnant as a result of one episode of sexual intercourse. They incorrectly believed that intermittent use of contraceptive pills was an effective control against pregnancy. Many also believed that being sexually active during adolescence enhanced their chances of fertility in later years (Seboni 1993). Again, this is incorrect. Recently Adjahoto et al. (2000) reported that only 72% of their sample in Togo knew about peak times for female fertility. Since over 90% claimed they had been given information about sex, the information they had received was clearly inadequate.

As a consequence of their lack of knowledge about sexuality African adolescents often have wrong ideas about sexual matters. Taboos against masturbation may be strong in some communities, reinforced by the teachings of some Christian churches, although there is no medical evidence that masturbation is harmful. In a study by Wanjohi (1987, as cited in Leshabari et al. 1988) boys were reported as believing that the only way to deal with the spontaneous erections that occur during male adolescent development was to have sexual relations with a girl. In fact, such erections disappear naturally without sexual release.

Ignorance of reproductive health and development makes it more difficult for adolescents to make informed choices about whether or not to become sexually active. Adolescents, both male and female, are subject to considerable pressure from their peers to become sexually active and to have multiple partners. This may be seen as a sign of modernity and sophistication (Nyanzi, Pool and Kinsman 2001). Various studies show that boys of this age reject the notion of fidelity (e.g. Courtois et al. 2001a 2001b; Nzioka 2001), and believe that having multiple partners is an indicator of adult manhood and virility. The adolescent males in Nzioka's study thought that getting a girl pregnant or having a sexually transmitted disease were both signs of successful male adulthood. These adolescent boys may boast about their sexual prowess to their friends. Despite this, the boys in Nzioka's study remained unwilling to talk openly to adults about sex and would not buy condoms unless they could do so anonymously, because they knew their sexual activity was not approved of by adults in their community.

Social pressure may mean that girls become sexually active before they really want to. Most would prefer to delay the onset of sexual activity, fearing pregnancy and HIV/AIDS. They also prefer to have sexual intercourse within the context of a longer-term relationship (Harrison, Xaba, and Kinsman 2001). Generally, they have had fewer sexual partners than their male peers. But they decide to become sexually active because doing so makes them feel good and grown up. It gives them a sense of belonging and acceptance among their already sexually active peer group and is seen as helping to maintain the friendship with their partner(s). Some want the monetary or other rewards they obtain from a rich or powerful partner, while others want a baby who will love them (Owuamanam 1982).

Sexually active adolescent women may not always have a choice about whether they have sexual intercourse or not. Courtois et al. (2001a) obtained data showing that 29% of the adolescent Congolese women in their study sample had had sexual intercourse under duress. Similarly, Magnani et al. (2002) mention the high level of sexual violence imposed on women in South Africa and Zambia, some of which arises from cultural requirements for female submissiveness to male demands. Other women who have sexual intercourse when they do not want to may be trying to meet survival needs for money, soap, food, or school fees. Adolescent women in this group are more likely than others to have intercourse with older partners (Leshabari et al. 1988; Nyanzi et al. 2001).

Knowledge about HIV

Reilly (2001, p.11) points out that '95% of African children under 15 [are] still HIV-free'. Unfortunately, many of these children and young people become infected with HIV within a few years of becoming sexually active.

Like studies of knowledge about sex and sexual relationships, studies of teenage knowledge and behaviours in relation to HIV/AIDS have concentrated on assessing adolescents in schools. The studies show variable knowledge in different countries. Sallah et al. (1999) reported that only 60% of 10 000 university students in Benin knew about HIV and AIDS. Very few of them knew how the infection was transmitted. Asuzu (1994) had found that 85% of a much smaller sample in Nigeria knew about AIDS, but only 68% knew how it was transmitted. As with more general knowledge about sexuality, adolescents reported learning about HIV/AIDS from radio and television, newspapers and classmates rather than teachers, parents, or other authority figures (Asuzu 1994; Ndlovu and Sihlangu 1992).

Even when adolescents have quite a lot of accurate knowledge about HIV/AIDS, they may still have some incorrect beliefs about transmission. This has been reported by Pattullo et al. (1994) and Courtois et al. (2001a), both of whom found that although adolescents generally had accurate knowledge about AIDS, some respondents still wrongly believed that AIDS could also be caught by sharing food, by mosquito bites, or by kissing. There is no evidence that this is so. Some of these secondary school students did not realise that the disease was fatal, or that a person who is infected with HIV can look healthy until he or she actually develops AIDS. Some, in studies by Caprara et al. (1993) and Courtois et al. (2000a), believed that magic and sorcery contributed to the spread of the disease. In this latter study, some believed HIV was a mutation of another STD and that the mutation had developed as a result of treatment for an initial STD infection.

The amount of knowledge about HIV, the kinds of sexual activity indulged in, and the number of partners all alter the risk of HIV transmission. Having more knowledge about HIV/AIDS is an advantage for young people, as it is often associated with delayed onset of sexual activity, fewer partners, and increased intent to use condoms (Magnani et al. 2002). These behaviours reduce the risk of HIV infection somewhat. Some relatively less common sexual practices can increase risk. For example, a small number of respondents in the Sallah et al. (1999) study acknowledged that they had participated in homosexual sexual intercourse, which often involved insertion of the penis of one partner into the anus of the other. Similarly, others had sexual relations with intravenous drug users. Both these activities carry high risk for HIV transmission.

The sense that one is personally at risk of becoming infected with HIV varies from one individual to another and this also alters behaviour. Adolescent males in Harrison et al.'s (2001) South African study felt less at risk than female respondents, but males in Nzioka's (2001) study were afraid of becoming infected. In Magnani et al.'s (2002) study in Zambia, young people acknowledged that HIV was transmitted sexually and worried about it in a general way, but indulged in risky behaviour. Most did not believe that they personally would become infected within the next 12 months. This sense of personal invulnerability was also reported by Lagarde, Pison and Enel (1996). These authors found that women who had sexual intercourse with casual partners felt less at risk than those who limited the number of partners. For men in the same study, a higher sense of personal vulnerability was associated with changes in behaviour to reduce risk. Sadly, the young males in Peltzer's (2001) study felt so vulnerable that they did not change their behaviour – if HIV/AIDS was inevitable, there probably seemed to be no point in trying to prevent it.

Condom use

Although many secondary school students know that using condoms is an excellent way of decreasing the risk of becoming infected with HIV, the great majority do not use them. Pattullo et al. (1994) for example report that although 41% of the males in their large sample of adolescent school students and 7% of females had multiple partners, just under 7% said they consistently used condoms. In all, 60% of the total sample said they had never used them. Similar low rates of condom use are reported in a number of other studies (Ahmed et al. 2001; Nyanzi et al. 2001; Volk and Koopman 2001).

Church rulings on the use of condoms may contribute to the decision not to use condoms in some parts of Africa, but many young people reject condoms because they associate using them with sexual promiscuity. The adolescent sense of invulnerability that is reported elsewhere (Legarde et al. 1996; Moore and Rosenthal 1991) may also play a role in the decision not to take actions designed to ensure safety. Courtois et al. (2001a) reported concerns that using condoms carried the risk of reduced fertility or reduction of the male's sexual virility. Young people living on the streets in South Africa claimed condoms 'smelled funny' and were 'good for balloons only' (Swart-Kruger and Richter 1997:962). Both men and women in the Courtois et al. study were concerned that women, who are not at risk of pregnancy when condoms are used correctly, might not be under social control without the fear of pregnancy. They feared this would contribute to the breakdown of traditional roles for each gender.

Condoms provide protection only if they are used every time a person has any form of sexual intercourse (vaginal, oral, or anal), but research to date shows that very few people use them consistently. Inconsistent use exposes everyone to the risk of infection with HIV and other sexually transmitted diseases (Ahmed et al. 2001). Some adolescents use condoms when having casual sex or in the early phases of a new relationship, but use decreases in longer-term sexual relationships as confidence in the partner's sexual fidelity increases (Courtois et al. 2001b). Because of taboos against discussing sexual matters, this confidence may be completely misplaced. When taboos are broken and sexual decisions are discussed, there may be increased use of condoms. Magnani et al. (2002) for example found that when such discussions had taken place, couples were five times more likely to use condoms than others who had not been able to talk openly about safe sex.

Sex roles

The patterns of behaviour expected of boys and girls, men and women over hundreds of generations continue to influence the behaviour expected today. Young women in many parts of Africa are still expected to be submissive to men. This can create problems for adolescent females when males exert pressure for sexual congress as the young men in various studies acknowledge they do (e.g. Mathews et al. 1995; Nzioka 2001). Adolescent males in the Mathews et al. study thought that seducing a virgin was proof of their virility and sexual potency. They admitted to losing respect for their partner once she had had sexual relations with them. These young men had difficulty with other aspects of relationships, and were concerned and confused about demands for non-sexual forms of intimacy.

Adolescent women in the same study group (Mathews et al. 1995) would have preferred to delay sexual activity but, because of cultural pressures to be submissive to men, agreed to sexual intercourse at an early age. The young women did not feel that they could ensure safe sex practices were followed, owing to lack of recognition in the culture of their right to make decisions for themselves. Similar results were obtained by Webb (1997), Harrison, Xaba and Kunene, (2001) and Magnani et al. (2002). All of these authors discuss the need for programmes to address gender inequalities and improve the negotiating skills and self-efficacy (sense of personal control) of girls and boys before children reach puberty.

Male circumcision

There is now consistent evidence that rates of HIV/AIDS are lower in ethnic groups where male circumcision has long been an established cultural practice. Various studies have shown that men who have *not* been circumcised are between two and eight times more likely to become infected with HIV than men who have been circumcised. They are also much more likely to have other sexually transmitted diseases than those who have been circumcised. Having an STD itself increases the risk of HIV infection (Halperin and Bailey 1999; Szabo and Short 2000).

Halperin and Bailey (1999) note that this discrepancy between infection rates is now recognised by some traditional healers who 'increasingly recommend circumcision' (1999:1814). They report that in Western Kenya as many as 60% of uncircumcised men said they would prefer to be circumcised. In a slightly later study, Bailey, Muga, Poulussen and Abicht (2002) assessed the attitudes towards circumcision of adults in a non-circumcising ethnic group, the Luo of Kenya. Both men and women who participated in group discussions indicated their willingness to accept male circumcision as a health-promoting behaviour.

They were concerned only about whether the procedure was painful, whether the men would bleed a lot, and how much it would cost. Some further research into circumcision may yield additional useful information, because in different traditional circumcision ceremonies different amounts of the foreskin are removed. This may have implications for variability in the rate of transmission of a range of STDs (Brown et al. 2001).

Education, social class, and gender

In general, adolescents and young adults who have higher levels of education have more knowledge about HIV/AIDS and its prevention than less educated people. They are therefore in a position to make more informed decisions about abstaining from sexual relations or using condoms when having sexual intercourse. A study of over 2 300 young people between the ages of 10 and 24 years showed for example that school attendance and knowledge of AIDS were associated with lower levels of sexual activity and more consistent use of condoms (Magnani et al. 2002).

Risk levels may also vary according to social class. In a study by Machel (2001) in Maputo, Mozambique, middle-class adolescent girls aged 14 to 20 years in two secondary schools had had fewer sexual partners and used condoms more often than girls from working-class families. Machel reports that the middle-class adolescents appeared more willing and able to challenge gender norms for behaviour and were more assertive than the working-class girls. Working-class girls were also more likely to be economically dependent on male partners. Therefore they were in a weaker position than middle-class girls when trying to negotiate for safe sex practices with their sexual partners. This made them more vulnerable to infection with STDs, including HIV/AIDS. It was not social class itself that provided the protection for middle-class women; instead the protection appeared to come from their greater economic independence and assertive negotiation about safe sex and use of condoms.

Irrespective of differences in education and assertiveness, women in Africa are generally much more vulnerable to HIV infection than men, especially during the early years of sexual activity. Glynn et al. (2001) for example report that between the ages of 15 and 19, young women in Kisumu (Kenya) and Ndola (Zambia) were six times more likely to be infected than men of the same age. This discrepancy in rates of infection decreases over time, so that by age range 25–49 years, men and women were equally likely to be infected, though men had had more sexual partners than women. Some authors (e.g. MacLachlan, Chimombo and Mpenba 1997) suggest that young women, who often form sexual relationships with older men, may be at risk because these older men are already infected. Glynn et al. suggest that the greater prevalence among women of genital herpes, another STD, may increase young women's susceptibility to HIV infection.

Religious beliefs

Thomas and Carver (1990) note that for American young people, having a personal religious commitment provides adolescents with both social controls and social support. Sexual abstinence for unmarried people is valued and there are known consequences for having intercourse, not only in the present life but also in the future. Mixing with a peer group that has the same value provides support for the young person who decides to remain sexually abstinent, even in communities where others of the same age may be sexually active.

A study in South Africa (Nicholas and Durrheim 1995) suggests that religious commitment has similar benefits there. Highly religious young adults in a study of over 1 800 first-year university students were less likely to engage in sexual intercourse and more likely to delay the onset of sexual relationships than students with low religious commitment. However, they were not more likely to engage in safe sex practices. Thus, the contribution of religion to sexual safety appeared to lie in the later onset of sexual activity and lower number of partners.

Health status

As noted earlier, infection with a number of other sexually transmitted diseases is associated with higher rates of HIV/AIDS infection (Halperin and Bailey 1999; Szabo and Short 2000). It is probable that the open sores (lesions) that occur when people have genital herpes or syphilis, or infection sites for gonorrhoea increase the risk that HIV infection will be transmitted between partners during sexual intercourse.

While rates of sexually transmitted diseases, other than HIV, vary considerably between urban and rural areas, and between regions within countries, the overall rate of non-HIV sexually transmitted diseases is fairly high in some parts of Africa. Buvé et al. (2001) found syphilis infection in over 10% of the population in a city in Zambia and rates above 3% in cities in Kenya and Cameroon. In addition, 4% and 9% of women in these same two cities were infected with chlamydia, an STD that causes female sterility. Ahmed et al. (2001), in a study of over 17 000 adults aged 15–59 years in Uganda, found lower rates of syphilis, chlamydia, gonorrhea, and HIV among those who consistently used condoms, but pointed out that inconsistent use of condoms was of no benefit in preventing these diseases. In this study only 4.4% of the sample reported consistent use of condoms, with a further 16.6% reporting inconsistent or irregular use.

Any sexual activity that causes bruising or tearing of the delicate tissues of the reproductive organs can permit HIV to be transmitted from one person to another. Forced sex, where the woman is reluctant and not sexually aroused, insertion of herbs or other objects to dry out the vagina, so that the male partner obtains greater pleasure, and anal intercourse all increase the risk that HIV will be transmitted from the male to his partner. The vulnerability of the foreskin to tearing is another factor that is now known to increase risk of HIV transmission.

Finally, people whose immune systems are weakened because of other chronic diseases (e.g. tuberculosis) or because of chronic low levels of malnutrition may not have enough natural resistance to prevent HIV from spreading through the body. Tuberculosis can be prevented by vaccination but, as Chapter Six showed, rates of vaccination remain low in some parts of Africa. Inadequacies in the diet are more difficult to deal with, but education programmes that promote growing and eating a wider range of foods than have traditionally been eaten may be of some assistance. Eating a wider range of foods can boost the immune system generally, although it cannot prevent HIV infection without other behaviour changes as well.

Conclusion

Research is slowly beginning to reveal the many factors that contribute to the spread of HIV/AIDS. HIV spreads rapidly in Africa because of long-standing cultural beliefs and attitudes about sexuality, patterns of sexual activity, and the general socialisation of boys and girls. As is shown later in the chapter, teachers can contribute to change in these areas of child and adolescent development. But the problem is much more complicated than that. Children need enough food, and a wide enough range of foods to develop healthy immune systems, but often do not receive the foods they need. Parents should have their children immunised against tuberculosis and other common illnesses, but they cannot be forced to do so. All children should get a good education, but not all countries provide this. These factors increase the risk of infection with the HIV virus.

Parents and teachers cannot change international and national political systems, the policies of agencies such as the World Bank or the International Monetary Fund, which limit access to funds that might otherwise be used to improve the general health status and levels of education of young people in each country. They can only offer young people more knowledge about sexuality, HIV and other STDs, and a chance to consider and re-evaluate the impact of culture on their behaviour.

Attitudes towards people with AIDS

Adolescents, like other members of their communities, stigmatise those who have HIV/AIDS. Stigmas arise when people are ignorant and afraid and when illness is defined in moral terms. People who are afraid of the disease blame others for becoming infected, as they try to convince themselves that differences between infected persons and themselves mean that they can remain safe. For example, some people might wrongly conclude that prostitutes get AIDS as a punishment for bad behaviour. Because they themselves are not prostitutes, they convince themselves that they will be safe. According to this way of thinking, the removal of prostitutes from the community will prevent the spread of HIV/AIDS and make it safe for others to continue to act as they have always done.

Suggestions for the removal of HIV positive people from the community can take extreme forms, as Webb (1997) found in his study of adolescent attitudes towards people with AIDS in South Africa. Webb asked adolescents in secondary schools in five different areas of South Africa what should happen to people with AIDS. He included a separate set of questions asking what should happen to relatives who had the disease. Up to 24% suggested people with AIDS should be killed, even when that person was a relative. Many others in each group (32-74%) suggested isolating infected persons from the community. Similar results have been obtained in a number of other studies (e.g. Kaplan and Worm, 1993; Macintyre, Brown and Sosler 2001).

This stigmatisation is worst in communities where less is known about HIV/AIDS and where people have not personally known anyone with the disease. A problem with the stigma attached to AIDS is that it makes it difficult for people to talk about the illness or to admit they might be at risk of catching it. Open discussion about HIV/AIDS in some of the programmes outlined in the next section has been shown to reduce stigma and to help young people recognise that people with AIDS need to be cared for.

Box 12 Hurtful attitudes harm children

'They (the neighbours) all know. They assume that we are also HIV positive. People used to really like my mother. Her brothers would help her – and through an NGO she was able to get free testing. That is how she found out she was HIV positive. She then had us tested because she was worried that we would also be infected. Thank God we are all negative. Our neighbours are not like before – they have distanced themselves. They should be distancing themselves from the virus, not from us.'

Ammanuel, 13, and orphaned by AIDS, Ethiopia

Source: UNICEF (2002:40)

Teachers and HIV/AIDS education

A few recent studies have trialled AIDS education programmes in schools. These have taken a number of different approaches. Some, such as that of MacLachlan et al. (1997), have focused on increasing knowledge about HIV/AIDS, successfully demonstrating that use of a simple board game was motivating and enjoyable for Malawian secondary school students. The students' knowledge increased during the few weeks when the game was played once a week. Most of this knowledge was retained at least one month after they stopped playing the game.

AIDS-specific programmes that require between 20 and 30 hours of teaching time have also been found to promote increased knowledge, changed attitudes towards people with AIDS, and changes in intentions about sexual activity and condom use. Most of these studies fail to include follow-up assessment of whether actual behaviour follows stated intentions, but a study by Ndeki, Leshabari, Hannan and Lyimo (1997) in Tanzania is an important exception. These authors provided material for a 20-hour AIDS education programme to teachers in 18 primary schools. A total of 1 063 pupils were involved in the study, with about half being taught the AIDS course. The average age of the pupils was 13.6 years.

Twelve months after the programme Klepp et al. (1997) obtained further data from the pupils. They found that the pupils who had been in the intervention group and had learnt more about AIDS had retained that knowledge. They were also more likely to have open and frequent discussion about AIDS than people who had not been taught the programme. Most importantly, they found that only 14% of boys who had been in the intervention group had become sexually active in the intervening year in contrast to the 35% of boys who had not received this education. A small number of girls had become sexually active, again fewer in the intervention group than in the comparison group (3% compared with 6%).

Other approaches have required more teacher training and more teaching time. Some have used materials developed by the local ministry of education or by United Nations agencies (Kinsman et al. 1999, UNICEF 2002). A curriculum in Uganda now places AIDS education within a broader life skills curriculum. In this life skills programme primary and secondary students are encouraged to develop skills in open communication, negotiating with others, solving problems together and other activities that promote a sense of self-efficacy and control over events. It is believed that such programmes will be beneficial in helping young adults to remain safe and healthy when they reach sexual maturity (Kinsman et al. 1999). A programme in Malawi also focuses on personal development in a range of areas. Children as young as eight years have two lessons a week throughout the school year using this curriculum material (UNICEF 2002).

Box 13 Young people reject aspects of AIDS education

'I think we young people don't listen to the elders because in most cases they preach water and drink wine, which I think is not fair.'

Youth, Africa

'Most of the campaigns don't involve young people in the design . . . maybe this is why they don't work, because they're just adult ministry of health campaign. They're just not cool!'

Youth, Africa

Source: UNICEF (2002:40)

A limitation of many of these short educational interventions is that they introduce knowledge about HIV/AIDS without fully dealing with the prevailing ignorance about the range of ways intimacy can be expressed without sexual relations or about normal sexual development and the range of normal sexual behaviours. The programmes may omit any discussion of other sexually transmitted diseases, such as chlamydia, syphilis and gonorrhoea, that are very common and that increase the risk of HIV transmission during sexual intercourse. They have also been criticised for failing to address such issues as anal intercourse, homosexual relations and transmission of HIV via hypodermic needles that have previously been used either by an injecting drug user with the infection or in the course of medical treatments. If asked, students may themselves mention concerns about these sources of infection (Sallah et al. 1999).

Halperin and Bailey (1999) note that AIDS education programmes have similarly failed to mention the protective effect of male circumcision. These researchers had a search carried out of over 30 000 health communication materials. Not one pamphlet, poster or flyer mentioned male circumcision in relation to HIV/AIDS. These are difficult issues for teachers, especially because cultural taboos against adolescent sexuality remain so strong. As long as discussing condom use is not allowed in some schools, it is extremely unlikely that discussion of STDs, anal intercourse and male circumcision will be permitted. But remaining free of STDs, using condoms, and practising male circumcision work together to reduce HIV risk. If these things are not all discussed, African adolescents will continue to become HIV positive and to die before they have had a chance of living out their lives.

Personal issues for teachers

Teachers in many education systems around the world are required to provide sex education to their pupils, and some teachers in most countries find this a difficult task (e.g. Hamilton and Gingiss 1993; Neubauer and Meltzer 1989).

African teachers are no different. Like other members of their ethnic group, community or country, teachers have certain knowledge and experiences, attitudes, inhibitions, and taboos in regard to sexual matters. This knowledge is intensely personal, in a way that other knowledge presented in the classroom is not.

Some teachers may find that they are comfortable with only parts of the reproductive health or life skills development curriculum. For example, some teachers, in a study by Kinsman et al. (1999) were willing enough to teach facts about sexuality and AIDS, but were not comfortable teaching about use of condoms as the best way, apart from abstinence, for protecting oneself against this disease. In the same study, some teachers were threatened with dismissal if they taught about condom use, thus their teaching reflected the values of their school principal. Some parents objected to teachers working with mixed groups of girls and boys. Teachers themselves may prefer to arrange for this material to be taught to single-sex groups.

The study in South Africa by Mathews et al. (1995) shows how important it is for curriculum developers to help teachers overcome their uncertainty, embarrassment or anxiety about teaching about sexual matters. In this South African study, the problem related to the religious requirement for premarital sexual abstinence, which teachers knew was at odds with adolescent behaviour. Discussions with religious leaders led to an increased emphasis on values in the programme and removal or reduced emphasis on some aspects that were incompatible with religious teachings. Teachers also changed their approach to teaching about values after reassessing their own values. They realised that they needed to help students think about and develop their own value systems, rather than try to impose their own values on adolescents who were unlikely to adhere to them.

Exploration of teachers' own beliefs, values and attitudes might also take place in informal discussion, more formal in-service programmes, personal discussion with health professionals at the local health centre or clinic or at other venues. In addition, teachers need to ensure they have sufficient factually accurate information about all aspects of sexuality before they begin teaching this curriculum. It is clear, from the research already cited, that pupils are likely to have misconceptions about sexuality that teachers can only correct if they themselves are well informed. If, having spent time trying to improve knowledge and insight into their own values, some teachers are still unable to deal with all the curriculum materials, they should teach those parts of the programme that they can manage, so that children obtain at least some knowledge. These teachers might be able to arrange for others to help out with material they find more threatening or difficult to teach.

Conclusion

African teachers do not need to be told that the AIDS epidemic demands urgent action. Adolescents and young adults become infected and die before their children have grown up. Their illness restricts the opportunities of their children and means that they are unable to contribute to the future economic development of their country. Teachers are in a particularly important position in relation to this disease. By introducing well-constructed material on normal development and sexuality and on sexually transmitted diseases, they can help adolescents develop sexual behaviours that will help them survive. Because so many adolescents become sexually active during their later primary school years and because relatively few pupils go on to secondary school in some countries, this task cannot be left to secondary school teachers. The role of primary school teachers in this aspect of education is crucial.

In your community (seven)

HIV/AIDS is a difficult subject for many people in Africa to talk about because of taboos about sexual matters. Choose one or more of the following activities. They have been selected to help you feel more comfortable about dealing with this topic.

1 Write confidential notes outlining what you know about sexuality and sexual behaviour. Check the accuracy of your understanding by reading a chapter in a book on human development, a basic text for nurses or similar material.

2 Check a medical dictionary, nurses' dictionary or general dictionary to ensure you know the correct name for various parts of the reproductive system. Say these words aloud (if necessary, while you are alone) a few times, to reduce the strangeness of saying them.

3 Spend time with a trusted friend, reviewing both your knowledge and that of your friend about sexuality, names and functions of reproductive organs, changes that occur during adolescence. Check texts if you are uncertain.

4 Write about the impact of HIV/AIDS on yourself, members of your family, your community. Check the accuracy of the facts you have listed. Discuss as much of this material as you feel comfortable talking about with one or two trusted friends, family members or health professionals.

5 Find and review any health education or personal development materials that have been prepared for use by teachers in schools in your country. What are the strengths of the programmes? What are their limitations?

Chapter Nine

Teacher values and beliefs

Introduction

When young people enter teacher training, they have beliefs and expectations about themselves and about the children and adolescents they will teach. These ideas reflect the folk theories about child development, teaching and learning, intelligence and knowledge that are found in the community. The aim of teacher training is to help the beginner teacher to develop a more informed, professional set of ideas and beliefs, so that folk theories are replaced by more developed understandings about the nature of teaching and learning. This chapter describes some commonly held values and beliefs and shows how they contribute to different approaches to teaching and learning.

Teacher motivations, beliefs and personal characteristics

Teachers sometimes believe that they do two important things in the classroom. They keep control of a group of students, and they convey information to them. But their approach to these things is influenced by each teacher's motivations, personality, values and beliefs in ways that are described in more detail in this section.

Intrinsic and extrinsic motivations

Like young people around the world, young adult Africans decide to become teachers from a mix of motivations and values. Extrinsic motivation is common in developing countries such as those in Africa. This means that the factors motivating a person to become a teacher come from outside the person. For example, some young Africans train as teachers because they cannot find other work in a country where unemployment is high, and they think they will always be able to earn a living as a teacher (Olasehinde 1972). Being able to have a lifelong job with a reasonable income may be a consideration. Some young people's parents may suggest that teaching is a good career and that they should train for this job. Others may think of the long holidays that come at planting time or allow them to earn extra money (Bastick 2000).

Pragmatic or practical reasons for becoming a teacher contrast with more idealistic, internal motivations. These are called intrinsic motivations and include such ideas as 'wanting to make a difference' or 'wanting to show young people that science is fascinating' that may also form part of the decision to become a teacher. It is important to understand that the two kinds of reasons for becoming a teacher, pragmatic and idealistic, tell something about the individual's values, but that neither kind of reason is better than the other, nor do most people have only one kind of motivation. A young person may be motivated to become a teacher partly for pragmatic reasons and partly for idealistic ones.

Box 14 The effects of high motivation

Teacher quality springs from individual teachers' motivations and capacities . . . [They] utilise a variety of teaching strategies . . . to control the tempo of learning [and] to meet the needs of individuals and groups. The classroom is a happy place, students are challenged, excited and motivated by the learning opportunities that surround them . . . these teachers work hard within and outside the lesson.

Source: Hopkins and Stern (1996:513)

Teacher beliefs about child development

In some education systems teachers are not well informed about child development. This is particularly likely in systems where young adults who have just completed secondary school can teach without further preparation for their task. These teachers have not had the opportunity to develop a professional level understanding about child development and its importance when planning and presenting school learning tasks. As a result, they continue to hold the kinds of beliefs about child development that are common in their community. They also have no real option but to teach in the way they were taught, since they have not been introduced to any other way of approaching the teaching task.

Other teachers may adhere to strongly valued cultural views of child development in spite of having been exposed to other information. For example, many teachers in sub-Saharan Africa do not believe that boys and girls are equal in value or ability, in spite of having completed courses of study addressing this issue. Harley, Barasa, Bertram, Mattson and Pillay (2000) cite the emphatic reply of a teacher whom they describe as knowledgeable about the rights of teachers and learners. When asked whether he personally believed in gender equality he responded, 'Never ever! As a man, I believe I am and will always be superior to a woman. Our culture is consistent with this view' (2000, p.295).

Male teachers who hold such beliefs describe girls, especially those girls who have reached adolescence, as stupid, lazy, lacking in ambition and competitive spirit and as having 'loose morals' (Davison and Kanyuka 1992; Lloyd et al. 2000). Some women teachers develop a kind of reverse discrimination in response to this traditional male view. In Guinea for example 56% of the women teachers in a study by Colclough et al. (2000) thought girls were more intelligent than boys and 67% said girls participated more than boys in class. Teachers may believe that there is not much point in trying to promote gender equality in schools because of entrenched community attitudes, and may therefore not encourage girls to develop their academic skills.

Some male teachers believe that once girls reach adolescence it is acceptable to think of them as being sexually available and to approach them as potential sexual partners (Jones 2001; Lloyd et al. 2000). In this, they are showing, once again, community attitudes towards adolescent females. Some parents consider that their daughter will be advantaged if she has a sexual relationship with a teacher and reportedly encourage daughters to form such relationships. As a result, sexual relationships between teachers and adolescent girls are not uncommon in some countries, and this can sometimes affect adolescent girls at primary school. A recent report from the Central Africa Republic notes for example that 'even primary school children have contracted the (AIDS) virus from their teachers. In some villages HIV infection is cited as the main reason for girls not finishing their education' (Jones 2001:3). Besides possibly infecting young females with a sexually transmitted disease, male teachers who take advantage of their special relationship with pupils to have sexual intercourse with them irreparably change the pupil-teacher relationship in ways that are detrimental to the young woman's concentration on her studies and future development.

Where negative attitudes towards ethnic groups other than one's own are common, teachers may believe that members of these groups (called out-groups) are less intelligent or less willing to learn than their own people. Tshireletso (1997) for example quotes teachers working with an ethnic minority group in Botswana who made such comments as 'compared with other children Basarwa children are slow to learn' (1997:182). Teachers blamed the parents for these children's educational problems, although their responses revealed their belief that these out-group children had different innate characteristics from other children.

The teacher's personality

Teachers sometimes believe that teaching is solely about the transmission of knowledge, but the knowledge always reaches the children having been filtered through the personality of the teacher. The ways in which teachers present material and manage children who are difficult or do not want to learn reflect aspects of personality. In times of change, as when a ministry of education decides that a new curriculum should be taught, teachers will also respond differently to the challenge, at least partly according to their personality. Thus, teachers who are often rather anxious will be likely to become more anxious, believing that they cannot manage the new curriculum. Like those with lower self-esteem, they may feel they should not have been asked to cope with new demands. Teachers who are more emotional in their reactions may respond with anger. If they usually express anger by resisting others' demands, they may make only minimal changes when introducing required new curriculum or teaching methods. Teachers who are less volatile emotionally may have a more moderate response to proposed changes in curriculum or school life.

Personal values

Each individual's values also influence the way that person teaches, so it is worth spending some time learning what psychology tells us about values and their relationship to behaviour. Recently Shalom Schwartz and various colleagues carried out many studies of psychological values. Schwartz (1994) defined values as goals that serve as guiding principles in a person's life. As goals, values serve the interests of the person or social group, motivate action and function as standards for judging and evaluating behaviour. Schwartz believes that values are acquired through interactions with groups of others and as a result of individual experiences. Some of the examples of values that he uses are 'Accepting my portion in life', 'Being honest', 'Being successful'.

Schwartz (1994) gathered data on values from 97 samples in 44 countries, including two in Africa – Zimbabwe and South Africa – and he presents evidence that many human values are universal. When gathering data, Schwartz presents a list of 30 nouns (e.g. creativity, authority) and 26 adjectives (e.g. curious, humble) and asks respondents to indicate the importance of each word as a guiding principle for them. Schzartz lists 10 different kinds of values that group together in various ways to form four bigger, more general clusters. The names given to the different values, and the kinds of values measured, are shown in table 14.

Table 14 Summary of universal values

Self-transcendence	Self-enhancement	Openness to change	Conservation
Universalism Protecting the environment A world of beauty Unity with nature Broad-minded Social justice Wisdom Equality A world at peace Inner harmony **Benevolence** Helpful Honest Forgiving Loyal True friendship A spiritual life Mature love Meaning in life	**Power** Social power Authority Wealth Preserving my public image Social recognition **Achievement** Successful Capable Ambitious Influential Intelligent Self-respect	**Self-direction** Creativity Curious Freedom Choosing own goals Independent **Stimulation** Daring A varied life An exciting life **Hedonism** Pleasure Enjoying life	**Tradition** Devout Humble Moderate Respect for tradition Detachment **Conformity** Politeness Honouring parents and elders Obedient Self-discipline **Security** Clean National security Social order Family security Reciprocation of favours Healthy Sense of belonging

Source: Adapted from Schwartz (1994:24, 31)

There are no right or wrong answers to questions about these values. Some people, because of their personality, their parents' values and the way they were brought up, will seek excitement and interest. Others will want to become powerful figures in the community, while still others will be concerned with being helpful and loyal in their relationships. As a trainee teacher you might like to think about these values. Which values do you hold? Do you think of yourself as valuing tradition, being conforming, being open to change?

Values are related to behaviours, although they do not allow us to predict behaviours precisely. For example, teacher trainees who accept their parents' decision about a career may be more conservative and hold more traditional values than others who freely made the decision to become a teacher. More conforming trainee teachers are likely to expect children to be obedient and also to respect tradition (because the values of conformity and tradition are closely associated). When these trainees become teachers, they are likely to think that young people should respect authority, because that has been a traditional value in the culture. These teachers will require pupils to show respectful behaviour towards them and towards other staff. In contrast, a teacher whose scores on the value scale show high levels of self-direction is less likely to have accepted his or her parents' advice about becoming a teacher, and once he or she has finished training may be more likely to take risks, approaching teaching in original and creative ways.

Teachers need to be aware of the ways in which their values may influence their lesson plans, their teaching and the ways they respond when children are difficult to teach. A teacher who values freedom and creativity might try to make all lessons very interesting and original, and not give sufficient emphasis to the children's need for social order. Or a teacher who is ambitious and wants to achieve the power that comes with holding a position of authority in the school may forget that children need to be aware of the beauty of the world, including the world of learning.

Culture level values

On a more general level, teachers' beliefs and preferred patterns of interaction reflect the culture in which they have been socialised. Hofstede (1986), whose work on cultural differences was discussed in Chapter Two, has written about the relationship between culture and the preferences of teachers as they work in their classrooms. As usual, he contrasts collectivist and individualist cultures, those with strong and weak uncertainty avoidance, and those with high and low power distance. Cultures that he describes as masculine, where male roles are tightly defined, are also contrasted with cultures referred to as feminine. Each of the contrasts is outlined below. Readers will recall the brief description of African cultures presented in Chapter Two that suggests that most are collective and masculine. There are probably differences between different ethnic groups in the degree to which people typically prefer to avoid uncertainty or have high power distance.

Collectivist versus individualist cultures

Hofstede (1986) states that in collectivist cultures teachers (and the children in their classes) value tradition. They expect children to speak only when called to do so by the teacher unless they are working in a small group. Teachers find it acceptable that children split into long-term work and social groups based on ethnicity. They are also willing to show a preference for some pupils in their class if someone in authority has recommended those pupils, or because of the pupils' ethnicity. Pupils are expected to learn how to do things.

All of these cultural values are the opposite of values that are common in individualistic cultures. In individualistic cultures teachers and pupils generally value what is new, children are expected to speak up in response to a general question, and will willingly speak out in the large group. Sub-groups vary for different activities, and teachers are expected to be impartial, not favouring one student over any other. Teachers expect pupils to learn how to learn, and design teaching materials and activities to encourage the development of problem-solving skills.

Power distance

Cultures where powerful people have much higher status than less powerful people are referred to as having high power distance in Hofstede's (1980) description of culture level values. In high power distance cultures the personal wisdom of the teacher is valued. Teachers are considered to merit the respect of their pupils, irrespective of their personal qualities, and older teachers are more respected than younger ones. Teachers and pupils expect that any communication will be initiated by the teacher, who will provide a teacher-centred education with the emphasis on order and on students knowing which path they must follow. Pupil achievement is believed to reflect the quality of the teacher, but even poor teachers are not criticised or contradicted.

In contrast, teachers in low power distance cultures have to earn respect through competence, and pupils may contradict or criticise poor teaching, whether from young or older teachers. Teachers and pupils generally believe that knowledge can be gained from anyone who is competent. Pupils are expected to develop their own competence by speaking up in class without being asked and by showing initiative in their own learning. Teachers and pupils have a much more equal relationship in low power distance cultures than in the high power distance ones that are more common in developing countries.

Uncertainty avoidance

Generally people in high uncertainty avoidance cultures try to avoid being unsure. Teachers are expected to have all the answers, to use academic language and to provide structured learning situations, with precise objectives. In these cultures teachers are more likely to reward pupils for accuracy in problem solving than for effort in finding ways of solving problems. If pupils publicly disagree with the teacher over some intellectual activity, the teacher may think the pupil is being disloyal. Teachers and parents typically believe the teacher is an expert. Parents do not think that they can provide any information about their child that will be useful for the teacher.

Again, teachers who are more comfortable with uncertainty generally behave in ways that contrast with those in high uncertainty avoidance cultures. Like teachers, the pupils in these cultures are generally comfortable with less structured learning situations, with saying 'I don't know', and with disagreement over intellectual questions. Teachers use plain language and reward students for finding novel solutions to problems.

Masculine and feminine cultures

In cultures in which the male role is tightly and clearly defined, teachers and pupils generally believe that it is acceptable for the teacher to praise good students openly, and to use their results as the norm against which they judge the performance of other pupils. Open competition between pupils is accepted, corporal punishment is also acceptable, and brilliance in teachers is admired. Boys avoid doing tasks or taking subjects that they see as belonging to girls.

In cultures where men have more choices, the so-called feminine cultures, teachers generally avoid openly praising the best, and they accept the average as the basis for assessing pupils. They encourage pupils to form more supportive relationships with their peers rather than competing with them. Teachers prefer to act in friendly ways towards pupils, and pupils can choose any task or subject to study, irrespective of whether they are boys or girls.

An African value

Makulu (1971) thought that Africans had a utilitarian view of education. He claimed that Africans generally had developed this view of education during colonial times. They saw that the educated white administrators did not have to do routine or physically demanding work and realised that education gave them their wealth and power. Naturally, Africans wanted wealth and power too and perceived that education would be useful in achieving this goal. People who believe that education has utilitarian value only are unlikely to value learning for its own sake. Where this idea about education is widespread, teachers also probably value education for its utility. Teachers who hold this view of education are unlikely to try to teach pupils that acquiring knowledge can be fascinating and amazing, to provide fun and recreation, or to expand their students' view of themselves in relation to others in their community or the wider world.

Teacher beliefs about their responsibilities as professionals

Teachers who have not had a lot of training often find it difficult to see themselves as having knowledge and skills that go beyond those of the general community. They believe they are responsible for transmission of culture, and do not realise that if cultural practices are harmful to child development and academic achievement they, the professionals, have a responsibility to take the actions that will be most beneficial for children. For example, teachers often believe that parents will protest when teachers change the way they teach, and this belief probably has some basis in reality. Parents around the world are routinely suspicious about new approaches to education, fearing that their children will be disadvantaged if new methods of teaching are less effective than known older methods.

Suspicion about new methods is probably greater in those African cultures where the links between past, present and future are valued and emphasised. In these cultures, looking to the past is seen as a way of coping with the problems of the present. Thus, parents who have been taught using teacher-centred methods probably believe that these methods from the past are the methods that should be used to solve the problems of the present and prepare their children for the future.

A narrow definition of the responsibilities of teachers means that teachers may not realise that they need to reflect on how their teaching influences learning outcomes. They prefer to explain the limited educational achievement of many of their pupils by referring to external problems. They state that limited physical resources (e.g. poor quality buildings, limited supplies of text books) are the cause of low achievement (Jessop and Penny 1998). If asked to explain why they personally use approaches that do not promote the greatest amount of learning, they might make comments such as:

- There aren't enough books.
- There isn't enough equipment.
- This way I can easily control the whole class.
- The class is too big for me to teach in any other way.

Teachers who do not want to change their approach to their tasks will comment as follows:

- If I let the children talk about the material, they will just waste time gossiping.
- If I let the children learn by discussion and activity, I will not get through the curriculum in time.

- If the children start to talk, it will be noisy and the principal or head of department will criticise me.
- If the parents hear that I am doing things differently, they will complain.

Some of these beliefs are probably correct. For example, one of the authors was told by a student, an experienced teacher, that she had been criticised by the principal of her school because, when children in her class were discussing some material, there was more noise than if she had been standing at the front telling the children things. This teacher was concerned that such critical comments might be recorded and adversely affect her career. Likewise, there will always be parents who will complain. But a narrow definition of professional responsibility limits teachers' ability to do their job really well.

Teachers' beliefs about knowledge and the ways children learn

Elliott (1989) points out that all teachers have implicit understanding of what education is and ideas about how children learn. These ideas can be clarified and expanded if teachers take time to reflect on their various beliefs about learning and knowledge and if they are willing to draw on ideas from more formal study in education, psychology and sociology in order to develop professionally. This section discusses different ways of thinking about knowledge and their implications for teaching.

Assumptions about children as learners

Bruner (1996) has described what he calls the 'folk pedagogy' of teachers. This folk pedagogy consists of the assumptions about children as learners and about knowledge that teachers bring to their task. The various assumptions and their implications for teaching method are summarised in table 15.

Table 15 Teacher beliefs about children and knowledge

Teacher belief	Assumptions about children	Assumptions about knowledge	Method used when teaching
Children learn by being told things	Children do not know the material being taught Children can learn by being told Children's minds are blank or empty and need to be filled up	Knowledge consists of rules and facts Knowledge exists somewhere - in books, maps, in the mind of the teacher Knowledge is evident when the children can apply facts or rules to solve problems. Knowledge can be measured by objective tests	Presentation of facts, principles, and rules to be learned
Children learn by imitation	Children do not know the material being taught Children want to know material being taught Children are ready to try to do what is being taught Children can learn by being shown how to do whatever is being taught	A knowledgeable person is one who has talents, skills and abilities to do things, rather than being a person who shows understanding Knowledge consists of learned habits.Children show they have learnt something by doing it Knowledge does not have to be supportedby theory, argument or negotiation	Teacher uses modelling and demonstration
Children learn by thinking about the world in which they live	Children are seen as attempting to understand the world, so can comprehend their experiences in it Through teaching children will come to have more informed, less one-sided views Children come to learning situation with history of learning and thinking Children are capablOe of thinking about their own thinking	Knowledge is the understanding of truths Truths are the product of evidence, argument and construction, these truths must be able to be justified on the basis of evidence and argument. They cannot be accepted solely on the basis of others' authority e.g. teachers or books.	Discussion of ideas, interaction with others in collaborations, expression of the views of children and teacher

Teacher belief	Assumptions about children	Assumptions about knowledge	Method used when teaching
Children bring useful past knowledge to the learning situation	Children have learnt much that is valued in their culture Children are capable of distinguishing between personal knowledge and more general cultural knowledge	Culture determines knowledge Culture can be broadened to include knowledge from elsewhere	Recognition and discussion of personal and broader knowledge

Source: Adapted from Bruner (1996)

The first two folk theories, which state that children learn by being told things and by imitation, have a long history. They have been used in countries around the world until recently. Traditional teaching in Africa used both these methods. Before the arrival of Europeans, children in African villages were expected to learn various tasks by observing others in the course of daily life. There was little direct instruction. However, at specified ritual times children might withdraw from the general community to be instructed in the ways of behaving during the next phase of life. At that time a more formal approach to teaching was used and children were expected to learn from being told certain facts and traditional stories. This commonly occurred around the age of puberty as young people were introduced to the responsibilities of adulthood. In some communities it also occurred at later stages in adulthood. When a person was being taught some specific skill, such as iron working, leather working, or pottery making, direct instruction was accompanied by learning by imitation (Mazrui 1986; Rodney 1982; Tabulawa 1997).

More recently, research into child development has shown that children start school with a long history of learning that teachers can draw on to promote the development of new knowledge and skills. Children are able to think about the way they think, and this meta-cognitive skill can be used in the classroom. Asking children to explain their thinking is particularly useful when teachers are trying to find out why a child is having difficulties with some task. So, although modern teachers might still occasionally find it useful to teach by telling or let children learn by imitation as happened in the past, a truly modern teacher who is basing his or her teaching on current knowledge about learning will use more interactive methods. These methods enable the pupils to make sense of their own world.

African teachers' assumptions about learning

An old saying stating that 'Teachers teach as they were taught' appears to be true of teachers in Africa, as elsewhere. Research in many countries in sub-Saharan

Africa has shown that teachers say they are using methods of teaching to which they were introduced as trainees. But when they are observed in the classroom, they are most likely to be using methods that come from the past. Observations of African teachers in various studies show that they generally spend a lot of time lecturing to children from a position at the front of the class. They generally expect one-word answers that are chorused by the whole class. Overall, teachers spend relatively little time monitoring pupils' written work (Chapman, Snyder and Burchfield 1993; Fuller and Snyder 1991).

The beliefs that underpin these teachers' behaviour in their classrooms probably come from traditional cultural ideas, both indigenous and imported, about the nature of teaching and learning. Some work by Fuller and Snyder (1991) and Tabulawa (1997) in Botswana is of interest here. Articles published by these authors suggest that in pre-colonial Tswana society children were perceived as empty vessels that had to be filled with information. They gained this information from people older than themselves, especially at ritual times when elders in the tribe provided direct instruction. Tabulawa also states that from the early days of colonial education in Africa the missionaries taught by telling and by demanding lots of rote learning. They used these methods because people everywhere thought that was the best way to teach in the nineteenth and early twentieth centuries.

Tabulawa (1997) argues that because the methods used by the missionaries and nineteenth-century educators were consistent with traditional beliefs among the Tswana, the methods of teaching used by the colonists were acceptable to Tswana pupils and teachers. The methods have been retained for the same reason. Teachers resist using the more varied and modern approaches to which they are introduced during teacher training and in-service programmes because they are inconsistent with traditional ideas. Tabulawa's explanation may apply widely across the African continent, since the traditional form of education in many African societies before contact with Europeans was also based on the idea of the expert elder conveying knowledge to an inexpert younger person. Comments by teachers in studies in other countries confirm that teachers may still hold this view. For example, Jessop and Penny (1998), who compared teaching in rural South Africa and Gambia, report teachers as saying that good teachers 'install [sic] knowledge to pupils' heads' or 'fill people with knowledge' (1998, p.397).

Teachers who believe that knowledge consists of having many facts probably encourage pupils to learn at a rather superficial level. This kind of superficial learning has been called surface learning and is contrasted by another approach that has been called deep learning (Biggs and Telfer 1987). Students who are using surface learning approaches do not think much about the meaning of the material they are studying. Instead they rely on teachers to define the learning task and then they use rote-learning methods. They are extrinsically motivated, valuing courses for the qualifications they offer. In contrast, students using a deep learning approach are interested in the meaning of the material they are studying. They try to relate new material to other knowledge they have, reaching conclusions based on evidence. These students are intrinsically motivated, that is, they study because they are interested in learning (Watkins and Regmi 1996).

Conclusion

For historical reasons and because of personal and cultural values teachers in sub-Saharan Africa are likely to believe that children's minds are empty and need to be filled up. Many probably also believe that knowledge consists of facts and rules. They encourage children to use surface learning approaches when studying. A problem arises when these teachers also believe that having enough facts in one's head enables pupils 'to confront all the problems which are around us' (Jessop and Penny 1998: 397). But problems are often solved by using facts in new combinations so that new ideas eventually emerge. Children will learn to solve problems by practising problem solving. Teachers need to adopt more flexible approaches to learning to ensure that children develop this skill.

Teacher beliefs about intelligence

Northern hemisphere investigators have struggled to find a satisfactory definition of intelligence, and debate about the components of intelligence continues (Elliott et al. 1996). Problems also arise when intelligence is thought to be 'what intelligence tests measure' because children's performance on an intelligence test can be influenced by variables such as self-esteem, tiredness, ill health, or lack of motivation. Most northern hemisphere authors (e.g. Borich and Tombari 1995; McInerney and McInerney 1998; Mouly 1982) define intelligence by referring to an ability to grasp relationships, skills in abstract reasoning, ability to learn, ability to solve problems, effectiveness in dealing with the environment, and an ability to manipulate symbols. Thus, intelligence is seen as a generalised adaptive ability that is used when individuals face the problems of daily life.

Cross-cultural researchers have known for a long time that folk theories about the nature of intelligence vary among ethnic groups (Kagitcibasi 1992). A number of early studies in sub-Saharan Africa showed that in this region folk theories about intelligence focused more on what Kagitcibasi has called the 'socio-affective' aspects of intelligence. This refers to the child's skills in dealing with the social and emotional aspects of village life. Berry (1984), in his review of a number of these studies, reported that social skills such as the ability to co-operate, conform, obey, and behave in a responsible manner were emphasised in definitions of intelligence offered by a number of different African ethnic groups. Some additional skills may also be included in certain groups as shown by Dasen (1984). This author reported that the Baoulé of Côte d'Ivoire thought that besides having the capacity to learn quickly, intelligent people showed good observation skills, memory and manual dexterity.

Socio-affective skills are not measured in common tests of intelligence, even those tests developed in Africa for use when assessing intellectual abilities. For example, Serpell (1974, as cited in Super 1983) asked adults in Zambia to rate the intellectual abilities of village children aged about 10 years. He used the local term for intelligence in this research. As in the African studies reviewed by Berry (1984), the adults thought the most intelligent children were the ones who were most responsible and had good social skills. The 42 children were then assessed using intelligence tests developed for use in Zambia. There was little relationship between the scores children obtained on the test and the ratings of intelligence given by the adults in their village.

Adults in various parts of Africa discriminate between home and school intelligence (Dasen 1988; Super 1983). A child who is 'intelligent at school' gets good marks for schoolwork, although he or she may not show the level of responsible behaviour that is referred to as being 'intelligent at home'. Dasen points out that the abilities that make one successful in school are perceived as being 'useless unless they are applied for the good and wellbeing of the social group' (1988:427). Once again this demonstrates the importance of the group above that of the individual.

A shift in the definition of intelligence appears to occur as people become more educated. Thus, Wober (1972), in a study in Uganda, stated that children who had been at school for several years thought that speed of processing was a component of ability. Unschooled adults in their community did not say this. Teachers, as well-educated people, are perhaps likely also to think that rapid processing of information is important, although they may still also believe that social behaviours are important indicators of a different aspect of intelligence.

Conclusion

More research is needed in Africa before it will be possible to reach any conclusions about the relationship between being socially responsible and having the kinds of problem-solving skills that have been described in northern hemisphere studies of intelligence. But it seems likely that children who develop the traditionally valued social skills earlier than others will generally also be the children who do well at school. Similarly many less responsible, less socially skilled children will probably have less developed reasoning skills than others of the same age, and will learn more slowly in school. However, because social skills development is especially likely to reflect the way parents have raised their children, the relationship between abstract reasoning and social skills is not likely to be very strong. Teachers, like other adults in their community, probably value the development of social skills and may emphasise these, not realising that helping children develop problem-solving and abstract reasoning skills is also an important part of their role. Both social skills and problem-solving skills can be developed in the classroom if teachers organise lessons in ways that permit children to practise these two kinds of skills.

Educational goals

Curriculum planners who are usually based in a centralised ministry of education are often the people who decide what children should learn in African schools. These people describe what material is to be covered in any given year. They often provide guidelines as to how the material should be taught. But much more learning goes on in schools than is included in the curriculum. So teachers need to be clear about all the sorts of learning that take place and have goals for teaching children other things besides those laid down in the curriculum.

As an important influence on child development, teachers also need to think about how children should interact with one another, with adults, and with the broader world. In other words, teachers need to have thought seriously about what characteristics a person requires in order to be seen as competent in his or her society. When thinking about this question, teachers need to take into account that African nations are still in the process of nation building and that this process is now occurring in the twenty-first century. If African nations are to interact with other nations without disadvantage, their people may need to have certain skills and characteristics that teachers have not necessarily considered before now.

Box 15 Aims of education: The UN Convention on the Rights of the Child

The aims of education must include the development of the child's personality and ability, preparation for a responsible life, respect for cultural identity and values, and respect for the natural environment.

Source: Save the Children (1990). Appendix

Teachers have been referred to as 'nation-builders' since the time of independence (Makulu 1971, Machel 1971, as cited in Gerdes 1997). Then, African educationists believed that teachers would help young people gain the skills and attitudes that were necessary if the many interest groups in the new nation were to be able to work together for the greater good of all. However, the goal of nation-building is too general to be helpful in terms of planning for the day-by-day, week-by-week, work of the school. On the other hand, a teacher without a goal is like a person who can drive a car, but does not have a map or any idea of where he or she wants to go. The driver might have all the skills he or she needs, but without a goal he or she can go round in circles and waste a lot of time and petrol.

Teachers without long-term educational goals can only take a narrow pragmatic view of their work. Some of the things that they might think are:

- If I present this material today, I will be closer to completing the curriculum before the end of the year.
- By the end of today I will be one day closer to the holidays (to retirement, to getting this month's pay).
- If I teach in this way, I will get a good assessment.
- Being rather harsh with the pupils teaches them to respect authority.
- When I have taught this material the children will be able to pass the test.

Their thoughts have little to do with helping the children in their class develop intellectually or socially, and more to do with getting through the time until something good happens for the teacher.

Teachers need to be aware of what they want for the long-term future of their pupils. They should be able to explain to others what personal characteristics, skills and knowledge they want the pupils to have by the end of the year or by the time they leave school. If they can state these goals, they can take a more long-term view of their work. They can ask themselves whether the way they are teaching helps children develop the characteristics, skills, and attitudes they think are needed for the future. Having goals provides them with a map, so they know where they are going.

The emphasis teachers place on the various goals reflects some of their personal and cultural values. For example, some years ago, one of the authors was working with teachers in Hong Kong and asked them to list the characteristics they thought children should have developed by the time they left primary school. The Chinese teachers emphasised moral characteristics (e.g. respect for older people, a sense of shame). These are highly valued characteristics in Chinese culture. While similar characteristics are also valued in northern hemisphere countries, it is unlikely that teachers from these countries would place these characteristics first. They would be much more likely to mention skills in literacy and numeracy as the top priority.

Problems arise when teachers say they have a set of educational goals, but do not teach in ways that allow pupils to acquire the skills they need to meet those goals. For example, teachers might say that they want children to become flexible thinkers and then teach in a way that requires lots of rote learning. Sometimes research into teaching describes this by saying that the rhetoric is that teachers want children to develop one way, but the practice does not support these statements. Reality is unconnected to rhetoric (Jessop and Penny 1998). Research tells us that children learn the 'hidden curriculum' (Alton-Lee, Nuttall and Patrick 1993; Wing 1997). If, despite the rhetoric favouring the development of problem-solving skills, the teacher's behaviour suggests that his or her real or hidden goals are for children to be able to produce lots of unrelated facts, children will learn to produce such facts. If science teachers emphasise correct English language, rather than the scientific approach, as some studies have shown (e.g. Cleghorn et al. 1989) then children will learn English language terms used in science. If teachers expect one-word correct answers children will learn to provide these, whether or not they realise that each correct answer has some relationship to other correct answers. In contrast, a teacher who genuinely wants children to learn how to solve problems with understanding should teach in such a way that children learn to solve problems. The teacher also needs to develop a range of types of questioning that will allow him or her to discover whether the child understands the requirements of the task.

At present teachers in sub-Saharan Africa are spending quite a lot of pre-service and in-service time learning the rhetoric of modern methods, but because this rhetoric is inconsistent with folk theories about the nature of knowledge and about the best ways of teaching, nothing changes in the classroom. In a recent study for example one teacher said that the reason she was being taught about curriculum was so that she would 'know what people are talking about when they use words like curriculum'. Because of her studies she expected to be able to 'explain what a curriculum is' (Modiba 1997:734). Clearly this teacher had no expectation that having better knowledge about the curriculum might help her to prepare a sequence of lessons that would help her achieve certain educational goals.

Changing beliefs, changing behaviours

In the general community most people believe that changing some aspect of thinking or behaviour is not really possible once a person is an adult. However, cognitive behaviourist theorists and therapists have repeatedly shown that behaviour can change as a result of changed beliefs. Equally importantly, they have shown that changes in behaviour may lead to changes in beliefs (e.g. Williams 1992: Scott, Williams and Beck 1989).

Trainees and other teachers need to discover and challenge some of their personal and culturally accepted ideas about what knowledge is, about how pupils' learn best, about the indicators of intelligence, and about how they should interact with parents. This is probably best done during training with friends, in small groups or teaching teams or, for teachers who are already qualified, during school-based in-service training. Very experienced teachers who have found a comfortable way of teaching and very inexperienced teachers, especially those who have had little or no post-secondary school training, may find this particularly demanding. Some teachers, like the one who told Modiba (1997) that the educational textbooks said she should not impose values, but her community expected her to, may also find that this exercise is not an easy one.

As professionals, however, teachers need to learn ways of thinking and acting that reveal their more complex and advanced understanding of child development, learning, individual and group behaviour than is common among adults in their community. Like lawyers, accountants or experts in the field of computing, teachers can be expected to have knowledge in their field that is more modern, broader, and deeper than is generally available. As professionals, they need to act in ways that show they have this knowledge.

In the many African cultures that acknowledge the importance of links between past, present and future, the idea that traditional teaching practice can change also poses problems. Thus, it may be necessary for trainee teachers and those with experience to consider some of these broader cultural values in their search for professionalism. Teachers may need to ask themselves questions such as the following:

- How central is this belief in my culture?
- Does holding this belief influence what I do in the classroom?
- Does holding on to old beliefs restrict the extent to which I can help pupils prepare for adult life in the twenty-first century?
- Can I hold on to old values and beliefs and just change my behaviour?
- How can I change the way I behave when teaching to reflect my knowledge of child development and learning without giving up my culture?
- Should I talk to parents about modern ideas so they can understand what I am trying to do and why it is different from the past?

Personal values are unlikely to change rapidly. Teachers who value tradition may always continue to do so, but they can reduce the extent to which they emphasise some traditional behaviours and observe what happens. This involves taking some risks, but it is also a professional response to some personal characteristics that might limit the development of the pupils. Similarly, values that prevail in the culture change only very slowly, but it is possible for teachers to modify the way they demonstrate their adherence to culture level values. For example, in collective cultures both teachers and pupils generally believe that the teacher is the expert and should control learning (Hofstede 1986). This does not mean that the teacher must always be in front of the class. A teacher can control learning by carefully selecting groups to work together, by giving them clearly defined tasks to do, by asking them to report back at the end of the lesson, or by monitoring the progress of individuals and the group as a whole. Teachers who have a clearer idea about the way their beliefs have influenced and limited their behaviour in the classroom might be more willing to use teaching aids, texts, and exercise books in a varied way.

Community values also change slowly. Parents in ethnic groups where there is high power distance or high uncertainty avoidance may not feel they can interact well with teachers who are figures of authority and expertise in the community. Naturally, parents with little or no education are also anxious and aware of their ignorance when they meet up with teachers. They may avoid meetings with teachers because of this. In addition, parents whose lives consist of a daily struggle for survival may not have the time or energy to become very involved with school projects. Teachers may need to reflect on ways of overcoming these problems. Parents who know what teachers are doing, and the reasons that teachers believe that they should change the way they teach are less likely to resist the proposed changes. This then makes it easier for teachers to feel comfortable about trying new methods.

Conclusion

Teachers learn what education is and what it ought to be during their own childhoods. They acquire certain beliefs about knowledge, how it is acquired, and who can best acquire it as a result of their enculturation into school life. They also learn these things from conversations and observations in their family and community. But like other professionals, teachers have the opportunity to incorporate more complex understandings about these things during their training.

As professionals, teachers need to change their behaviours to reflect this more advanced understanding about children and the ways they learn. This task is not easy. People everywhere take commonly held beliefs for granted. To become really effective in their classrooms, teachers need to reflect on these widely accepted beliefs and work towards an integration of modern knowledge and traditional beliefs. Truly professional teachers will lead their communities towards better understandings. They can do this only if they are aware of, and have thought seriously about, the impact of their beliefs on their behaviour in the classroom.

In your community (eight)

Exploring your own educational goals

Read the list of characteristics that teachers in your community might hope children will have by the time they leave school. If there is something else that you think is important, write it at the end. Next, rank the characteristics from 1 to 21 in order of their importance to you.

.... Can read complex documents with understanding
.... Knows and uses practical procedures that promote health
.... Obeys persons in authority
.... Perseveres when faced with a difficult task
.... Has a sense of humour
.... Reads the newspaper or listens to radio or TV news regularly
.... Is polite
.... Treats all people as equals
.... Accepts others who are different
.... Is able to evaluate important social and political issues
.... Can present logical argument in support of his or her beliefs and values
.... Able to work well with others
.... Takes responsibility for own actions
.... Seeks information from a variety of sources (e.g. books, parents, other community members)
.... Helps others in community if they are in need
.... Understands and uses scientific knowledge (e.g. uses scientific facts when trying to improve productivity)
.... Lives by well-developed moral code
.... Can solve disagreements with others without resorting to violence
.... Can communicate clearly in writing.
.... Shares material wealth with extended family
Other: ....

When you have decided what you think is important, look at your selection again. Do the items with high rankings measure academic skills only, or are some social skills included? Do you rank skills in assessing social and moral problems highly or is it important that pupils should have learnt to do as they are told?

Talk to two or three friends who are also teachers or trainee teachers. Do they have the same goals for their pupils as you do? Try to persuade them that your goals for children will be more likely to enhance their happiness and success than theirs will. Will the skills you emphasise help in nation-building? Will they help people from your nation to interact as equals with those from other nations?

Talk to your parents, other adults, or students who are not training to become teachers. Do these people have the same ideas about educational goals as you do? If not, ask them to explain why they have different goals.

Chapter Ten

Teachers and groups of children

Introduction

African nations, like other modern nations, are made up of people from different ethnic backgrounds. The number of ethnic groups may be extremely large. Nsamenang (1992a) for example cites research showing that there are more than 200 ethnic groups in Nigeria and over 239 in Cameroon, a country with a very much smaller population than Nigeria. In some nations this tribal and ethnic group makeup is recognised and valued at the socio-political level; in others it may be rejected, denied, or ignored.

The preceding chapters have pointed out that broadly based values in the culture and individual beliefs, attitudes and behaviours influence the ways in which each person perceives and interacts with the world. A strong commitment to one's own beliefs and culture is a source of psychological wellbeing. However, devaluing others' cultures can be detrimental both to the development of the nation as a whole and to individuals within that nation. Devaluing some people may mean that the devalued people end up with limited human rights and access to justice. The restriction may be based on ethnicity, gender, socio-economic status or religion (Banaji and Greenwald 1994). Some members of minority groups in countries around the world are adversely affected for all of these reasons.

Teachers in African countries need to be aware of the ways in which they may help all children develop a strong positive identity, as members of both their ethnic group and the broader national group. To achieve this goal, teachers need to understand the importance of identity, and how they might have developed prejudices against certain groups. They also need to know what they can do to reduce or eliminate their own tendency towards discriminatory behaviours. This is important at a time that members of different ethnic groups are moving away from tribal lands and traditional lifestyles into bigger towns and cities where they are required to mix with people from other tribes and countries of origin, both in school and in the broader community. The present chapter discusses these issues.

Identity and the in-group

Each individual has a personal, private identity and a social identity. The private identity forms as a result of individuation. Each person develops a sense of himself or herself as separate from others in his or her social world (Reykowski 1994; Yamaguchi 1994). This contrasts with social identity, which is based on a sense of oneself as a member of a social group. In the latter instance the similarity between oneself and others is valued (Tajfel 1978). Social identity is, therefore, the sense of oneself as having a recognised place in the family, school and community. This sense of belonging develops during childhood, as children come to recognise that they share physical, social, cognitive, and other characteristics with members of their family and the broader community. Children's delight when told 'You look just like your Dad' or 'Your Mum used to laugh and jump about when she was a little girl, just like you do' shows how much they like being reminded of their place in the family, their primary social group. Unacceptable behaviours, too, can help in identity formation. A parent who says, 'No-one in this family behaves in that way' excludes certain possibilities, and again contributes to identity formation.

The social identity is so strong among Africans that they have been described as 'conceiving of the self as coming into being as a consequence of the group's being' (Nobles 1995:177). According to Nobles, an African's self-identity is always a people-oriented identity. He also calls this an 'extended identity' or 'extended self'. Among Africans, the separation of the private self from the group is much less strong and less important in daily life than this social identity. Thus, an important part of the identity of African children is their sense that they are valued members of the larger extended family, clan, and tribe. Learning about and participating in community events and activities contributes to the growing child's extended identity.

People want to spend time with others with whom they identify, those whose ideas and behaviour resemble their own. This is their in-group. Other people, with different histories, values and behaviours, form the out-group. In African countries, members of other tribes and ethnic groups may be labelled the out-group. In collectivist cultures the in-group is often rather fixed and stable (Hofstede 1980; Triandis 1995b; Smith and Bond 1993). Thus, in Africa a member of any one tribe may spend all his or her time with other members of the tribe, regardless of what activity is going on. In rural villages and communities where members of only one tribe live close together, a person may have little choice about whom to spend time with. However, in larger towns and cities where there are more mixed groups of people from other tribes, some people still chose to spend their time with others from their own ethnic group.

Besides the sense of belonging to an ethnic group, people belong to other groups, and these also contribute to their identity. In collective cultures these subgroups are formed within the stable larger in-group. Thus for example a woman who is interacting with other women feels a sense of in-group membership based on shared gender. Teachers working together form a group of educationists and value their social identity as professionals in that in-group. Membership of some in-groups may include more than one aspect of identity, for example when a Chewa woman who is also a Christian interacts with others of her gender, ethnic, and religious groups. But membership of some in-groups excludes memberships of others. In a religious context, for example, it is impossible to be a member of both the Christian and Moslem in-groups, although Moslems and Christians may be members of the same in-group when participating in non-religious activities. Finally, the aspects of social identity that influence action depend on which in-group the individual identifies with at that moment.

As is common in collectivist cultures, African people have wide-ranging obligations to members of their stable in-group. They have been described as being bound by mutual obligation. Obligations may continue over long periods, even generations. Among traditional Dowayo people in Cameroon for example a man's unsettled debts are remembered over many years and may even be inherited (Barley 1986). This is also true in traditional communities in other ethnic groups (Onwuejeogwu 1975).

Besides the general obligations that exist in collectivist cultures, other obligations may arise out of specific traditional relationships. Thus, in matrilineal societies, those in which the husband moves to the wife's place of residence on marriage, the woman's brothers have traditionally had a lot of responsibility for helping her to raise her children. Uncles in particular have had an important relationship with nephews. Similarly, in some societies in Uganda, the highest-ranking man in the community (the kabaka) had traditional obligations to his sister. He was required to act in ways that enhanced her status and wealth (Boulding 1992). In traditional societies where statehood had been established, the way in which one tribe viewed another was partly determined by the wealth of the chief. Members of the tribe had a social as well as an enforceable obligation to contribute to chiefly wealth. These long-standing obligations towards the wellbeing of others in the in-group continue to influence the behaviours of African peoples today.

Interactions between in-groups and out-groups

In collectivist cultures there is generally a marked difference between the way people perceive and treat members of their in-groups and the way they respond to out-groups (Triandis 1995a). Members of a collectivist in-group perceive members of their own group as nurturant and respectful of others, and they automatically obey their authority figures. They distrust and are unwilling to cooperate with members of out-groups whom they see as wanting to manipulate them. They will also do anything to maintain the integrity and survival of their own in-group, to the extent that they will fight and die for its survival. This can cause difficulties for out-groups in collectivist multiethnic nations where in-groups remain narrowly defined. This is the true of much of Africa.

Expanding the concept of the in-group to include all who live in one's country requires a cognitive shift on the part of citizens that may still be evolving in many parts of Africa, as Marshall Segall and some colleagues discovered not long after independence. The study was later cited by Berry et al. (1992). It reportedly showed that in 1976 Banyakore men in Uganda said, 'I'm a Banyakore', when asked 'What are you?' However, when they were asked 'How *should* the Banyankore think of themselves?', they were more likely to say they should think of themselves as Ugandans. The authors reportedly concluded that these men had not yet come to see themselves as Ugandans, despite recognising that they should think of themselves in this way. This identity confusion may still be contributing to civil wars across Africa today.

In the many African countries where one group holds power, other groups are typically treated as out-groups. The powerful in-group devalues the experiences, values and beliefs of out-groups, holding prejudicial beliefs about them, acting in oppressive ways and discriminating against them. As powerful figures in the classroom, teachers may help perpetuate these patterns when they are unaware of their own preferences toward their in-group. They may behave in discriminatory ways towards children and colleagues who are out-group members. But teachers can promote individual development of the children in their class and the development of the idea of the nation as an in-group when they act in non-discriminatory ways. To do this they need to understand what stereotypes, prejudices, and discrimination are and how they influence behaviour. They also need to know about psychological outcomes of discriminatory practices and what they can do to minimise the damage to children that comes when teachers act in discriminatory ways.

Stereotypes and prejudices

Stereotypes and prejudices are so similar that the two terms are often used almost interchangeably in psychological literature. However, some authors do define these terms in ways that show where they are different. For example, Simons, Kalichman and Santrock (1994) define a prejudice as 'an unjustified negative attitude toward an individual based on the individual's membership in a group'. These same authors define a stereotype as 'a generalization about a group's characteristics, which does not take into account any variation from one individual to the next' (1994:213). Both prejudices and stereotypes are beliefs about a group of others that are 'overgeneralized, inaccurate, and resistant to new information' (Myers 1990:332; Ponterotto 1991). They are based on limited information.

Although stereotypes and prejudices may be positive or negative, negative stereotypes and prejudices are more commonly investigated. Thus, Africans may be described as 'lazy' and Chinese as 'hard-working' by people who know little about them, and are unwilling to learn about how much variation there is within each broad group. People who have formed a stereotype about the different groups resist the idea that some Chinese might be lazy, as some Africans and some Europeans are, while others from all groups are hard working and energetic.

Various kinds of prejudice have been defined. For example, an individual may have a prejudice against members of certain ethnic groups, against those with different religions from his or her own, against very young or very old people. All of these prejudices arise from fearfulness and a sense that those against whom one is prejudiced might threaten some aspect of one's life. Stephan, Diaz-Loving and Duran (2000) have pointed out that fear and threat appear to be the basis of much negative ethnic prejudice. They describe four kinds of threats that can contribute to the development of ethnic group prejudice. It is important to note that these 'threats' are perceived threats only; they influence behaviour because the perceiver *thinks* something bad will happen, not because it is necessarily going to happen. Threats of this kind, described by Stephan et al., have been summarised and are shown in table 16.

Table 16 Characteristics of perceived threat in situations involving prejudice

Type of threat	Characteristics of threat
Realistic	Perceived threat to the economic wellbeing, political and economic power of the in-group
Symbolic	Perceived threat to the in-group's worldview. Differences in values, goals, patterns of relationships of the out-group are seen as a threat to the survival of in-group values and goals
Threat to emotions	Embarrassment, anxiety and discomfort during interaction with out-group members. Leads to dislike of out-group as a whole
Threat of harm	Fear of out-group because of stereotypes that they will harm in-group (e.g. all members of out-group perceived as aggressive)

Source: Adapted from Stephan et al. (2000:241)

These perceived threats can occur quite commonly in the social and political life of modern nations. For example, when the leader of a politically powerful in-group seems likely to lose political power, members of that ethnic group may feel threatened by the potential loss of status of their group in general. In the same situation they may believe that their values and way of life are at risk if members of another ethnic group come to hold power. More generally, intergroup anxiety is increased when people live in close proximity to members of other ethnic groups and are obliged to interact with them. This often occurs when rural people from different ethnic groups move to towns and cities. Members of each ethnic group may fear interactions with members of other ethnic groups because they have notions that members of those groups are dishonest, aggressive, will use witchcraft to harm them, or will try and force them to change their religious practices.

Similarly, when in-group and out-group are defined because of gender, there is typically a difference in power and status between the two genders. Men may feel that their economic power is threatened when women gain financial independence through employment outside the home, or they may think that their status in the community is diminished when women ask them to contribute more to household chores. Some women may find interacting with men in senior positions in the workplace embarrassing. However, because they feel anxious about this, they may form a prejudice against these men as a group. Prejudices against other groups are formed in the same way.

Discrimination

Having prejudices appears to be a normal human characteristic. As such, a prejudice is probably of only limited importance, even when it is negative. However, once a negative prejudice influences behaviour, as commonly occurs, it is referred to as discrimination, and discriminatory acts are harmful. In countries around the world people translate their preference for their own group and their negative generalisations about members of out-groups into overt acts that are detrimental to members of the out-group. At the broadest level discriminatory behaviours limit the access of out-groups to the nation's resources. The United Nations Human Development Report 2000 (UNDP 2000) shows for example that minority groups in some countries are likely to have to travel further than others to use a variety of public services, such as the post office, hospital, school, or district centre.

Various forms of discrimination have been named. Discrimination against people who belong to an ethnic group that is different from one's own is called racism. The term *sexism* is used where people are discriminated against on the basis of their gender, and the terms *religious intolerance* or *religious prejudice* are used when people discriminate on the basis of religious beliefs. Discrimination based on social class is likely to become more prevalent as modern African societies become more clearly stratified into social classes with competing interests.

Racism

Ridley (1989) defines racism as 'any behavior or pattern of behavior that systematically tends to deny access to opportunities or privilege to one social group while perpetuating privilege to members of another group' (1989:60). Ridley emphasises that racism is not the sole responsibility of any single ethnic group, but that anyone can act in racist ways. This author points out that the question of whether an act is racist or not can be judged only by the consequences of the behaviour. It is no use for members of the privileged group to say that they did not mean to harm members of the other group, they may still have acted in a racist way. Finally, Ridley points out that racism is perpetuated by power. If one social group has no power over the other, then racism loses its force. In this context, however, power includes the ability to make others feel unimportant, sad or angry, as well as control over resources such as clean water, telephones, or quality education that are denied to the out-group when others in the nation are able to obtain these things.

Box 16 Minority group rights: The UN Convention on the Rights of the Child

Children from minority or indigenous communities have the right to enjoy their own culture, religion and language.

Source: Save the Children (1990). Appendix

In Africa, racism often takes the form of tribalism, a preference for one's own tribe that is accompanied by negative evaluations of the characteristics and behaviour of members of other tribes and acts that are harmful to them. However, other expressions of racism also occur. Thus, when Idi Amin, as president of Uganda, expelled the people of Indian descent from the country, he was acting in a racist way, but not showing the tribal form of racism. Similarly, when (as witnessed by one of the authors) young men of Indian descent used derogatory language when talking to much older African men who were senior members of their social club in Malawi, they were also acting in a racist manner, but not one that could be described as being based on a preference for a particular local clan or tribe. White racist behaviour towards Africans often occurs and is widely recognised, but black racism towards white members of the community also occurs and is less widely recognised as a behavioural expression of prejudice.

These various expressions of racist prejudices arise out of the history of interactions between ethnic groups on the continent. Where there was a tradition of oppression, with members of one ethnic group defeating another in war and holding power over them by conquest, racism is obviously of long standing. Most African countries can provide examples of this source of racism from somewhere in their history. The racist attitudes held by some black Africans towards whites, and the attitudes of some whites towards black Africans have arisen out of the fears generated by the interactions between these groups in the last 150 to 300 years. Racism may also develop where it did not exist in the past. It may develop in times of economic hardship when one group is perceived as having economic advantage over others, or when people who would never have met in the past begin to live in close proximity in towns in modern Africa.

Sexism

Sexism is the gender-related expression of prejudice. Again, people who behave in a sexist manner are damaging others in psychological ways that are reported later in the chapter. Both men and women can act in sexist ways, but because men usually have more power than women, they are more likely than women to be able to use that power consciously or otherwise to control others and reduce the quality of women's lives. This social power is the outcome of traditional cultural beliefs and practices in many parts of Africa and more recent events. Traditional practices across the continent have resulted in the separation of male and female roles with some, but by no means all, societies allocating the major decision-making roles primarily to men. For example, in Islamic communities the father traditionally decided whom his daughter should marry (Dirie 1998). The powerful position of men in regard to life-influencing events was accepted by women whose roles, though often still esteemed, had only a more private power within the family.

The modern relationship between men and women also developed partly in response to the impact of colonialism. During that period men's roles changed as a result of decreased dependence on their capacities as hunters and warriors. This has required some psychological adjustments for African men, who traditionally showed their care and concern for the group, for wives and children, and for security of property through these activities. At the same time the impact of decisions by colonial administrators in Africa reduced the independence and, therefore, the public power of women in some ethnic groups. In East Africa traditional patterns of land tenure gave women control over the land they farmed, to the extent that they were able to decide who should inherit. During the colonial period the European pattern of male ownership of land was imposed (Okeyo 1980). Similarly, in West Africa, markets that were traditionally managed by a woman appointed by the women who had stalls came under the control of men appointed by the white male administrators during colonial times (Boulding 1992).

Events such as these sometimes resulted in permanent shifts in cultural beliefs and practices, especially when the changes were written into the law at the time of the change. Only the African men and women whose lives were directly altered by these imposed patterns of behaviour knew that things had been different in the past, although folk stories and songs might still refer to old ways of doing things. For subsequent generations the belief that 'this is the way we do things in our culture' becomes established and is difficult to change. Those who have gained power are reluctant to give it up, and others became permanently disadvantaged. As a result of these shifts in culture some people lose their identity. They may struggle to retain self-esteem and to find an acceptable new identity. Some will attempt to retain previous power through new means or through excessive use of behaviours such as wife-beating that had been culturally acceptable, but only within certain limits, in the past.

Discrimination on the basis of religion

Because religion is closely aligned to ethnicity in many African countries, it is sometimes difficult to know which kind of prejudice underpins the actions of members of various religious groups when they act in discriminatory ways against members of other faiths. In particular, this is an issue where poorly educated believers from one faith and ethnic group physically attack others in their community who belong to a different ethnic group and have different religious beliefs. Thus, if members of one ethnic group who are also Christians attack members of a different ethnic group who are Moslems, they may have done this because they feared the threat to their values that the Moslems represented, or they may have done it because they held stereotypical views about the other group that had little to do with religion (e.g. that all group members are thieves).

Moslems may, of course, be as likely to have instigated the violence. A third possibility is that ethnic and religious prejudices combined to motivate the first group to attack the second.

Prejudices about members of different faiths, and the discriminatory acts that flow from prejudice, are important in Africa because religious beliefs are a major social force on the continent. Individuals who hold prejudicial views emphasise the differences between faiths, rather than acknowledging the similarities. In fact, there are many similarities among the three faiths, Islam, Christianity and traditional animism. Each faith provides a sense of the continuity of life, from the past to the future. Each also provides security in times of stress through the teaching that events in this world have meaning in relation to past behaviour and possible future behaviours. All emphasise believers' obligations to others and to one or more higher powers. They describe the characteristics of a moral person and encourage believers to lead a moral life. They also offer the reward of continuation of life after death. The better-educated Moslem clerics and Christian ministers of religion understand that only the core message matters, but others in their religious communities may continue to hold prejudices against out-group faiths and to express these in discriminatory actions against others.

Some other characteristics of the two imported faiths also confuse the picture. Both came to Africa with ideas drawn from the cultures in which they developed. These ideas may have little to do with core religious values. These accretions (or additions) continue to influence African life. Islam arrived early and brought the social isolation of women, who were required to wear veils and live hidden from men as much as possible (Ruthven 1994). Once Islam became established, some pre-Islamic beliefs and practices also became associated with the faith. For example, the practice of female genital mutilation, which pre-dates the rise of Islam, is now strongly associated with Islamic beliefs. Some people justify damaging women in this way by referring to the Koran, even although it is not mentioned there (Dirie 1998). Later, the nineteenth-century Christian missionaries brought racist beliefs that they were superior to indigenous peoples. These beliefs almost certainly had the same damaging psychological effects that racism has today. Socially, missionaries brought sexual taboos that had not previously existed, they required local people to dress according to nineteenth-century Christian definitions of decency, and they rejected the widespread practice of polygyny.

Conclusion

Interactions between individuals and between different groups can be affected adversely by ignorance and prejudice, especially once the prejudice becomes translated into discriminatory acts. Each of the various forms of discrimination is harmful to social justice and harmony. Each is also harmful in other ways that are outlined in the following section.

Social and psychological outcomes of various forms of discrimination

While the various forms of discrimination may have a powerful effect on the physical lives of those who are discriminated against, this section of the chapter will focus on the psychological impact of discriminatory behaviours. It is important to realise that the impact of the discrimination is much the same, irrespective of whether the discriminatory behaviour reflects racist or sexist beliefs or other forms of intolerance. Thus, the discrimination practised by oppressive, powerful tribally based political leaders, the more personal racism expressed by one person towards another, the sexist behaviours of powerful men against women, and the intolerance of members of one ethnic group towards another work in the same way to prevent the wellbeing of all people. Both the people performing the discriminatory acts and those being discriminated against are harmed.

The perpetrators of discrimination

Little is known about the psychological characteristics of discriminators in sub-Saharan Africa. Clearly, the tendency to act in ways that are harmful to members of out-groups is learned in Africa, as elsewhere. However, studies from the individualist cultures of the northern hemisphere are unhelpful when considering issues of discrimination in the collective cultures of Africa. This is because of general differences between the individualist cultures of the north and collectivist cultures of Africa in social identity, in the strength of the in-group, and in the dislike of out-groups.

In many nations the freedom to act in discriminatory ways reflects the political culture. Leaders in the multiethnic northern hemisphere nations moved towards a culture of pluralism in the last part of the twentieth century. They want all people, including immigrants from many countries, to believe that their culture is valued. Hence, they have written laws that acknowledge the rights of all people to be safe from discriminatory acts on the part of others. In the recently formed nations of Africa, the political shift towards pluralism is still evolving. Consequently, the expression of racist views is still acceptable. Persons who behave in discriminatory ways are less likely to be seen as maladjusted, and more likely to have their behaviours accepted as normal expressions of their culture.

There is a range of general evidence, however, to suggest that acting in discriminatory ways limits the full development of the perpetrators and of the communities in which they practise their discriminatory behaviours. Paulo Friere (1972), who worked in the developing countries of South America, argued that people who discriminate against others are dehumanised by their actions. He described the restricted view of what it means to be human that is held by people who maintain their power or status at the expense of others. He states that, to maintain their wealth and power, such people give up any capacity to love others in the broad general way that promotes the social wellbeing of all. They see out-group members as likely to restrict their capacity to acquire more wealth, power and status and, because they do not love them, are able to justify acting in ways that harm others. They give up the freedom to develop intellectually and socially because they have to spend all their time and energy protecting their position of power. They lose the capacity to empathise with others, which is necessary, in the long term, for the survival of communities and nations.

Using examples from politics, Friere stated that in the struggle against oppression (which in Africa in the twentieth century was initially the struggle against the colonists), 'the oppressed, instead of striving for liberation, tend themselves to become oppressors'. Like other writers (e.g. Berry et al. 1992; Rogoff 1990) Friere believed that the ways in which people think are the result of the situation in which they find themselves. Men (and, although he does not mention them, this includes women) who have grown up under an oppressive regime learn that 'to be a "man" is to be an oppressor. This is their model of humanity . . . For them, the new man is themselves become oppressors' (Friere 1972, p.22–23).

Oppressive and arbitrary kinds of leadership have existed everywhere throughout time. In Africa, the willingness of some chiefs to become wealthy by selling their people to slave traders in the nineteenth century instead of keeping them safe provided a model that leadership meant the acquisition of wealth (Fage and Tordoff 2002). Some of the powerful administrators of the colonial past also modelled an oppressive kind of leadership (e.g. in what was then the Belgian Congo). The colonial administrators who selected individuals to be chiefs in the previously leaderless 'stateless' societies, or set a member of one ethnic group over other ethnic groups (Barley 1986) were modelling a pattern of arbitrary decisions about who should lead.

In today's world, oppression may be the result of corruption. Mazrui (1986) states that initial corruption may occur because of 'cultural confusion'. He points out that the widespread traditional obligation for individuals who have some advantage to help other members of their ethnic group to a better life can easily become problematic when one member of the group holds public office or wealth, and others in the group seek help in meeting their needs for jobs, money, education and so on. Village traditions based on notions of reciprocity no longer hold in the modern economy – it is unlikely that the recipient of a 'gift' will ever be in a position to assist the already more powerful donor. In addition, the 'gift' in modern economies often does not genuinely belong to the giver (e.g. giving a position in the public sector to a relative, in spite of his or her unsuitability in terms of the necessary skill or knowledge deprives the community of the skills of a more qualified person).

Mazrui (1986) also discusses problems with misappropriation of funds, another form of corruption in the public sphere. He points out that during the colonial era and, more particularly, during the struggle for independence, an African who was able to misappropriate government funds or property was often admired. He or she was seen as contributing to the struggle against the oppressors. This view of public wealth may continue to influence ideas about public morality and about who should help whom today.

Alan Boesak, who portrayed the behaviours of Christians during the apartheid era in South Africa, described a failure of morality in the kinds of harmful actions taken by leaders in the Christian churches in that country. This failure contributed to the extremes of discrimination that occurred in South Africa. Boesak pointed out that Christians had 'justified slavery, violence and war [and] sanctified racism'. He described how leaders in African churches had encouraged discrimination against women, keeping them servile 'whilst [hiding] our fear of them behind claims of "masculinity" and sanctimonious talk about Adam and Eve' (Boesak 1984, p.38). Finally he pointed out that powerful Christians had also often become rich through exploiting the poor. Boesak acknowledges that these practices are harmful to all Christians, since their faith requires them to value all people, and includes a specific demand to help the poor.

People who are discriminated against

People who are discriminated against are typically referred to as 'victims' of discrimination in social psychology texts. The use of this term has been rejected in some other spheres of psychology (e.g. in studies of people who have been sexually abused) because it implies a helplessness and lack of ability to cope, to change either one's own response to the event or to do something to change the situation. But many people whose lives have been harmed by the discriminatory activities of others have the courage and strength to try to effect change in their society. These people do not feel helpless and defeated. For this reason the term 'victim/survivor' will be used in this text.

People who are discriminated against may respond in any of a variety of ways. Their response includes both emotional and cognitive components, and may be active or passive. Crocker and Major (1994) have suggested that the kind of psychological response to being discriminated against depends on whether victim/survivors believe that they can control the characteristic identified as undesirable by the person who is discriminating against them. Ethnic group and gender cannot be changed, and religious beliefs are only changed rarely, so these characteristics fall into the uncontrollable category. Crocker and Major have shown that victim/survivors' reactions to discrimination based on uncontrollable characteristics include anger, dissatisfaction and protest.

Self-esteem, defined as the extent to which individuals believe themselves to be capable, significant, successful and worthy (Coopersmith 1967) may or may not be altered because of being discriminated against. This depends on whether victim/survivors accept the negative stereotype of themselves. Self-esteem may not be altered if the victim/survivor blames the other person for being unreasonable, insensitive or unfair. However, if they accept the negative stereotype, self-esteem will be lowered. This latter outcome may be more likely when the general cultural belief and practice confirm the stereotype, rather than when it is held by only some individuals. For example, in African communities there is a widespread belief that women are less intellectually able than men. Research has shown that in some societies both men and women believe this (Davison 1993; Modiba 1997; Stephens 2000). In these societies a woman who is discriminated against may believe that the discrimination is justified and this will contribute to lowered self-esteem.

Behaviourally, a number of different kinds of responses to discrimination also occur. Some people respond passively, doing nothing to improve their situation. They may show the stress symptoms of anger, anxiety or depression that reflect low self-esteem and a sense that they are helpless to change the situation. Others are more active, choosing either individual or group action such as political protest or other activity that has a goal of improving society. To some extent, the action taken depends on whether the victim/survivor believes that the discrimination is 'institutionalised' discrimination. Institutionalised discrimination may be discrimination that is written into the laws of the country, or it may just be discrimination which is routinely shown by members of powerful agencies such as those allocating public housing or school funds.

Lalonde and Cameron (1994) point out that where there is institutionalised discrimination, the victims/survivors are more likely to take group action. Importantly, they are more likely to take extreme action such as resorting to violent acts against society. Such violence may be aimed at the perpetrators of discrimination, but individuals who are very damaged by discrimination may act in self-destructive ways, using drugs, becoming sexually promiscuous, or using violence in their personal relationships. This has sometimes been referred to as horizontal violence. Unable to express their anger and distress towards people who control their lives in hurtful ways, they lash out at those around them who are also suffering. Consequently, there may be high rates of violence, including assault and murder, within communities that are routinely discriminated against.

Teachers and discrimination

Like other members of any community, African teachers are at risk of acting in discriminatory ways. They have been exposed to cultural beliefs and practices that emphasise obligations to a select in-group and hostility towards out-groups, including those who are members of different ethnic groups in their own country. In many countries they have observed leaders, including politicians, law enforcement agents, bureaucrats and possibly even other teachers, modelling a lack of concern for individuals from out-groups. They have witnessed the political corruption and the failure to acknowledge that political power requires the powerful person to treat all members of the nation as an in-group. They have seen powerful people offer favours to their kin at the expense of others.

As a result of having witnessed corrupt behaviours on the part of some or all role models in the community, some teachers will come to believe that such behaviours are acceptable and will also start behaving in similar ways. Thus, for example, in Mauritius in the 1980s many teachers demanded that parents pay for so-called private tuition that they provided after school hours to pupils in their class. Children whose parents could not or would not pay these fees were doubly disadvantaged, because the teachers paid little attention to them during the school day. Similarly, there have been more recent reports of corrupt practice on the part of teachers in Uganda and Angola (Carlsson 2000; Jeter 2001). In Uganda many parents who were asked why they did not send their children to government primary schools indicated that they could not afford school fees. But officially there were no school fees for primary schooling in the region where the survey was done. Teachers were demanding the fees illegally.

Teachers may justify behaving in discriminatory ways to themselves. A wide range of explanations can be used to justify their harmful behaviour, but these are all examples of prejudiced and stereotypical thinking. They may think or say the kinds of things that are listed in table 17.

Table 17 Examples of prejudicial and stereotypical thinking

Basis for comment	Example of comment
Tribalism/racism	Those people from . . . tribe are all rubbish anyway. They deserve anything that happens to them I can't think why those people don't behave the same as we do, the correct way. They must all be completely dumb
Sexism	Everyone knows that girls (women) are stupid Girls (women) over the age of about 14 should be at home with kids
Religious prejudice	If we aren't careful those Moslems (Christians) will insist we live the way they do If we don't get in first, those Christians (Moslems) will destroy our mosque (church). It's really important to get rid of them, one way or another

Teachers may justify demands for extra money by saying to themselves, 'Teachers are well educated and should be paid more than others in the community. The education department pay isn't enough to show it recognises this. So, it is all right to obtain extra "pay" from the community.' Or they may think, 'If the leaders in the community take extra money, it must be all right to do so.' Another problem is that teachers often learned these prejudicial beliefs and behaviours while they were quite small children themselves. By observing the behaviours of adults in the community and listening to their comments, they learned culturally accepted ways of thinking about members of out-groups and ways that they should behave towards them. They have not questioned these beliefs because they 'seem' right.

Teachers will begin to give up being perpetrators of racism, sexism, and other forms of discrimination only when they recognise that the ways they think about and behave towards members of out-groups are limiting the progress of the very students that they have been employed to assist towards maximum development. A difficulty is that, like members of other collectivist cultures, many teachers value the way things were done in the past. For them, the thought of doing something in a way that has not been traditional is associated with the belief that their culture is being damaged or changed in ways that are undesirable. In addition, many people across Africa have seen African values and beliefs destroyed, denigrated, and damaged as a consequence of interactions with peoples from the North. Some now believe that it is important to hold on to what remains and state that 'We've always treated other people this way' when in-group culture seems to be under threat.

Re-assessing some beliefs

Teachers who do want to stop acting in harmful ways need to reassess their thinking and change it if they discover that they are making faulty overgeneralisations that influence their behaviour. They need to consider the extent to which they think about 'us' and 'them' as opposed to thinking about 'me as a teacher' in relation to 'this pupil'. Generalisations about groups of pupils are more likely to include elements of stereotyping and prejudice. Even when thinking about their own in-group, whether it be their ethnic group, gender, or religious group, people tend to think in a prejudicial manner. In this instance the prejudice is often a positive one (e.g. New Zealanders don't tell lies, Australians are egalitarian). Depending on who makes the statement, there is often an implied negative prejudice against some other group (e.g. New Zealanders don't tell lies, but Australians tell many; Australians are egalitarian, but the British treat people differently according to how wealthy they are).

Teachers who want to discover some of their prejudices might listen carefully to what members of their in-group say about out-groups. Teachers frequently make negative comments about out-groups of various kinds in the staffroom. Alternatively, a teacher might ask others in the in-group what they think are the characteristics of some out-group. If some comments are made frequently, and these comments are negative and refer to the characteristics of a large group, they probably reflect prejudices to which the teacher has been repeatedly exposed and which they may have acquired.

Looking for evidence of discriminatory behaviours

Because thinking and behaving are closely connected, teachers who are re-evaluating their thinking also need to consider their behaviours. To find out if their prejudicial attitudes are influencing the way they interact with children in their class, they need to ask themselves a number of questions. Because it is easy to overlook one's own behaviour, asking a trusted colleague to comment on it might also be helpful. Questions to ask are:

- Do I speak more impatiently (rudely) to some children in my class, according to the ethnicity (gender, religion) of the child I am talking to?
- Do I make negative (rude, hurtful) general comments about the tribe of certain children?
- Do I more often choose children from my own clan (tribe, religious group) to do the fun things?
- Do I mostly (regularly, routinely) give boring chores to children who are not from my clan (tribe, religious group)?
- Do I help children from my in-group more than others?

- Do I punish children who are not from my in-group more than others for the same misdemeanour?
- Do I avoid some children because of the group to which they belong?
- Do I award higher marks for assignments to children from my in-group?

More senior teachers and educational administrators need to ask additional questions, including, for example:

- Do more children from one ethnic (or clan or religious) group drop out of school before completing? Why is this? What can I do about this problem?
- Are more children from one ethnic group, clan or religion required to repeat a year's work? Why is this? What can I do about this problem?
- Do more girls than boys (or more boys than girls) fail to complete schooling? Why? What can I do about this?
- Do some or all teachers in my school show a preference for children from one group over others? What can I do about this?

Senior teachers and educational administrators also need to think about the questions listed for teachers in the classroom. But in this instance they need to consider whether they treat certain members of their staff in some of these ways. Teachers or school administrators who answer 'yes' to these sorts of questions are discriminating against some in the school community.

Teachers who want to change the way they interact with out-groups

To overcome the tendency to think in prejudicial ways and to act in a discriminatory fashion teachers need to do some or all of the following:

- **Look for alternative explanations for behaviours of out-group children:** A teacher who thinks 'All people from . . . tribe are stupid' needs to consider the evidence more carefully. Children who behave 'stupidly' in school may be unable to concentrate because they are constantly hungry. They may be tired because of an excessive out of school workload, or in poor health because their family cannot afford medical treatment. Or such children may be behaving in ways that indicate competence in their own tribe, but which the teacher does not recognise because of his or her ignorance about behaviour in cultures other than his or her own. This sort of problem is recognised in research by Tshireletso (1997). This author found that Basarwa children's high level of autonomy led to them to make independent decisions about school attendance. Their teachers, from other ethnic groups, thought that the children's independence showed that Basarwa parents were incompetent. If a behaviour is culturally competent, children will show that they are not stupid in other situations, outside the classroom. Finally, teachers need to look at children in the class who are from the preferred group. Inevitably, when they do this, they will find that some children in the preferred in-group also show evidence of stupidity.

- **Try to find out what purpose out-group behaviours serve:** Children's behaviour is not random. Like adults, they act purposefully. If teachers can see out-group children's behaviour as functional, they will be able to respond to it in more appropriate ways. Simons, Kalichman and Santrock (1994) suggest trying to look at things as if one was a member of the different group. For example, teachers who are trying to understand some children's behaviours might ask themselves 'If I was an X, what experiences might I have had? How would I feel if I was a member of X group? How would I think and behave if I had grown up in their world?'
- **Spend time getting to know adult members of the out-group:** Teachers need to get to know members of the out-group personally. Taking this approach will be successful only if the interaction is voluntary and the individuals are interacting in mixed groups as equals, making complementary contributions to an activity (Duckitt 2001). Thus, trying to get to know parents of pupils when still in the teaching role is unlikely to result in reduced prejudice on either side because of differences in status. However, when the teacher plays social sport in a mixed team, or joins a mixed group who are working together on a community project, there is a better chance for the kind of interaction that helps members to get to know people from out-groups as individuals. In this way, teachers can learn that out-group members of the community, like others, are all different, and have both positive and negative aspects to their personalities and social skills.
- **Take responsibility as a professional for changing own behaviour:** Teachers who hold prejudices can begin to challenge their own ideas in discussion with others, reading, interactions with members of out-groups and in other ways. As professionals, they need to recognise that the behaviours they show because of their prejudices are limiting the development and happiness of the children in their care. The idea of the teacher as being 'in loco parentis', which is basic to the view that teachers in the north have of their role, is relevant here. The term means that teachers are in the place of parents, and should treat the children in their care in the way that a really concerned and caring parent would do. Competent parents do not discriminate between their children; competent teachers should not do so either.
- **Recognise that change takes time:** It is difficult to change patterns of thought and behaviour that have been practised over many years, and a change in behaviour will occur only if the teacher is motivated to behave in a professional manner. Mistakes and slips will occur as with any other learning. However, these will become less frequent over time as new habits of thinking and behaving replace old ones.

Thinking about sexism and equality

Because research cited elsewhere in this book has repeatedly demonstrated that the educational development of girls in Africa is limited as a result of cultural beliefs that girls are not equal to boys, it is important to address this issue specifically. Male and female teachers differ in their views about equality. Women teachers want equality for girls and women because they can generally see the advantages in terms of freedom to develop intellectually and socially, to have the right not to be beaten, to negotiate with partners and husbands about use of family finances and so on. Thus, women who aspire to equality see that it brings positive gains for them. This contrasts with a common male view. Some male teachers probably hold onto their belief that girls and women are inferior to boys and men because they can see equality only in terms of loss of own power and prestige.

A new way of thinking about equality could be to list advantages for men that arise when males and females are equal. For example, when gender equality exists:

- Men as well as women have more choice. They do not have to keep to pre-determined roles according to their gender. A husband can help his tired wife with the weeding. She can help him break in the land when a new garden is needed. Both can work to get seeds planted before the storm breaks. Both get time to rest when chores are done together. The woman is less likely to get sick if she is not overwhelmed with work.
- Men can gain genuine respect through their kind and helpful actions. They know that this respect is real, not just the token respect accorded to them because they are more powerful than women.
- A man's daughters can grow up with high self-esteem if they are treated as equal to their brothers.
- A daughter can reach her highest potential if she has high self-esteem. Like her brother, she is then in a better economic position. Like her brother, she can help her parents financially when they are old.
- A son can learn that it is all right to express his feelings instead of having to lock them away because it is 'unmanly' to acknowledge that there are times when he is afraid or sad.
- Male teachers can gain the satisfaction of knowing they have behaved in a truly professional way by ensuring that all pupils, not just boys, have been encouraged to develop all their skills to the highest level they can manage. (Similarly, female teachers can gain the satisfaction of knowing they have helped boys as much as girls.)
- Men do not have to take total responsibility for all the difficult decisions. For example, a man might be offered a job that means he will have to work

away from home. The family might be better off economically, but worse off in other social and emotional ways if he works away from home. Such a man might reach one conclusion when he thinks only about the job and its implications for him, and another conclusion if he and his wife can freely discuss the effect of his absence on the family.

Male teachers who do not believe in gender equality can still change their behaviour in the classroom and, acting as social scientists, can observe what happens when girls are treated *as if* they had the same abilities, rights, and responsibilities as boys. Some early work in the United States, in which teachers were told that certain children in their class could be expected to make rapid intellectual growth while others would not, produced the predicted outcome. The children who were expected to make significant cognitive gains did so, and those whom teachers did not expect to learn much lagged behind (Rosenthal and Jacobson 1968). Later studies showed that this result came about because teachers treated the so-called slower learners in ways that reduced their chances of learning. Among other differences in treatment, they were less likely to ask children of whom they had low expectancies to answer questions; they waited for a shorter period before asking someone else; they accepted lower standards from these pupils; and they were more likely to criticise them, (Good and Brophy 1997). African teachers who think girls are less intelligent or less interested probably do the same. On the other hand, girls who are treated as intelligent responsible people with equal rights to learn, to feel safe and cared for will almost certainly show good levels of academic achievement.

It is important to realise, however, that both men and women often behave in ways that show they do not believe everyone is equal. Women who claim equality cannot then argue that girls are more intelligent than boys, and they cannot go on teaching only their daughters to cook, care for children, or take up occupations that are less valued in the community than the positions they recommend for their sons or for male pupils in their classes.

Conclusion

One of the difficulties facing African teachers is that identifying with one's own tribe is a source of psychological strength and wellbeing, but at the same time may become a block to the personal development of others and to national development. When they make decisions based on obligations to a narrowly defined in-group, such as their own tribe, politicians and leaders are failing in their duty to develop the nation for all. As leaders in the community, teachers are also in a position where decisions favouring members of their own group may limit the full development of some children and adolescents. Through prejudicial beliefs, racist, and sexist practices teachers may unfairly penalise and harm some students.

It is possible for teachers to give up prejudicial beliefs and discriminatory behaviours if they have a deep commitment to the wellbeing and development of all pupils. To do this, teachers need to change both behaviour and thinking. Without a change in thinking, changes in behaviour will not be long lasting. Some teachers may work scientifically at this by observing their own behaviour and that of their students very closely. Others may find it useful to read more about out-groups, or to interact socially with adults from out-groups. By becoming better informed about the behaviour of others, teachers will no longer need to act in unthinking and harmful ways in the classroom.

In your community (nine)

Being discriminated against is unpleasant and can be harmful if it occurs frequently. Choose one or more of the following activities to explore this issue more fully:

1 Recall an incident when someone discriminated against you. Tell a group of friends or colleagues about it. Explain how you felt as well as what happened. What did you do to cope with the situation?

2 Read as much as you can about minority tribes within your country or talk to someone from a minority group about discrimination. What sort of discrimination is common in your community?

3 Talk to four or five children in the age range 6–12 years about children from an out-group. What stereotypes do they hold? Do they all hold these stereotypes? Report back to members of your class.

4 Listen to teacher talk in a school staffroom. Make some brief notes (afterwards if you cannot do so at the time) of the kinds of stereotypical statements teachers make about children. Discuss the probable impact of these teacher beliefs on the children with a colleague.

5 Collect jokes and cartoons by locals about people in your country. Do they show evidence of prejudice, stereotypes or discrimination? Present your material to your group.

Chapter Eleven

Improving learning outcomes

Introduction

Many children in sub-Saharan Africa do not learn much at school. The high number of children who must repeat any given year of schooling inflates class sizes and increases the cost of education, often without increasing the amount of learning that has taken place (Cooksey 1981; Motala 1995). While there are many reasons for these problems, one factor that may be contributing to the current low levels of pupil achievement is the reluctance of teachers to accept imported knowledge about child development and education, and to incorporate it into their professional practice. This resistance to imported ideas can be seen as an indicator of the strength of local cultures and, as such, merits respect.

Another view, which has been discussed since the 1970s, is that African teachers can maintain cultural values while still accepting ideas from outside the continent. This was the view of African educators such as H. F. Makulu and politicians such as Samora Machel, both of whom were interested in what has been called the retraditionalisation of African education. Samora Machel, who later became the president of Mozambique, stated that:

> 'Education must give us a Mozambiquan personality which, without subservience of any kind and steeped in our own realities, will be able . . . to assimilate critically the ideas and experiences of other peoples, also passing on to them the fruits of our thought and practice.'

A few years later he wrote: 'Long suppressed manifestations of culture have to regain their place' (Machel 197, 1978, both as cited in Gerdes 1997: 223).

Earlier, Makulu (1971:31) had stated that 'education should sharpen the child's awareness of his (sic) cultural heritage and be a means by which this culture is revitalised'. Neither of these authors believed that a return to the pre-colonial past was possible or desirable. But both recognised that Africans need to develop approaches to educating children that recognise the social environment, traditions, and beliefs that have formed African cultures over long periods.

Teachers can begin the task of retraditionalising African education by taking the findings from northern hemisphere research and working out ways in which this knowledge can be adapted to meet the needs of teachers and pupils in schools in Africa. The present chapter discusses some issues that arise for teachers who want to improve the quality of education they can offer to their pupils through this process.

Characteristics of African children and their teachers: a review

A quick review of information in previous chapters will show some of the factors that need to be considered when thinking about how best to retraditionalise African education.

The children

The social interactions of African children show that:

- They are almost certainly deeply connected with their social group.
- They are largely autonomous (independent in what they do) from an early age.
- They show concern for others by helping them.
- They are moderate in their expression of emotion.
- They believe that boys and girls have quite different roles in life, with boys holding more status than girls.
- They will do almost anything to ensure the wellbeing of their in-group and are prejudiced against out-groups.

African children have also established preferred ways of learning:

- They learn by observation.
- They do much of their learning within the peer group.
- They learn without a lot of verbal input.
- They practise without direct oversight, except for some input from slightly older children.
- They learn to do things when the practical need arises.
- They act co-operatively rather than competitively (in many ethnic groups).

When adults are involved in children's learning:

- Children learn without much adult praise, but with quite severe punishment for failure.
- They expect to follow adult instruction without question.
- They know that adults do not ask questions unless they genuinely do not know the answer.
- They show respect towards all adults.

The children's health is not good:

- They are almost certainly mildly malnourished and have poor immune systems.
- They are likely to be affected by chronic and acute health problems.
- They are frequently absent from school because of ill health.
- They are unlikely to have received the full range of vaccinations available to protect them from common infections.
- They are likely to have been adversely affected by social disruption such as war or the presence of HIV/AIDS in their family.

Finally, the majority of African children come from homes where there is either no history of literacy, or only a very recently established history of limited literacy. Books and newspapers are a luxury that many families cannot afford.

African children from rural villages are more likely to have learnt to behave in ways that have long been traditional, while urban and peri-urban children may have had learning experiences that show an influence from other cultures. But even these more advantaged children will have absorbed some values, attitudes, and behaviours that come from the past and continue to form part of their African heritage. Teachers need to be aware of the influence of the past, and to accept long-established approaches to learning when they have a positive or even a neutral effect for the pupils' future. But cultural practices that hinder learning need to be re-evaluated.

The teachers

Besides having had broadly similar cultural experiences to the children in their classes, African teachers have many school-based experiences that influence their classroom behaviour. Some of these experiences are incompatible with out-of-school cultural values:

- They were taught in classes where the whole group did the same activity at the same time.

- They were taught that education was about rote learning and the ability to pass tests.
- They learned how to succeed in schools, even if the teaching was of low quality and resources were limited.
- They learned whether teaching is a valued profession in their community.

Teachers have beliefs about intelligence, learning and knowledge that they acquired as they grew up. These beliefs come partly from their own school experiences and partly from others in the broader community. In addition, they are partly acquired during any period of training for a teaching career that the teachers might have experienced.

Teachers have learnt the behaviours required to be perceived as competent in their ethnic group. Because of their own schooling, they have also developed an idea of what is defined as teacher competence in the culture. In school, therefore, they show the following behaviours:

- They do not allow children to work with their peers.
- They lecture for long periods.
- They provide close oversight of all activities.
- They do not show how material learned has any connection to practical needs or daily life.
- They constantly ask questions to which they clearly know the answer.
- They expect children to show respect.
- They may punish children quite severely for minor misdemeanours and failures.

The children they teach are at first confused by the irrelevance of the classroom to everyday life and then become resigned to it.

The pre-service and in-service training of teachers in much of sub-Saharan Africa emphasises ideas about learning and teacher behaviours that are inconsistent with the teachers' experiences and with cultural and historical beliefs. This is because knowledge from northern hemisphere studies is often being introduced. This northern hemisphere-based training emphasises that primary-school-age children learn best when:

- They can explore and discover rather than having to rote learn.
- They work in groups rather than as a whole class.
- Marks on tests are not emphasised.
- Praise is offered frequently and to individuals.

- Teachers do not impose their values, but allow children to discover their own.
- Teachers act as facilitators or guides rather than as instructors.
- Teachers understand that learning is about acquiring problem-solving skills, not memorising thousands of unrelated facts.
- Teachers spend time reflecting on their teaching with the goal of improving their personal competence.

Teachers need to find ways of 'Africanising' the information they are given, adapting knowledge to which they are introduced during training to obtain a closer fit with their own cultural practices and beliefs. Three important aspects of this problem, teacher preparation and planning, teacher management of pupil behaviour, and teaching behaviours, are discussed in the remainder of this chapter.

Preparation and planning

At present most teachers in Africa use curriculum material that has been developed by outside experts at their local ministry of education, often in conjunction with others from the teacher training centres or universities in their country. Sometimes there has been input from outside aid agencies from northern hemisphere countries (e.g. Fuller and Clarke 1994; Harley et al. 2000). Studies of teachers' thinking about curriculum and of the ways they teach modern curricula have mostly been done in junior high schools, but the issues raised are still relevant to the present discussion. Studies in primary schools would be useful, however, and need to be undertaken to obtain a better understanding of African schooling overall.

Preparing for lessons

Often curriculum material comes with sets of prepared lessons for teachers to use. This makes it easy for teachers to avoid preparing their own lesson plans. But the essential nature of personal preparation is shown in research by Cleghorn et al. (1989). Cleghorn and his colleagues observed a small number of trained and untrained teachers. They found one untrained teacher who was actually teaching more effectively than trained teachers. He was also the only teacher in the study who regularly previewed the lesson plan that had been provided by the ministry of education.

Box 17 Poor preparation, poor teaching

We are now in our English lesson and are all bending over our exercise books filling in the blanks - we are always filling in the blanks. To most of us, the whole exercise is ridiculous guesswork. The new teacher doesn't seem to know what he is about. That's why the blanks are so many. He won't explain anything, he won't lead us to discover anything. He just comes into class with 'blanks' written all over his face. I cannot see the difference between 'then' and 'when' and I am filling the blanks in a most unusual way: I have *then* and *when* written up on two pieces of paper, which are rolled into tight balls, and the whole exercise is performed the way our current politicians go about their secret ballots: I juggle the two paper balls in my hands, smell them, dance them under the desk to confuse the whole issue of identity, pick one up, unroll it and fill in a blank. I have filled in number eight in the list and it reads, 'I shall go home *then* the school is closed', and I get punished for this mistake . . .

Source: David Mulwa (1979:35–36)

Teachers should remember that the lesson plans provided are only guides to teaching for inexperienced or poorly trained staff. Others can be free to adapt material – teachers who want to be most effective and professional will take the kinds of plans provided by the ministry of education and use them as a starting point for their own thinking. On the other hand, teachers who do not believe they can or should write their own lesson plans can still improve their teaching by previewing the lesson material provided. Effective teachers do this some time before the lesson, so that they can prepare or collect teaching aids. Some examples of the kinds of things teachers need to think about when using pre-prepared curriculum and lesson plans are:

- How can I link this material to what the children already know?
- Is this material presented in such a way that my pupils will understand it or should I change the way I present it?
- How difficult are the ideas that are presented in this material?
- Is this the best way of presenting this material to my particular class, in view of their abilities, interests, and experiences?
- How else might I teach this material?

When teaching children who are learning in their second or third language some questions are:

- Do the children in my class have sufficient language skills in their second (or other) language to be able to understand these concepts when I present them in that language?

- What words am I not sure about myself? How can I explain clearly in my second (or other) language? Do I need to check my dictionary to make sure I have the correct vocabulary?
- How much should I emphasise correct language, and how much should I focus on understanding? Does it matter if children use simple everyday language instead of the correct jargon of the subject to respond to questions?

Teachers who do not use pre-prepared lesson plans should always have a lesson plan that they have prepared, with approximate times for each part of the lesson, sample questions and prepared examples for pupils to work. These sorts of lesson plans are usually discussed in detail in courses on teaching methods. Without lesson plans teachers are likely to present material in much the same way day after day, as is common in many classrooms in sub-Saharan Africa (e.g. Chapman et al. 1993; Fuller, Snyder, Chapman and Hua 1994; B. Vlaardingerbroek, personal communication, June 1998). Repeated use of the same method soon reduces its motivating effect.

Other planning for improved outcomes

Other kinds of planning can also influence learning outcomes, simply through increasing or decreasing the amount of time available for learning. This is sometimes called the opportunity to learn. Fuller and Snyder (1991) point out for example that teachers need to limit the amount of time spent on simple administrative tasks, such as giving out and collecting textbooks and teaching materials used in a lesson. Others note that pupils' opportunities to learn may be reduced when teachers are consistently late to class, or when teacher absenteeism is high and relief teachers are either unavailable or ill prepared (Lloyd et al. 2000). Jessop, in unpublished work cited by Harley et al. (2000), concluded that in primary schools where staff were completely demoralised, the minimum definition of professionalism – that teachers should be 'sober, present and punctual' – did not give rise to any real expectation that much would be taught or learnt.

Box 18 What happens when teachers do not teach well

I *am* studying the words on page . . . (of the dictionary) but they don't mean anything to me. There's a word called 'gargoyle' – which sounds rather funny. We make no attempt to *learn the words or even define them.* They come from the dictionary into our heads and evaporate with the evening air at the end of the lesson.

Source: David Mulwa (1979:36)

Managing pupil behaviour

Managing groups of children and keeping them focused on their learning task is extremely demanding, even when most of the children are reasonably well adjusted. But groups of children in schools will always include some who are difficult to manage. These children are often referred to as acting out, maladjusted or emotionally disturbed. Their problems may occur because they come from families where parenting has been inconsistent or overly punitive. They may occur because of some innate characteristics of the child, or they may occur because the child's earlier experiences in school and with teachers have not been satisfactory. Whatever the reason for the difficult behaviours, teachers can take action to improve these children's behaviour. Effective management of these pupils leads to an improved general classroom environment, provides better opportunities for learning for all pupils, and enhances the wellbeing of the troubled or difficult pupils who might otherwise continue to disrupt lessons.

Reward

Children who are difficult to manage can be dealt with by attending to them on the few occasions when they do behave in acceptable ways or by punishing them on the frequent occasions when they behave badly. Northern hemisphere psychological research from a behaviourist theoretical framework has shown that attending to and rewarding desired behaviours increases the probability that they will recur (Elliott et al. 1996; Kazdin 1989). The behaviourists have also shown that attending to undesirable behaviour also increases the probability that it will happen again.

Other research by these authors has shown that children come to fear the person who punishes them excessively, and find it difficult to learn when they are feeling anxious and afraid. As a result of all these studies, researchers recommend reward for good behaviour. Individual reward for behaviour is acceptable in the northern hemisphere norm and so behaviourists from that region recommend that teachers provide individual rewards. Thus, northern hemisphere texts encourage teachers (and parents) to make favourable comments such as 'That's great!' 'What a wonderful drawing!' 'You're a really good helper.' Teachers also learn to provide treats (outings, toys, food, free time in class) when children behave in culturally defined acceptable ways.

A range of strategies for managing 'bad' behaviour include ignoring it, briefly removing the child from the peer group, and taking away some privileges. Behaviourists suggest that only behaviour that is harmful to others should be punished in more severe ways. Even then, they do not recommend the use of physical punishment (Alberto and Troutman 1995; Kazdin 1989).

Although these principles for behaviour management are based on a very extensive body of research, parents and teachers in collectivist cultures in Africa may reject them for a number of reasons. Some characteristics of traditional African cultures that have been discussed in previous chapters make it unlikely that much verbal attention has ever been given to desirable behaviours. First, African parents, busy ensuring the survival of the family, were not expected to be involved in children's learning in a way that might provide opportunities for praise and reward. Second, in many cultures, the tradition of not drawing attention to positive characteristics of the child for fear this will attract misfortune is widespread. The concept of the 'evil eye', for example, is common in Muslim communities, although it is not part of formal Islam. Fear of attracting witches and other evil spirits by drawing attention to the positive characteristics of the child also limits the extent to which African parents are willing to single out their child for praise. The collective nature of African cultures is the third feature of the child's environment that reduces the likelihood that personal attention will result from success. Singling out one person in cultures where the wellbeing of the group is paramount reduces group cohesion and can be a source of conflict within the group.

Punishment

All children, everywhere, are punished by parents and teachers when they behave in ways that are unacceptable. The kinds of punishments used reflect both the adult's personal history and the cultural norms. For example, parents may hit their child because that is the way they were punished when they were children, or because hitting a naughty child is seen as the normal way of responding when children have misbehaved in their ethnic group and culture.

In traditional cultures around the world corporal punishment has been used to eliminate undesirable behaviours. Beliefs about the use of corporal punishment and the actual use of this technique for disciplining children probably vary widely between ethnic groups in Africa, as they do elsewhere. Matchinda (1999:246) for example states that the 'way of thinking of Cameroonian parents is influenced by the ancient conception of education, which is inseparable from punishment. For them, only punishment and corporal punishment for that matter helps to make children assume responsibility for their actions', but in Malawi a Chewa employee of one of the authors objected strongly to corporal punishment.

There are also cultural differences in deciding whether a certain punishment is acceptable or abusive. At present, this evidence comes from countries outside Africa. Studies from Singapore (Elliott, Tong and Tan 1997) and the Pacific Ocean island of Palau (Collier, McClure, Otto and Polloi 1999) have shown that teachers and parents there believe some behaviours are acceptable if the original intention is to discipline the child, even when the adult's behaviour causes real harm (e.g. during punishment the child is thrown against the wall; the child's arm is pulled to the extent that his or her shoulder is dislocated). Singaporean parents in the 1997 study by Elliott et al. also took account of the frequency with which physical punishment was inflicted when deciding whether punishment was abusive or not.

In some countries even the law permits a degree of harm to children that would not be accepted if the same harm was done to adults. For example, in one state in Mexico the law acknowledges the right of parents to inflict punishment that might cause injury, provided that the injury heals up in fewer than 15 days (Corral-Verdugo, Frias-Armento, Romero and Munoz 1995). This contrasts with the view of Australians and New Zealanders. In these countries any behaviour that results in physical harm is seen as abusive, irrespective of the caregiver's intent or the frequency with which it occurs.

In general, international research suggests that adults living in more traditional cultures talk less to their children and accept the need for physical punishment more than those in modern, technological cultures (Kagitcibasi 1996). In communities where parents, mothers especially, are illiterate or have had very few years schooling, interactions between parent and child are likely to be physical rather than verbal. This will naturally include interactions when the child is being punished. Studies by Youssef, Attia and Kamel (1998) in Egypt showed that characteristics of the parents that were associated with greater use of corporal punishment included low levels of education, parental illiteracy, and father's unemployment or employment in an unskilled or semi-skilled occupation. Families with few social contacts were more likely to use corporal punishment. In these conditions verbal praise for good behaviour and rewards in the form of treats are also less likely, the latter because of poverty.

African teachers, reward and punishment

African teachers are often in the confusing situation of being taught during their pre-service and in-service programmes to reward individuals for 'good' behaviours and ignore their bad behaviour, but this is the reverse of their own experience and what is generally expected within their culture. Teachers who have not realised they can modify pupil management techniques developed outside Africa continue to behave in traditional, culturally consistent ways. This means that they do not praise pupils individually and continue to use quite a lot of punishment, even although behaving in these ways may not be helping children to learn as much as they could. Teachers need to ask, therefore, if there are any things they can do that are culturally acceptable, but which will still show whether African children also learn best when rewarded for desired behaviours and when their undesirable behaviours are ignored.

Among ethnic groups, differences in what is acceptable almost certainly exist, but in general it seems likely that rewards for whole groups of children will be more acceptable than individual rewards, and that individual rewards, when used, might best be non-verbal. Group rewards might include:

- Positive comment for groups of children. For example, praise for the row or cluster of children who work quietly or efficiently. Or positive comment about general behaviour that relates to classroom organisation. Comments such as these could be made: 'Children in the third row are working well today.' 'Children in the back two rows started work very quickly in this lesson.' 'Children on the left side of the class have their area very neat and clean.' 'The five boys (girls) sitting near the windows are tidying their books away very quietly.'
- Group reward for good behaviours. For example, when the class as a whole has worked well during a lesson, the teacher might decide to stop five minutes early and do a fun activity, such as playing Hangman or Simon Says, reading or telling a story, letting children chat quietly for a few minutes.

Non-verbal rewards for individuals might include a nod, a wink, a smile. Teachers need to ensure that all children receive individual and group reward at about the same rate. Children will soon observe differences in the amounts of attention they receive. The risk of social dissension is then high and there is a possibility that, if unrewarded children do not do so well, parents may accuse teachers of ill-wishing their child in some way. Teachers need to find ways of rewarding children who are less successful academically. A teacher who believes that children's achievement is the only thing that matters will not recognise the effort that is also worthy of positive attention, so a re-consideration of the value of pupils' efforts might be helpful.

Ignoring undesirable or 'bad' behaviours may be difficult for teachers who believe that punishment is an important part of child-rearing. Most will have experienced quite a lot of punishment themselves. This increases the probability that they will think it does no harm or is even beneficial, despite all the research evidence to the contrary (Alberto and Troutman 1995; Kazdin 1989). African teachers need to be quite scientific in their approach to the question of punishment, testing the findings of research from the northern hemisphere in their own classroom. They can try ignoring minor undesirable behaviours. If, at the same time, they increase their attention to 'good' behaviours of the identified child and children sitting near him or her, they may find that the child's unacceptable behaviour decreases over time. If they take this approach, teachers need to be aware that there may be a temporary increase in unacceptable behaviour, as the child attempts to use old techniques to gain attention.

If unacceptable behaviours are rewarded by attention from other children, the teacher may need to try some of the other approaches to managing behaviour that have been described in many northern hemisphere textbooks on behaviour management, modifying them according to what they know about their own culture. For example, in collectivist cultures where children are socialised towards the group, imposing social isolation for a short period of time is probably a more powerful, more extreme form of punishment than it is in the individualist cultures of the northern hemisphere. Thus, although it is routinely recommended in northern hemisphere textbooks, African teachers need to think carefully about when and whether they should impose this social isolation on disruptive pupils.

Conclusion

Like teachers everywhere, African teachers need to think carefully about reward and punishment. In cultures where punishment has historically been used quite a lot, they may need to re-evaluate their ideas about how effective it is, and when and how it should be used. Appropriate reward may be more effective with children because they will generally work hard when their efforts and achievements are obviously valued by their teachers.

Changing teaching practices

Teachers who want to increase the amount children learn while in their class need also to think about what they do when they are teaching, what they want to keep from traditional practices, and how they can modify their use of these practices. They also need to think about how they can use introduced knowledge effectively, while retaining their right to behave in African ways.

Changing common teaching practices

Policy statements prepared by staff at various ministries of education in countries across sub-Saharan Africa emphasise introduced ideas about teaching (e.g. Fuller, Snyder et al. 1994; Harley et al. 2000). However, the rate of change is slow and many teachers continue to teach as they always have. Since most teachers want to help children learn, there must be reasons that they do not follow the directives of advisors and other experts. This may be because there is often unspoken but clear consensus among teachers as to the nature of the teaching task which is different from that being proposed by outsiders (Chapman et al. 1993). Resistance to change probably has its origins in both the general culture and in the culture of the school and education system. While individual teachers cannot individually change broad cultural practices, they may change their own behaviours in order to promote higher educational achievement among their pupils. To do this they may need to change current practices. Some examples of changes are presented in the remainder of this section, but changes can be made in any teaching task where modern knowledge is at odds with traditional practice.

Reducing use of chanted responses

Communicating in chanted chorus has long been part of many African cultures (e.g. Sarno 1993; Somé 1999). Stories, riddles and other forms of verbal activity often require chorused responses. African-style songs, sung in a wide range of situations, rely on the willingness of singers to repeat rhymes that sound good, but that may have little coherent meaning (Hudson 1989). Very young children living in African villages repeatedly hear these kinds of chorused responses. They willingly accept the continuation of this practice when they reach school.

In school, children commonly give group responses in two different kinds of situations. First, they may chant when there are fixed rules for responses, such as when children are learning spelling or times tables or are reading in a group from the same text. Second, children may respond as a group to questions posed by the teacher. Northern hemisphere educators and African teacher trainers do not believe that a chanted response is useful in either situation, because the teacher does not find out who knows the answer and who does not. Therefore they cannot help the children who are struggling. Chorusing one-word answers to questions also encourages rote learning. It does not help children to learn to solve problems and is demotivating for pupils because many children are not challenged to think.

African teachers in general appear to agree that asking children to chorus responses is the correct way to teach. Such an agreement may not have been explicitly discussed and chosen, but forms part of the school culture in much of sub-Saharan Africa (Chapman et al. 1993; Fuller and Snyder 1991). Fuller and Snyder suggest that teachers who elicit chorused answers may be trying to animate the children, to obtain some response from them. Lack of animation among the children may arise because they are not motivated towards learning, because they are over-anxious, tired, hungry or unwell. These problems can all be dealt with in better ways. In particular, increased variety in teaching methods and activities for children can contribute to greater participation by increasing pupil motivation. High levels of motivation are required if children are to overcome the lethargy that accompanies health problems and lack of food.

It is also possible that the children from the collective cultures of Africa are reluctant to give individual answers because they do not want to stand out from the group. In cultures where uncertainty avoidance is high, children may not be comfortable with the risk involved in offering an individual response. In classes where boys and girls are taught together, girls may find that offering an individual response elicits critical comment from male peers. Teachers need to consider all these possibilities when they think about why they continue to ask for group answers, and why children seem more willing to answer questions by chorusing the response. Changes teachers make should reflect the conclusions they have reached about the cultural, historical, personal and social factors that are influencing their practice and children's behaviours.

Because chorusing and rote learning are both culturally acceptable, teachers may find it easier to change their practice bit by bit. An easy way to introduce change is to reduce reliance on chorusing, using choruses for relaxation and fun, only after children have shown they have understood new concepts. For example, in mathematics, teachers should not expect children to chant addition or multiplication facts (1 + 1 = 2, 1 + 2 = 3; or 2 x 0 = 0, 2 x 1 = 2, 2 x 2 = 4) until they have shown that they understand the mathematical concepts underlying addition and multiplication. Rote learning of number facts then allows children to manipulate the numbers easily.

Some possible times and situations when rote learning and group chorusing of answers may be used are listed below, but teachers may want to think of other options, or discuss this issue in teams or in school-based in-service.

- **Use rote learning and chants for fun or for brief periods of rest from other activities.** For example, instead of the whole class chanting some spelling or number facts, divide the class into two. Randomly point to one half of the class and let them chant one or two responses, then point to the others to get them to continue. This requires children to remain alert and do not just 'switch off' during rote drills.
- **Use rote learning to enable pupils to check their own knowledge**. Get one row, one group or one half of the class to chant the spelling of a word, ask individuals or groups in the rest of the class whether the first group spelled the word correctly.
- **Find, or make up, rhymes and rhythms that put number facts, correct spelling, rules about spelling (e.g. 'i' before 'e' except after 'c') into song, poetry or dance**. (Children often remember such patterns for the rest of their lives – one of the present authors can still chant the alphabet backwards after being taught the rhythm needed for recall about 45 years ago.) Children might be able to make up some rhymes and rhythms

themselves. Small groups might be able to present their rhyme as a brief 'entertainment' break from more intense periods of study.

To avoid chorused answers at other times, teachers need to think about how they ask questions. It is impossible for children to chorus answers to open-ended questions. For example, 'What do you think happened next in the story?' will elicit a range of possible answers, as do the questions 'How can we solve this problem?' 'How does X happen?' But if individual children do not answer these questions, teachers may find that they can elicit an answer if they let pupils talk in groups of two to four for one to two minutes, working out the answer, and the reasons that their answer is a good one. Then a pre-selected spokesperson for the group can present the answer. Teachers who introduce this method may find they need to teach pupils how to interact within their group, so that all pupils get a chance to contribute to the discussion. This approach can overcome some of the difficulties for individuals in schools in collective, high uncertainty avoidance and masculine cultures, such as are widespread across Africa.

Increasing opportunities for problem-solving practice

Children develop competence in any skill when they practise it and this is true of problem-solving, as for other skills. Before teachers move from teaching facts to helping children practise problem-solving skills, they need to have thought about the kinds of issues discussed in Chapter Nine. A teacher who thinks that an educated child is one who can recite lots of facts, or whose educational goal is to impart many facts, is unlikely to spend a lot of time teaching children how to solve problems. Even teachers who understand that knowledge changes very rapidly, and that the best way of preparing children for the future is to help them develop skills in understanding and interpreting information may still not know how to teach problem-solving skills.

In the northern hemisphere teachers often use open-ended questions to encourage problem-solving or they set problems for which various answers are possible (e.g. In how many ways can we use these containers to raise water from a well?). The limited research on open and closed questions in Africa has been done in junior secondary schools. Studies by Fuller and his colleagues showed that teachers asked a ratio of about three closed questions, requiring one-word answers, to one open-ended question in English and science. In mathematics the ratio was about 7 to 1.

Gender differences in the amount learned by boys and girls whose teachers ask more open-ended questions suggest that boys learn more when questions are more open-ended (Fuller, Hua and Snyder 1994). This may reflect the greater risk for adolescent girls when they are asked to reveal their thinking in cultures where they do not have equal status with boys and where expectations about girls' abilities are typically low. Alternatively, it is possible that teachers direct the more complex open questions at boys, with the result that they learn more than girls who may be asked to answer simpler questions. The greater cognitive demand of open questions would then enhance boys' learning. These possibilities also need to be considered by primary school teachers who want to increase their use of open questions.

Another aspect of traditional culture may slow the rate at which pupils begin to use problem-solving approaches when first introduced to problem-solving in hypothetical situations. Some research from Africa and elsewhere suggests that when children are living a traditional lifestyle they learn context-specific problem-solving skills. As reported in Chapter Five, Cole et al. (1971) found that unschooled people were unwilling to talk about hypothetical events. They preferred to refer to the concrete situation in which they found themselves. Within this context they were competent problem-solvers. Teachers in Australia have found that Aboriginal children living in traditional communities learn to solve specific problems, but do not generalise knowledge gained in solving one problem to similar situations (Partington and McCudden 1992). In these communities children also learn a great deal by observation, with little direct verbal instruction. This is similar to the way children in much of Africa learn skills. Together, the results from these studies of traditional communities suggest that African teachers may need to teach skills of generalisation, giving pupils opportunities to practise generalising from one task to another similar one. At the same time pupils need to become aware of the limits to which they can safely generalise. These important skills can help pupils to solve new problems efficiently and quickly.

Using key knowledge from northern hemisphere studies

Teachers need to think about how they can adapt their teaching practice to incorporate the use of introduced knowledge in their classrooms. To encourage teachers to begin this task, a few of the key northern hemisphere findings are listed below. Some of the difficulties that teachers might face when they think about these northern hemisphere findings are discussed, together with advantages that arise from adapting the findings to meet the needs of pupils in African schools. The suggestions are offered as a starting point for discussion and reflection, not as absolutes that teachers must accept without analysis and discussion.

According to a great number of northern hemisphere studies children learn best:

- when teachers teach from the known to the unknown
- when children are offered 'individualised' programmes
- when competition is reduced and co-operation increased
- when testing is reduced and monitoring of pupils' work during class is increased
- when anxiety is fairly low and motivation is high
- when they are taught how to study effectively.

Making small changes

Some small changes can be made quite easily. For example, telling and re-telling traditional stories may make the transition from home to school easier for young children. In this instance the teacher is working from the known to the unknown if he or she also writes the story in simple words on large sheets of paper, ties the pages together to make a book, and uses these books as aids when teaching reading. This is likely to be especially useful in schools where there are not enough basic readers. Teaching aids for mathematics can be made from bottle tops or buttons or from twigs tied in bunches of ten or one hundred. Children are already familiar with these objects in their environment.

It is possible that some teachers already do these things. However, some may not, perhaps because they believe it is the ministry of education's responsibility to provide teaching aids, or they think that only stories about modern life are useful, or they are not entirely sure how to differentiate between basic vocabulary that children need to learn and other 'interest' vocabulary that is less important in the early stages of reading. Other teachers may think they should not have to gather up odds and ends from their environment for use when teaching mathematics. In an ideal situation all of these beliefs may be reasonable, but many African teachers are not working in an ideal educational environment. However, if teachers keep in mind that their prime responsibility is to ensure that children learn as much as they can, the follow-on responsibility is easily recognised. As far as possible, teachers must overcome the weaknesses of their educational system to ensure children do well academically.

A second small change that will improve learning outcomes is to ensure that pupils do lots of practice examples of newly introduced material in their exercise books, and do not spend any significant part of the day merely copying from the blackboard. Fuller and Clarke (1994) found, for example, that the majority of teachers in Soweto did not ask pupils to practise examples in their exercise books. Instead these books were used solely for recording what teachers had written on the board or what they said when lecturing the whole class. This activity results in very little, if any, learning.

Making changes where issues are more complex

Two other changes require more intense re-evaluation of beliefs and practices. These are, first, changing from teacher-centred to more child-centred approaches and individualising the programmes offered. Second, the cluster of related issues concerned with competition and testing need careful consideration.

- **Individualising programmes:** Individualising programmes requires some thought and effort on the part of northern hemisphere teachers who generally have only around 30 pupils in their class. In contrast, there are more than 60 or 70 pupils per teacher in many parts of Africa. How can African teachers provide material at all different levels? The answer is that they cannot. But African teachers could try using various methods of grouping children so that, at any one time, they are actively involved with smaller numbers of pupils, while others in the class work independently. Grouping pupils in this way shows that the teacher has taken account of individual differences to some degree, perhaps as much as is possible when teaching large numbers of pupils.

  Working with a split class may be difficult at first and teachers who are trying it out should not think they have to teach in this manner for the whole day. Instead, they could try the approach for part of a lesson only, later using grouping only in one subject area, and later still, when they are more confident, having children work in groups for much of the day. Planning for group work also involves teaching all children about the rules for working without direct supervision. Some of these might include the following: Do not interrupt the teacher when he or she is working with the other group, Work independently, It is (or is not) acceptable to talk quietly about the task to the child sitting nearby.

Some examples of how group work might be introduced:

- The teacher works with half the class to introduce some new reading skill or to provide some practice in reading aloud. Each pupil is asked to read a few sentences, while others in the teaching group listen and read the same passage silently. Comprehension questions are answered orally. The children in the other half of the class work quietly at their desks doing some reading-related activity that does not require immediate supervision.
- The teacher asks most children to work in pairs to practise times tables, while he or she spends a few minutes reviewing some multiplication concepts with

children who are having difficulty. Then the teacher provides the whole class with some activity involving use of tables.

- The teacher asks half the class to work on mathematics examples from the blackboard, while she or he teaches new material to the other children for 10 or 15 minutes. This can then be reversed, so that the second group works with the teacher on new material and the others practise what they have just learnt.

The advantages to the children are obvious. If they are placed in groups according to approximate ability when learning basic skills, and use texts suited to their abilities, they do not waste time doing work that is too easy or too difficult. Less able pupils will experience less anxiety and will learn more. More gifted children will experience just enough anxiety to increase their motivation to learn. Because the teacher is working with only half the class, each child gets more teacher attention when learning new concepts, vocabulary or skills. When the teacher is working with the other part of the class, children working independently learn to work without direct supervision and to continue to learn from and with their peers. This kind of independent study with peer interaction is consistent with traditionally valued ways of learning where parents do not provide constant oversight, and children spend much of their time learning from siblings and peers (Teachers should note that ability grouping for only parts of the day does not lower self-esteem, as long as children work in mixed ability groups at other times.)

When there is a shortage of texts, this method also improves learning outcomes. Research in developing countries has shown that when children share one book between two pupils, they learn a great deal more than if they have to share among many children (Farrell 1993; Rama 2001). Using the group teaching method outlined above, for example, it would be possible for a class of 60 children to have reasonable access to reading material even when there were only 15 reading texts available. Each child would be taught in a group of 30, sharing with one other child.

Learning to use new methods involves taking risks and breaking with general and school-based tradition. The teachers' willingness to take risks may vary according to how much they personally value tradition and how much the culture of the school emphasises traditional ways of doing things. Teachers who are more conservative, who value continuity with the past or who have a high need to avoid uncertainty may all fear change. They may need to think about how they can cope with these aspects of their personality and values, so that they can try new methods without too much distress and anxiety. For new teachers there is also the question of control. They may fear that the group they are not working with will just waste time. This can be overcome by spending some time discussing the rules that will apply when pupils are working without direct supervision. Teachers may also need to develop the habit of quickly scanning the independent group and attending to those who are working well with some brief comment.

More experienced teachers may feel that they are being 'de-skilled' (rather than 're-skilled') because ways of teaching that have worked for them can no longer be used. These teachers may believe that they are no longer in control once pupils are working without their direct supervision. But because teachers have made all the decisions about group members, about what children will do in groups, and about how long the group work will continue, they are still the controlling force in deciding what happens in their classrooms. To reduce feelings of discomfort, teachers can initially divide the class into two groups. They can also use this kind of group work for only a small part of one lesson at first, until they and their pupils are comfortable with the method. Doing this also keeps the risks associated with change rather small.

An advantage for teachers who take the risk of getting children to work in groups may be that they develop a new sense of professionalism. (For example, the teacher might think, 'As a professional, I must try new things to discover whether they improve learning outcomes in my class. Research from elsewhere suggests they might.') Teachers who introduce group work may want to reassess what is learnt. Naturally, they need to ensure that children learn what is required in their curriculum, but when children are working without direct teacher control, they are probably also learning many other things, and teachers might want to assess development of social and personal skills as well. For example, children working with less direct supervision may learn to work independently without being distracted from the task, may become more willing to help others who are in difficulty when the teacher is not available, and may learn to cope with the frustration of not being able to solve occasional problems. Thus, teachers can learn that they are contributing to the development of the whole child, not just instilling many facts into his or her head.

Teachers who are developing as professionals may find adults in their community who think that challenging tradition is potentially harmful. Parents and other adults who have been to schools where everything was teacher-centred may believe that this is the best way for their children and grandchildren to learn. (This is also true around the world and can be a source of difficulty for all teachers who are changing their teaching methods with a goal of improving learning outcomes.) Teachers who plan to introduce new methods will need to deal with parents' responses. They may need to discuss their plans with members of the community, explaining the nature of the proposed change in action and reasons for change. They may want to point out that children learning together has a much longer history in Africa than children learning in a controlled way from adults.

It may be difficult to talk directly to parents in ethnic groups where uncertainty is avoided. As noted elsewhere, both teachers and parents in these groups generally believe that teachers are the experts. By becoming more available to parents, teachers in high uncertainty avoidance cultures may be acting in ways that are inconsistent with their culture. In this instance, it may be necessary for teachers to present new information in very formal ways, maintaining their role as the expert on education matters during the information session. Teachers in high power distance cultures, where there is an expectation that authority figures have much higher status than other people, may need to have initial discussions with village elders, chiefs or other powerful members of the community. If these people can be convinced, they may be of vital assistance in educating others. Young teachers in high power distance cultures and women teachers in the so-called masculine cultures might find that educating parents is not easy, because of their perceived lower social and professional status relative to others. They may need the assistance of more senior staff who already approve the use of new approaches. All teachers may need to reassure parents that the approach will be tried in some minimal way for a fixed period before its effectiveness is reviewed.

Competition and testing

Competition and testing were introduced into African schools by missionaries in the schools of the nineteenth century. Teachers at that time mistakenly emphasised test results, posting results on the walls and punishing children who had not done well. They thought this would increase children's motivation to learn. Since that time, northern hemisphere studies have shown that excessive competition and frequent testing reduce learning by inducing anxiety, taking up learning time and reducing the self-esteem of children who constantly receive low marks.

The continued emphasis on high levels of competition in sub-Saharan African schools is inconsistent with the cultural valuing of co-operation that has long helped many families and tribes across the continent to survive. On the other hand, teachers cannot manage without testing pupils; some testing is always necessary. The most useful tests are the quick tests given while teaching a unit of work. These provide the teacher with feedback that informs subsequent teaching (formative assessment), unlike the terminal assessments that are made once a complete unit of work has been studied. Terminal assessments have little positive impact on teaching.

Teachers can learn a great deal about children's skills without testing if they monitor children closely as they work on exercises following instruction. But many sub-Saharan African teachers still teach almost entirely from the front of the classroom (Chapman et al. 1993; Fuller and Snyder 1991). The effect of close monitoring, in which the teacher moves around the class while children are practising new skills, may vary from one country to another. Lockheed and Komenan (1989) found that in Nigeria that teachers in schools rated as high performing did more monitoring and evaluation of pupils' work than teachers in less successful schools. But in Swaziland the reverse was true. Female and male teachers may also differ in the extent to which they monitor deskwork (Fuller, Snyder et al. 1994). Reasons for these variations in teacher behaviour are unknown at present. In some instances, the extent of monitoring may reflect the amount of formal teaching within each culture prior to contact with missionary teachers. Alternatively, between-nation differences may have developed because nineteenth-century missionary teachers taught in slightly different ways according to their own cultures.

Ethical issues

The research from the northern hemisphere raises some ethical issues. As professionals, teachers are responsible for providing the best, most up-to-date education possible for their pupils. Failure to do so becomes a moral and professional issue. For example, only very few African children pass the relevant examination at the end of primary school and progress on to secondary school (UNICEF 2000a). If children have not been taught using the best practices, a gifted child can miss out on the opportunity for further schooling. Thus, teachers who do not apply current knowledge about learning are potentially depriving some pupils of their right to reach their fullest potential through completing their education. These teachers are not meeting their moral obligation to ensure that children do achieve as well as they might. This does not imply that teachers must accept northern hemisphere research without thought. As usual, teachers need to think about how northern hemisphere research findings might be adapted to meet African preferences.

Conclusion

If teachers are willing to think about how they can adapt northern hemisphere knowledge to meet both their own need to behave in culturally acceptable ways and the needs of their pupils for culturally relevant education, they can become much more effective educators. However, teachers need to spend time thinking about what stops them from using this imported knowledge. When they are clear about the reasons that they do not want to change, there is a much greater likelihood that they will find the courage to face their fears and gradually modernise and retraditionalise the ways they teach.

Reflective teachers

In their study of rural primary school teachers in Gambia and South Africa, Jessop and Penny (1998) investigated the teachers' perceptions of their role. They found two different emphases. Many teachers emphasised what the authors called the 'instrumental role'. These teachers perceived their role as consisting largely of instilling information. In discussions about their role, such teachers expressed interest in knowledge and results and in their own conditions of service. They mentioned salary, holidays and free time, job security, and status as aspects of their role that they valued. The responses of the other teachers emphasised the importance of their relationship with their pupils. The researchers called this a 'relational' approach. Teachers who made responses that fitted them into this group talked about loving and caring for their pupils. They were concerned about having friendly relationships with pupils and being able to show sympathy and support for them, encouraging them and influencing their development through the strong relationship.

Jessop and Penny expressed concern that although teachers in both of these countries were being exposed to new curricula and new methods of teaching by officials from their ministries of education, they had not accepted these ideas or made them their own. In interviews they did not talk about how they could best promote pupils' understanding of concepts, or the ways the new curricula might influence their teaching. Teachers did not seem to realise that it was their responsibility to reflect on their own teaching and discover ways in which they could improve it. Thus, there was a gap in their understanding of their role – they had not developed the personal sense of responsibility for learning outcomes that would lead them to try the new ways of teaching to which they had been introduced.

Jessop and Penny (1998) thought that teachers' inability and reluctance to change arose because in-service courses were short and imposed from outside. This may be one reason for lack of change. But being faced with change, especially change imposed from outside, is threatening, and some are naturally reluctant to enter a threatening situation. As stated earlier, teachers may feel that by doing some things in a different way they are being de-skilled in a some general sense. Some may want to change the way they teach, but thoughts and beliefs such as those listed below may make it difficult for them to take the risk.

- I have only been teaching a little while. More experienced teachers don't teach the way I'm supposed to. It would be better to do as they do.
- I have been teaching for many years. I know how to do it. Who does this so-called expert think he (she) is, telling me how to do my job?
- If I change my ways of teaching I will have to spend a lot more time on preparation. I don't have that time.
- I could change if only the ministry of education supplied the equipment or extra staff. Until then, I'm stuck with limited resources and can't manage any other way.
- If I change my ways of teaching, I won't be able to get through the curriculum. There just isn't enough time for all this chat about problems and how to solve them.
- If I change my ways of teaching, I will be the only one in the school doing things differently. That's too scary.
- This just isn't the way we do things in this country. Why should we do things the way they do in other parts of the world?

Box 19 A teacher speaks

'I think that professional development is something that a person in a profession should seek out without waiting for somebody to bring it to his or her doorstep, because really, if you are in something, and you want to progress in what you are doing, I think you must find all the necessary means . . .'

South African primary school teacher

Source: Jessop and Penny (1998:397)

Outside experts often fail to take account of these beliefs. They do not recognise the strength of the school culture (e.g. In our school we do things this way) or the isolation of individual teachers who have attended in-service courses may experience after they return to their schools. Changes are more likely to occur when these sorts of issues have been discussed within the school and strategies for change have been thought through. It is not enough solely to change the curriculum or required teaching methods.

In African cultures where the preference for avoiding uncertainty is strong, resistance to the uncertainty that goes along with changing one's ways of teaching is likely to be even higher than elsewhere. Teachers from such cultures need to find ways of feeling certain that they are doing the right thing when they decide to change the way they teach. These teachers may be more comfortable with change when there is consensus in their team or school that everyone will try new methods, or that everyone will teach one subject or one lesson per day using the new methods. They may be happier if a respected colleague helps them to change, perhaps discussing and approving lesson plans, observing occasional lessons and making positive comment about parts of the lesson that were especially successful. In egalitarian cultures teachers may also be pleased to receive help and advice from a more experienced, senior colleague. On the other hand, teachers in high power distance cultures may be more comfortable working with their peers than being monitored by a more senior staff member. Women teachers may find it easier to work with other women in schools where traditional male and female roles continue to be imposed. Teachers who feel anxious about change for any reason need assistance in their struggle to ensure that they are doing their best to prepare pupils for the future.

Teachers who are beginning to reflect on their teaching might want to ask themselves some of the following questions when thinking about one lesson, or at the end of the day when reviewing their teaching:

- How well did I explain new concepts in lessons today? Could I have explained more clearly? Exactly what could I have said that would have been clearer?
- How well had I prepared for this lesson? Do I need to spend more time planning lessons?
- How well did I monitor pupils as they were doing their exercises? Did I move around the class observing and checking for pupils who were having difficulties? Did I re-teach when it became obvious that several pupils were struggling? Why did I need to re-teach?
- Did I give the pupils adequate feedback about their work? Should I make more specific comments, instead of just saying 'Good work?' Is my marking up to date?
- What about the test I gave pupils today? Is there any evidence that pupils were confused by the question itself? Did the test measure the most important concepts I have been teaching in the last week or month? Did the test require rote learning or did I include some opportunities for pupils to show they can solve problems?
- Was there a particular group of pupils that I did not teach well today? For example, children from another ethnic group? Girls? Boys? What do I need to do to teach these children effectively? Do I need to observe more closely and see if they learn best when I teach in certain ways? Do they learn best alone? In groups?
- Was I fair and kind to all pupils or only some? Which pupils was I kind to? Why these pupils? What do I need to do differently so that other pupils realise I care about them and about how much they learn? Do I need to change the way I speak to them, the number of times I ask them questions, the kinds of questions I ask them?

- What can I do about the fact that I don't like teaching this subject? Do I need to learn more about it? Can I overcome my personal fear (hatred) of it? Who can I ask for help with it?
- Overall, how do I feel about my teaching? What did I do well today? Am I getting better at teaching? Am I bored? Do I hate it? What can I do about these feelings? If I change some aspect of my work, will I enjoy it more?

The examples of questions that teachers might ask themselves show that some intensive thought is required. Taking responsibility for one's own actions is also necessary. Some teachers in individualist cultures have found it useful to keep a diary recording their thoughts about what they did and how it influenced children's learning (e.g. Holt 1982,1984). Teachers in the collectivist cultures of sub-Saharan Africa might find it easier to plan to discuss some of these questions with one or two trusted colleagues regularly. In spite of cultural taboos against saying what they have done well, teachers also need to be able to identify the best aspects of their teaching in order to be able to do those things again. If it is difficult to talk about these good things, teachers who have formed discussion groups may find it easier to write them down on a scrap of paper, re-read them silently and save them somewhere private. Colleagues who have observed others' effective work, even in passing, might be able to comment positively on what they saw, either privately or within the group.

Conclusion

Despite the many problems in educational systems in much of sub-Saharan Africa, teachers can make a difference. They need to consider many issues when trying to adapt imported knowledge to enhance children's academic achievement. Teachers who have analysed the teaching task are likely to have more motivation to accept changes required by their ministry of education. This is because, when analysing their task and their responsibilities, they have also had the opportunity to explore their fears and hesitations and to find ways of overcoming these in their search for greater professionalism.

Some of the suggestions probably sound as if the authors believe that the 'facts' discovered by northern hemisphere researchers will all be proved true of African children. It does seem probable that this will be so if such knowledge is interpreted in ways that are culturally acceptable to teachers and pupils. However, teachers can only find out what is best for African pupils if they are willing to experiment with new ideas, modify practice and experiment again. In this way they will find out when, how, and even if, they can successfully incorporate northern hemisphere knowledge into their teaching. In the long term, some northern hemisphere knowledge may prove not to be useful, but with thoughtful teachers who are willing to accept the strengths of their traditional ways and eliminate those parts of tradition that are harmful or useless in today's world, children in sub-Saharan Africa can receive an education that is retraditionalised, African and modern.

In your community (ten)

Trainee teachers need opportunities to observe experienced teachers in action. But they need to remember that not everything an experienced teacher does is necessarily the best, so they should also feel free to experiment with doing things differently during their teaching practice. Choose one or more of the following activities that are designed to help trainee teachers become more willing to try new ways:

1. Observe teachers as they interact with children in any number of situations. Try to discover what the teacher who gets the most relaxed and compliant reaction from the children does well.
2. Go to class with a lesson plan that includes a fun activity that you can use to give the children a short break from serious work. Use this activity if children seem to be losing interest, or at the end of the lesson for a reward.
3. When students are working on prepared exercises, spend five minutes moving around the classroom, making group praise comments while at the same time monitoring pupil progress on their task.
4. Make notes on the way the class teacher presents a lesson. Prepare an alternative lesson plan for the same material. Discuss this with other teacher trainees or with the college supervisor.
5. Obtain some lesson plans that have been prepared by staff at the ministry of education. Evaluate these with reference to the knowledge and skills of the pupils in your practicum class. Modify them according to what you know of the pupils and then teach this material.

References

Aboud, F. 1988. *Children and Prejudice*. Oxford: Basil Blackwell.

Adjahoto, E. O., Hodonou, K. A. S., DeSouza, A. D., Tété, V. K. and Baeta, S. 2000. 'Information des Jeunes en Matière de Sexualité'. *Santé* 10:195–199.

Ahmed, G. (ed.). 1990. *Perceptions and Facts on Population Issues in Kweneng District: A Report on the Findings of the District Level Survey on Attitudes towards Population and Development Issues*. Gaborone, Botswana: University of Botswana.

Ahmed, S., Lutaol, T., Wawer, M., Serwadda, D., Sewankambo, N. K., Nalugoda, F., Makumbi, F., Wabire-Mangen, F., Kiwanuka, N., Kigozi, G., Kiddubavu, M. and Gray, R. 2001. 'HIV Incidence and Sexually Transmitted Disease Prevalence Associated with Condom Use: A Population Study in Rakai, Uganda'. *Aids* 15:2171–2179.

Ainsworth, M. D. S. 1977. 'Infant Development and Mother-Infant Interaction among Ganda and American Families'. In P. H. Leiderman, S. R. Tulkin and A. Rosenfeld (eds.). *Culture and Infancy: Variations in the Human Experience*. New York: Academic:119–149.

Ainsworth, M. D. S., and Wittig, B. A. 1969. 'Attachment and Exploratory Behavior in One-Year-Olds in a Strange Situation'. In B. M. Foss (ed.). *Determinants of Infant Behavior IV*. Toronto: Allyn & Bacon:111–136.

Airhihenbuwa, C. O. 1995. *Health and Culture: Beyond the Western Paradigm*. Thousand Oaks, Calif.: Sage.

Akinboye, J. O. 1997. *Psychological Foundations of Education in Africa*. Ibadan, Nigeria: Stirling-Horden.

Alberto, P. A. and Troutman, A. C. 1995. *Applied Behavior Analysis for Teachers*. Englewood Cliffs, N.J.: Merrill.

Alton-Lee, A., Nuttall, G. and Patrick, J. 1993. 'Reframing Classroom Research: A Lesson from the Private World of Children'. *Harvard Educational Review* 63(1):50–84.

Altshuler, J. L. and Ruble, D. N. 1989. 'Developmental Changes in Children's Awareness of Strategies for Coping with Uncontrollable Stress'. *Child Development* 60:1337–1349.

Astill, J. 2001. 'The Terrible Truth about The Ship of Slaves'. *Guardian Weekly* April 26–May 2:7.

Asuzu, M. C. 1994. 'Sexual Beliefs, Attitudes and Knowledge of Adolescent Youth in Ibadan concerning Aids'. *West African Journal of Medicine* 13:245–247.

Bailey, R. C., Muga, R., Poulussen, R., Abicht, H. 2002. 'The Acceptability of Male Circumcision to Reduce HIV Infections in Nyanza Province, Kenya'. *Aids Care* 14:27–40.

Ball, A. 1988. *Family Planning for Youth in Botswana: Information Source and Availability Draft Report*. Ontario, Canada: School Rural Planning and Development.

Banda, M. A. 1995. 'Future Strategies Regarding Children Affected by HIV/Aids'. In Y. Shiokawa and T. Kitamura (eds.). *Global Challenge of Aids: Ten Years of HIV/Aids Research*. Tokyo: Kodansha:211–217.

Barker, P. 1995. *Basic Child Psychiatry*. Oxford: Blackwell Science.

Barley, N. 1986. *A Plague of Caterpillars: A Return to the African Bush*. Harmondsworth, England: Viking.

Barley, N. 1994. *Smashing Pots: Feats of Clay from Africa*. London: British Museum Press.

Barnartt, S. N. and Kabzems, V. 1992. 'Zimbabwean Teachers' Attitudes towards the Integration of Pupils with Disabilities into Regular Classrooms'. *International Journal of Disability, Development and Education* 39:135–146.

Bastick, T. 2000. 'Why Teacher Trainees Choose the Teaching Profession: Comparing Trainees in Metropolitan and Developing Countries'. *International Review of Education* 46:343–349.

Bastos, I., Mallya, J., Ingvarsson, L., Reimer, A. and Andreasson, L. 1995. 'Middle Ear Disease and Hearing Impairment in Northern Tanzania. A Prevalence Study of Schoolchildren in the Moshi and Monduli Districts'. *International Journal of Pediatric Otorhinolaryngology* 32:1–12.

Baumrind, D. 1971. Current Patterns of Parental Authority. *Developmental Psychology Monograph* 4 (no 1 pt 2):1–103.

Bejiga, A. and Alemayehu, W. 2001. 'Prevalence of Trachoma and Its Determinants in Dalocha District, Central Ethiopia'. *Ophthalmic Epidemiology* 8:119–125.

Berlinsky, E. B. and Biller, H. B. 1982. *Parental Death and Psychological Development*. Lexington, Mass.: Lexington.

Berndt, T. J. 1992. *Child Development*. Fort Worth, Tex.: Harcourt Brace Jovanovich.

Berk, L. E. 2000. *Child Development* (5th ed.). Boston: Allyn & Bacon.

Berry, J. W. 1976. *Human Ecology and Cognitive Style: Comparative Studies in Cultural and Psychological Adaptation*. New York: Sage/Halstead.

Berry, J. W. 1984. 'Towards a Universal Psychology of Cognitive Competence'. *International Journal of Psychology* 19:335–361.

Berry, J. W. 1994. 'Ecology of Individualism and Collectivism'. In U. Kim, H. C. Triandis, C. Kagitcibasi, S-C. Choi and G. Yoon (eds.). *Individualism and Collectivism: Theory, Method and Applications*. Thousand Oaks, Calif.: Sage:77–84.

Berry, J. W., Poortinga, Y. H., Segall, M. H. and Dasen, P. R. 1992. *Cross-Cultural Psychology: Research and Applications*. Cambridge: Cambridge University Press.

Berry, J. W., Poortinga, Y. H., Segall, M. H. and Dasen, P. R. 2002. *Cross-Cultural Psychology: Research and Applications* (2nd ed.). Cambridge: Cambridge University Press.

Biddlecombe, P. 1993. *French Lessons in Africa*. London: Abacus.

Biggs, J. B. and Telfer, R. 1987. *The Process of Learning* (2nd ed.). Sydney, Australia: Prentice Hall.

Bledsoe, C. and Isiugo-Abanihe, W. 1989. 'Strategies of Child Fosterage among Mende Grannies in Sierra Leone'. In R. J. Lesthaege (ed.). *Reproduction and Social Organization in Sub-Saharan Africa*. Berkeley, Calif.: University of California Press:442–473.

Bloch, M. N. and O'Rourke, S. 1982. 'The Nonsocial Play Behavior of Young Senegalese Children: Sex Differences and the Effect of Maternal Employment'. In J. W. Loy (ed.). *The Paradoxes of Play: Proceedings of the 69th Annual Meeting of the Association for the Anthropological Study of Play*. West Point, N.Y.: Leisure Press:150–159.

Bloom, M. 1990. 'The Psychosocial Constructs of Social Competency'. In T. P. Gullotta, G. R. Adams and R. Montemayor (eds.). *Developing Social Competency in Adolescence*. Newbury Park, Calif.: Sage:11–27.

Boesak, A. A. 1984. *Walking on Thorns: The Call to Christian Obedience*. Grand Rapids: Eerdmans.

Boothby, N. 1996. 'Children of War: Survival as a Collective Act'. In M. Mccallin (ed.). *The Psychological Wellbeing of Refugee Children: Research, Practice and Policy Issues* (2nd ed.). Geneva: International Catholic Child Bureau:136–149.

Borich, G. D. and Tombari, M. L. 1995. *Educational Psychology: A Contemporary Approach*. New York: HarperCollins.

Borke, H. 1973. 'The Development of Empathy in Chinese and American Children between Three and Six Years of Age'. *Developmental Psychology* 9:102–108.

Bornstein, M. H. and O'Reilly, A. W. 1993. Editors' Notes. In M. H. Bornstein and A. W. O'Reilly (eds.). *The Role of Play in the Development of Thought*. San Francisco: Jossey-Bass:1–3.

Bornstein, M. H., Gaughran, J. M. and Homel, P. 1986. 'Infant Temperament: Theory, Tradition, Critique and New Assessments'. In C. E. Izard and P. B. Read (eds.). *Measuring Emotions in Infants and Children* (vol. 2). Cambridge: Cambridge University Press:172–199.

Boulding, E. 1992. *The Underside of History: A View of Women Through Time* (rev. ed., vol. 1). Newbury Park: Sage.

Brandes, P. J. and Ehinger, D. M. 1981. 'The Effects of Early Middle Ear Pathology on Auditory Perception and Academic Achievement'. *Journal of Speech and Hearing Disorders* 46:301–306.

Brazelton, T. B., Koslowski, B. and Tronick, E. 1976. 'Neonatal behavior among urban Zambians and Americans'. *Journal of the American Academy of Child Psychiatry* 15:97–107.

Brislin, R. W. 1990. 'Applied Cross-Cultural Psychology: An Introduction'. In R. W. Brislin (ed.). *Applied Cross-Cultural Psychology*. Newbury Park, Calif.: Sage:9–33.

Bronfenbrenner, U. 1979. *The Ecology of Human Development: Experiments by Nature and Design*. Cambridge, Mass.: Harvard University Press.

Bronfenbrenner, U. 1988. 'Interacting Systems in Human Development. Research Paradigms: Present and Future'. In N. Bolger, A. Caspi, G. Downey and M. Moorhouse (eds.). *Persons in Context: Developmental Processes*. Cambridge: Cambridge University Press:25–49.

Brown, J. E., Michenai, K. D., Grant, E. M., Mwenda, J. M., Muthuri, F. M. and Grant, A. R. 2001. 'Varieties of Male Circumcision: A Study from Kenya'. *Sexually Transmitted Diseases* 28:608–612.

Brown, R. 1995. *Prejudice: Its Social Psychology*. Oxford: Blackwell.

Bruner, J. 1996. *The Culture of Education*. Cambridge, Mass.: Harvard University Press.

Bruner, J. S., Goodnow, J. J. and Austin, G. A. 1956. *A Study in Thinking*. New York: Wiley.

Buvé, A., Weiss, H. A., Laga, M., Van Dyck, E., Musonda, R., Zekeng, L., Kahindo, M., Amagonou, S., Morison, L., Robinson, N. J., Hayes, R. J. 2001. 'Study Group on Heterogeneity of HIV Epidemics in African Cities. 2001. The Epidemiology of Gonorrhoea, Chlamydial Infection and Syphilis in Four African Cities'. *Aids* 15, Supplement 4:S79–88.

Caldwell, J. C., Caldwell, P. and Quiggin, P. 1994. 'The Social Context of Aids in Sub-Saharan Africa'. In I. O. Orubuloye, J. C. Caldwell, P. Caldwell and G Santow (eds.). *Sexual Networking and Aids in Sub-Saharan Africa: Behavioural Research and the Social Context*. Canberra, Australia: Health Transition Centre, Australian National University:129–162.

Cammish, N. K. and Brock, C. 1994. 'State, Status, and the Status Quo: Factors Affecting the Education of Girls in Cameroon'. *International Journal of Educational Development* 14:233–240.

Caprara, A., Seri, D., DeGregorio, G. C., Parenzi, A., Salazar, C. M. and Gozé, T. 1993. 'The Perception of Aids in The Bété and Baoulé of The Ivory Coast'. *Social Science and Medicine* 36:1229–1235.

Carlsson, C. 2000. 'Invisible Burdens'. *Guardian Weekly* June 8–14:24.

Cartwright, G. P., Cartwright, C. A. and Ward, M. E. 1995. *Educating Special Learners* (4th ed.). Belmont, Calif.: Wadsworth.

Cassidy, C. M. 1980. 'Benign Neglect and Toddler Malnutrition'. In L. S. Greene and F. E. Johnston (eds.). *Social and Biological Predictors of Nutritional Status, Physical Growth and Neurological Development*. New York: Academic Press:109–139.

Chapman, D. W., Snyder, C. W. and Burchfield, S. A. 1993. 'Teacher Incentives in The Third World'. *Teaching and Teacher Education* 9:301–316.

Chinese Culture Connection 1987. 'Chinese Values and the Search for Culture-Free Dimensions of Culture'. *Journal of Cross-Cultural Psychology* 18:143–164.

Cleghorn, A., Merritt, M. and Abagi, J. O. 1989. 'Language Policy and Science Instruction in Kenyan Primary Schools'. *Comparative Education Review* 33:21–39.

Cleland, J. G. and van Ginneken, J. K. 1988. 'Maternal Education and Child Survival in Developing Countries: The Search for Pathways of Influence'. *Social Science and Medicine* 27:1357–1368.

Cliff, J. 2003. TAN, *Cassava Cyanide Diseases Network* News 2:4.

Cliff, J. and Noormahomed, A. R. 1993. 'The Impact of War on Children's Health in Mozambique'. *Social Science and Medicine* 36:843–848.

Cole, M., Gay, J., Glick, J. A. and Sharp, D. W. 1971. *The Cultural Context of Learning: An Exploration in Experimental Anthropology*. London: Methuen.

Colclough, C., Rose, P. and Tembon, M. 2000. 'Gender Inequalities in Primary Schooling: The Roles of Poverty and Adverse Cultural Practice'. *International Journal of Educational Development* 20:5–17.

Collier, A. F., McClure, F. H., Collier, J., Otto, C. and Polloi, A. 1999. 'Culture-Specific Views of Child Maltreatment and Parenting Styles in A Pacific-Island Community'. *Child Abuse and Neglect* 23:229–244.

Cooksey, B. 1981. 'Social Class and Academic Performance: A Cameroon Case Study'. *Comparative Education Review* 25:403–418.

Coopersmith, S. 1967 *The Antecedents of Self-Esteem*. San Francisco: W. H. Freeman.

Corral-Verdugo, V., Frias-Armenta, M., Romero, M. and Munoz, A. 1995. 'Validity of A Scale Measuring Beliefs Regarding The 'Positive' Effects of Punishing Children: A Study of Mexican Mothers'. *Child Abuse and Neglect* 19:669–679.

Courtois, R., Mullet, E. and Malvy, D. 2001a. 'Approche De La Sexualité Au Congo Dans Le Contexte Du Sida'. *Santé* 11:43–48.

Courtois, R., Mullet, E. and Malvy, D. 2001b. 'Comparaison des Comportements Sexuels de Lycéens Congolais et Francais dans le Contexte du Sida'. *Santé* 11:49–55.

Crocker, J. and Major, B. 1994. 'Reactions To Stigma: The Moderating Role of Justifications'. In M. P. Zanna and J. M. Olson (eds.). T*he Psychology of Prejudice: The Ontario Symposium* (vol.7). Hillsdale, NJ: Lawrence Erlbaum:289–314.

Cummings, E. M. 1987. 'Coping With Background Anger in Early Childhood'. *Child Development* 58:976–984.

Cummings, J. S., Pelligrini, D. S., Notarius, C. I. and Cummings, E. M. 1989. 'Children's Responses To Angry Adult Behavior As A Function of Marital Distress and History of Interparent Hostility'. *Child Development* 60:1035–1043.

Dasen, P. R. 1984. 'The Cross-Cultural Study of Intelligence: Piaget and the Baoule'. *International Journal of Psychology* 19:407–434.

Davis, T. L. 1995. 'Gender Differences in Masking Negative Emotions: Ability Or Motivation?' *Developmental Psychology* 31:660–667.

Davison, J. 1993. 'School Attainment and Gender: Attitudes of Kenyan and Malawian Parents Toward Educating Girls'. *International Journal of Educational Development* 13:331–338.

Davison, J. and Kanyuka, M. 1992. 'Girls' Participation in Basic Education in Southern Malawi'. *Comparative Education Review* 36:446–466.

Denham, S. A., McKinley, M., Couchoud, E. A. and Holt, R. 1990. 'Emotional and Behavioral Predictors of Preschool Peer Ratings'. *Child Development* 61:1145–1152.

Devlieger, P. 1995. 'Why Disabled? The Cultural Understanding of Physical Disability in an African Society'. In B. Ingstad and S. R. Whyte (eds.). *Disability and Culture*. Berkeley, Calif.: University of California Press:94–106.

De Vries, M. W. 1994. 'Kids in Context: Temperament in Cross-Cultural Perspective'. In W. B. Carey and S. McDevitt (eds.). *Prevention and Early Intervention: Individual Differences in Risk Factors For the Mental Health of Children: A Festschrift For Stella Chess and Alexander Thomas*. New York: Bruner/Mazel:126–139.

De Vries, M. W. and Sameroff, A. J. 1984. 'Culture and Temperament: Influences on Infant Temperament in Three East African Societies'. *American Journal of Orthopsychiatry* 54:83–96.

Dirie, W. 1998. *Desert Flower*. New York: Virago.

Dixon, S. D., Levine, R. A., Richman, A. and Brazelton, T. R. 1984. 'Mother-Child Interaction Around A Teaching Task: An African-American Comparison'. *Child Development* 55:1251–1262.

Dixon, S., Tronick, E., Keefer, C. and Brazelton, T. B. 1981. 'Mother-Infant Interaction among the Gusii of Kenya'. In T. M. Field, A. M. Sostek, P. Vietze and P. H. Leiderman (eds.). *Culture and Early Interaction*. Hillsdale, N.J.: Lawrence Erlbaum:149–170.

Dodge, C. P. 1990. 'Health Implications of War in Uganda and Sudan'. *Social Science and Medicine* 31:691–698.

Dolin, P. J., Faal, H., Johnson, G. J., Ajewole, J., Mohamet, A. A. and Lee, P S. 1998. 'Trachoma in The Gambia'. *British Journal of Ophthalmology* 82:930–933.

Draper, H. H. 1977. 'Biological, Cultural, and Social Determinants of Nutritional Status'. In P. H. Leiderman, S. R. Tulkin and A. Rosenfeld (eds.). *Culture and Infancy: Variations in the Human Experience*. New York: Academic Press:189–209.

Dyregrov, A. 1991. *Grief in Children: A Handbook For Adults*. London: Jessica Kingsley.

Ejiofor, L. U. 1981. *Dynamics of Igbo Democracy*. Ibadan, Nigeria: University Press.

Elliott, E. S. and Dweck, C. S. 1988. 'Goals: An Approach to Motivation and Achievement'. *Journal of Personality and Social Psychology* 54:5–12.

Elliott, J. 1989. 'Educational Theory and the Professional Learning of Teachers: An Overview'. *Cambridge Journal of Education* 19:81–101.

Elliott, J. M., Tong, C. K. and Tan, P. M. E. H. 1997. 'Attitudes of the Singapore Public to Actions Suggesting Child Abuse'. *Child Abuse and Neglect* 21:445–464.

Elliott, S. N., Kratochwill, T. R., Littlefield, J. and Travers, J. F. 1996. *Educational Psychology: Effective Teaching, Effective Learning* (2nd ed.). Dubuque, IA: Brown & Benchmark.

Emerson, P. M., Bailey, R. L., Walraven, G. E. and Lindsay, S. W. 2001. 'Human and Other Faeces As Breeding Media of the Trachoma Vector Musca Sorbens'. *Medical and Veterinary Entomology* 15:314–320.

Epanchin, B. C. 1987. 'Childhood and Adolescent Depression'. In B. C. Epanchin and J. L. Paul (eds.). *Emotional Problems of Childhood and Adolescence*. Columbus, Ohio: Merrill:198–214.

European Collaborative Study 1991. 'Children Born to Women with HIV-1 Infection: Natural History and Risk of Transmission'. *Lancet* 337(8736):253–260.

Fage, J. D. and Tordoff, W. 2002. *A History of Africa* (4th ed.). London: Routledge.

Fang, F-X. and Keats, D. M. 1989. '"The Master and the Wolf". A Study in the Development of Social Perspective Taking in Chinese and Australian Children'. In D. M. Keats, D Munro and L. Mann (eds.). *Heterogeneity in Cross-Cultural Psychology*. Amsterdam: Swets and Zeitlinger:419–425.

Farley, J. 1991. Bilharzia: *A History of Imperial Tropical Medicine*. Cambridge: Cambridge University Press.

Farrell, J. P. 1993. 'International Lessons For School Effectiveness: The View From the Developing World'. In J. P. Farrell and J. B. Oliveira (eds.). *Teachers in Developing Countries: Improving Effectiveness and Managing Costs*. Washington, D.C.: The World Bank:25–37.

Ferraro, G. P. 1993. 'Marriage and Conjugal Roles in Swaziland: Persistence and Change'. In M. S. Das (ed.). *The Family in Africa*. New Delhi: M. D.:89–128.

Fletcher, A. C., Darling, N. E., Steinberg, L. and Dornbusch, S. M. 1995. 'The Company They Keep: Relation of Adolescents' Adjustment and Behavior to their Friends' Perceptions of Authoritative Parenting in the Social Network'. *Developmental Psychology* 31:300–310.

Friere, P. 1972. *Pedagogy of the Oppressed*. London: Penguin.

Fuller, B. and Clarke, P. 1994. 'Raising School Effects While Ignoring Culture? Local Conditions and the Influence of Classroom Tools, Rules and Pedagogy'. *Review of Educational Research* 64:119–157.

Fuller, B., Hua, H. and Snyder, C. W. 1994. 'When Girls Learn More Than Boys: The Influence of Time in School and Pedagogy in Botswana'. *Comparative Education Review* 38:347–376.

Fuller, B., Snyder, C. W., Chapman, D. and Hua, H. 1994. 'Explaining Variation in Teaching Practices? Effects of State Policy, Teacher Background, and Curricula in Southern Africa'. *Teaching and Teacher Education* 10:141–156.

Fuller, B. and Snyder, C. W. 1991. 'Vocal Teachers, Silent Pupils? Life in Botswana Classrooms'. *Comparative Education Review* 35:274–294.

Gerdes, P. 1997. 'On Culture, Geometrical Thinking and Mathematics Education'. In A. B. Powell and M. Frankenstein (eds.). *Ethnomathematics: Challenging Eurocentrism in Mathematics Education*. Albany, N.Y.: State University of New York Press:223–247.

Glynn, J. R., Carael, M., Auvert, B., Kahindo, M., Chege, J., Musonda, R., Kaona, F., Buvé, A; Study Group on the Heterogeneity of HIV Epidemics in African Cities. 2001. 'Why Do Young Women Have a Much Higher Prevalence of HIV than Young Men? A Study in Kisumu, Kenya and Ndola, Zambia'. *Aids* 15 Supplement 4:S51–60.

Goldberg, S. 1977. 'Infant Development and Mother-Infant Interaction in Urban Zambia'. In P. H. Leiderman, S. R.Tulkin and A Rosenfeld (eds.). *Culture and Infancy: Variations in the Human Experience*. New York: Academic:211–243.

Goldschmidt, W. 1975. 'Absent Eyes and Idle Hands: Socialization for Low Affect among the Sebei'. *Ethos* 3:157–163.

Good, T. L. and Brophy, J. E. 1997. *Looking in Classrooms* (7th ed.). New York: Longman.

Goodnow, J. J., Cashmore, J., Cotton, S. and Knight, R. 1984. 'Mothers' Developmental Timetables in Two Cultures'. *International Journal of Psychology* 19:193–205.

Goodyer, I. M. 1990. *Life Experiences, Development and Child Psychopathology*. Chichester, England: John Wiley & Sons.

Graber, J. A., Brooks-Gunn, J. and Petersen, A. C. (eds.). 1996. *Transitions through Adolescence: Interpersonal Domains and Context*. Mahwah, NJ: Lawrence Erlbaum.

Gray, C., Baudouy, J., Martin, K., Bang, M. and Cash, R. 1990. *Primary Health Care in Africa: A Study of the Mali Rural Health Project*. Boulder, Colo.: Westview Press.

Greenberg, A. E., Nguyen-Dinh, P., Mann, J. M., Kabote, N., Colebunders, R. L., Francis, H., Quinn, T. C., Baudoux, P., Lyamba, B., Davachi, F., Roberts, J. M., Kabeya, N., Curran, J. W.

and Campbell, C. C. 1988. 'The Association between Malaria, Blood Transfusions, and HIV Seropositivity in a Pediatric Population in Kinshasa, Zaire'. *Journal of The American Medical Association* 259:545–549.

Halperin, D. T. and Bailey, R. C. 1999. 'Male Circumcision and HIV Infection: 10 Years and Counting'. *Lancet* 354:1813–1815.

Hamilton, G. and Gingiss, P. L. 1993. 'The Relationship of Teacher Attitudes to Course Implementation and Student Responses'. *Teaching and Teacher Education* 9(2):193–204.

Harkness, S. and Super, C. M. 1983. 'The Cultural Construction of Child Development: A Framework for the Socialization of Affect'. *Ethos* 11:221–231.

Harkness, S. and Super, C. M. 1985. 'The Cultural Context of Gender Segregation in Children's Peer Groups'. *Child Development* 56:219–224.

Harkness, S. and Super, C. M. 1991. 'East Africa'. In J. M. Hawes and N. R. Hiner (eds.). *Children in Historical and Comparative Perspective: An International Handbook and Research Guide.* New York: Greenwood Press:217–240.

Harkness, C., Super, C. M. and Keefer, C. H. 1992. 'Learning To Be An American Parent: How Cultural Models Gain Directive Force'. In R. G. D'Andrade (ed.). *Human Motives and Cultural Models.* Cambridge: Cambridge University Press:163–178.

Harkness, S. and Super, C. M. 1996. Introduction. In S. Harkness and C. M. Super (eds.). *Parents' Cultural Belief Systems: Their Origins, Expression, and Consequences.* New York: Guilford.

Harley, K., Barasa, F., Bertram, C., Mattson, E. and Pillay, S. 2000. '"The Real and the Ideal": Teacher Roles and Competences in South African Policy and Practice'. *International Journal of Educational Development* 20:287–304.

Harrison, A., Xaba, N. and Kunene, P. 2001. 'Understanding Safe Sex: Gender Narratives of HIV and Pregnancy Prevention by Rural South African School-Going Youth'. *Reproductive Health Matters* 9:63–71.

Hatcher, J., Smith, A., Mackenzie, I., Thompson, S., Bal, I., Macharia, I., Mugwe, P., Okoth-Olende, C., Oburra, H., Wanjohi, Z., Achola, N., Mirza, N. and Hart, A. 1995. 'A Prevalence Study of Ear Problems in School Children in Kiambu District, Kenya, May 1992'. *International Journal of Pediatric Otorhinolaryngology* 33:197–205.

Helander, B. 1995. 'Disability as Incurable Illness: Health, Process, and Personhood in Southern Somalia'. In B. Ingstad and S. R. Whyte (eds.). *Disability and Culture.* Berkeley, Calif.: University of California Press:73–93.

Herskovits, M. J. 1948. *Man and his Works.* New York: Knopf.

Hess, R. D., Kashiwagi, K., Azuma, H., Price, G. G. and Dickson, W. P. 1980. 'Maternal Expectations for Mastery of Developmental Tasks in Japan and The United States'. *International Journal of Psychology* 15:259–271.

Hetzel, B. S. 1990. 'The Iodine Deficiency Disorders'. In G. A. Harrison and J. C. Waterlow (eds.). *Diet and Disease in Traditional and Developing Societies.* Cambridge: Cambridge University Press:114–136.

Hewlett, B. S. 1992. 'Husband-Wife Reciprocity and the Father-Infant Relationship among Aka Pygmies'. In B. S. Hewlett (ed.). *Father-Child Relations: Cultural and Biosocial Contexts.* New York: Aldine De Gruyter:153–176.

Heyneman, S. P. and Loxley, W. A. 1983. 'The Effect of Primary-School Quality on Academic Achievement across Twenty-Nine High- and Low-Income Countries'. *American Journal of Sociology* 88:1162–1194.

Hirschfeld, L. A. 1996. *Race in the Making: Cognition, Culture, and the Child's Construction of Human Kinds*. Cambridge: Mass.: MIT Press.

Hofstede, G. 1980. *Culture's Consequences: International Differences in Work-Related Values*. Beverly Hills, Calif.: Sage.

Hofstede, G. 1986. 'Cultural Differences in Teaching and Learning'. *International Journal of Intercultural Relations* 10:301–320.

Hollins, E. R. 1996. *Culture in School Learning: Revealing the Deep Meaning*. Mahwah, N.J.: Lawrence Erlbaum.

Holt, J. 1982. *How Children Fail*. Harmondsworth, England: Penguin.

Holt, J. 1984. *How Children Learn*. Harmondsworth, England: Penguin.

Hopkins, D. and Stern, D. 1996. 'Quality Teachers, Quality Schools: International Perspectives and Policy Implications'. *Teaching and Teacher Education* 12:501–517.

Howell, E. R. and Peachey, G. T. 1990. 'Visual Dysfunction and Learning'. In S. R. Butler (ed.). *The Exceptional Child: An Introduction to Special Education*. Sydney: Harcourt Brace Jovanovich:223–238.

Hsu, C-S., Soong, W-T., Stigler, J. W., Hong, C-C. and Liang, C-C. 1981. 'The Temperamental Characteristics of Chinese Babies'. *Child Development* 52:1337–1340.

Hudson, M. 1989. *Our Grandmothers' Drums*. London: Secker & Warburg.

Hughes, F. P. 1995. *Children, Play, and Development* (2nd ed.). Boston: Allyn & Bacon.

Hunter, S. S. 1990. 'Orphans as A Window on the Aids Epidemic in Sub-Saharan Africa: Initial Results and Implications of a Study in Uganda'. *Social Science and Medicine* 31:681–690.

Illingworth, R. S. 1991 *The Normal Child: Some Problems of Early Development and Their Treatment* (10th ed.) Edinburgh: Churchill Livingstone.

Irwin, M.H. and Mclaughlin, D. H. 1970. 'Ability and Preference in Category Sorting by Mano Schoolchildren and Adults'. *Journal of Social Psychology* 82:15–24.

Ijzendoorn, M. H. Van and Kroonenberg, P. M. 1988. 'Cross-Cultural Patterns of Attachment: A Meta-Analysis of the Strange Situation'. *Child Development* 59:147–156.

Jackson, S. and Rodriguez-Tomé, H. 1993. 'Adolescence: Expanding Social Worlds'. In S. Jackson and H. Rodriguez-Tome (eds.). *Adolescence and Its Social Worlds*. Hove, England: Lawrence Erlbaum:1–14.

Jareg, E. 1996. 'Basic Therapeutic Actions: Helping Children, Young People and Communities Cope through Empowerment and Participation'. In M. Mccallin (ed.). *The Psychological Wellbeing of Refugee Children: Research, Practice and Policy Issues* (2nd ed.). Geneva: International Catholic Child Bureau:168–175.

Jayasuriya, L. 1993, October. 'Transcultural Psychiatry: Some Emerging Issues'. Paper Presented at The First Asian Psychology Conference, Singapore.

Jefferson, T., Herbst, J. H. and McCrae, R. R. 1990. 'Associations between Birth Order and Personality Traits: Evidence from Self-Reports and Observer Ratings'. *Journal of Research in Personality* 32:498–509.

Jessop, T. and Penny, A. 1998. 'A Study of Teacher Voice and Vision in the Narratives of Rural South African and Gambian Primary School Teachers'. *International Journal of Educational Development* 18:393–403.

Jeter, J. 2001. 'Angola Handicapped by a Culture of Corruption'. *Guardian Weekly* November 29 – December 5:33.

Jones, D. P. H. 2000. 'Editorial: Mental Health Problems among Children Living in War Zones'. *Child Abuse and Neglect* 24:289–290.

Jones, L. 2001. 'Teachers Blamed for Aids Crisis in Schools'. *Guardian Weekly* August 30–September 5:3.

Kagitcibasi, C. 1992. 'Research in Child Development, Parenting and the Family in a Cross-Cultural Perspective'. In M. R. Rosenzweig (ed.). *International Psychological Science: Progress, Problems, and Prospects*. Washington: American Psychological Association:137–160.

Kagitcibasi, C. 1996. *Family and Human Development across Cultures: A View from the Other Side*. Mahwah, NJ: Erlbaum.

Kaplan, M. E. and Van Den Worm, Y. 1993. 'The Relationship between South African Adolescents' Knowledge and Fear of Aids and Their Attitudes toward People Who Have Aids'. *Journal of Social Psychology* 133:581–583.

Kastenbaum, R. 1992. *The Psychology of Death* (2nd ed.). New York: Springer.

Kayongo-Male, D. and Onyango, P. 1984. *The Sociology of the African Family*. London: Longman.

Kazdin, A. E. 1989. *Behavior Modification in Applied Settings*. Pacific Grove, Calif.: Brooks/Cole.

Keefer, C. H., Tronick, E., Dixon, S. and Brazelton, T. B. 1982. 'Specific Differences in Motor Performance between Gusii and Americans and a Modification of the Neonatal Behavioural Assessment Scale'. *Child Development* 53:754–759.

Khoo, S. E. and Price, C. A. 1996. *Understanding Australia's Ethnic Composition*. Canberra, Australia: Australian Government Publishing Service.

Kilbourn, P. 1995a. 'The Impact of War on Children: A Kaleidoscope of Experiences, Emotions and Traumas'. In P. Kilbourn (ed.). *Healing the Children of War: A Handbook for Ministry to Children Who Have Suffered Deep Traumas*. Monrovia, Calif.: MARC:7–30.

Kilbourn, P. 1995b. 'An Introduction to the STOP Sign Model'. In P. Kilbourn (ed.). *Healing the Children of War: A Handbook for Ministry to Children Who Have Suffered Deep Traumas*. Monrovia, Calif.: MARC:133–146.

Kilbride, J. E. and Kilbride, P. L. 1975. 'Sitting and Smiling Behavior of Baganda Infants'. *Journal of Cross-Cultural Psychology* 6:88–107.

Kilbride, P. L. 1980. 'Sensorimotor Behavior of Baganda and Samia Infants: A Controlled Comparison'. *Journal of Cross-Cultural Psychology* 11:131–152.

Kilbride, P. L. and Kilbride, J. E 1974. 'Sociocultural Factors and the Early Manifestation of Sociability Behavior among Baganda Infants'. *Ethos* 2:296–314.

Kilbride, P. L. and Kilbride, J. E. 1983. 'Socialization for High Positive Affect between Mother and Infant among the Baganda of Uganda'. *Ethos* 14:232–245.

Kilbride, P. L. and Kilbride, J. C. 1990. *Changing Family Life in East Africa: Women and Children at Risk*. University Park, Pa.: Pennsylvania State University Press.

Kilbride, P. L. and Leibowitz, H. W. 1975. 'Factors Affecting the Magnitude of the Ponzo Perspective Illision among the Baganda'. *Perception and Psychophysics* 17:543–548.

Kinsman, J., Harrison, S., Kengeya-Kayondo, J., Kanyesigye, E., Musoke, N. and Whitworth, J. 1999. 'Implementation of a Comprehensive Aids Education Programme for Schools in Masaka District, Uganda'. *Aids Care* 11:591–601.

Kirk, S. A. and Gallagher, J. J. 1983. *Educating Exceptional Children* (4th ed.). Boston: Houghton Mifflin.

Kivilu, J. M. and Rogers, W. T. 1998. 'A Multi-Level Analysis of Cultural Experience and Gender Influences on Causal Attributions to Perceived Performance in Mathematics'. *British Journal of Educational Psychology* 68:25–37.

Klepp, K. I., Ndeki, S. S. Leshabari, M. T., Hannan, P. J. and Lyimo, B. A. 1997. 'Aids Education in Tanzania: Promoting Risk Reduction among Primary School Children'. *American Journal of Public Health* 87:1931–1936.

Kohn, M. L. 1969. *Class and Conformity: A Study in Values*. Homewood, Ill.: Dorsey.

Konner, M. 1977. 'Infancy among the Kalahari Desert San'. In P. H. Leiderman, S. R. Tulkin and A. Rosenfeld (eds.). *Culture and Infancy: Variations in the Human Experience*. New York: Academic Press:287–328.

Kunii, O. and Shibuya, K. 1999. 'Women's Beliefs About Breastfeeding and Transmission of Aids in Rural Côte d'Ivoire'. *Journal of The American Medical Association* 282:733.

Kyrios, M., Prior, M., Oberklaid, F. and Demetriou, A. 1989. 'Cross-Cultural Studies of Temperament: Temperament in Greek Infants'. *International Journal of Psychology* 24:585–603.

Lagarde, E., Pison, G. and Enel, C. 1996. 'Knowledge, Attitudes and Perception of Aids in Rural Senegal: Relationship to Sexual Behaviour and Behaviour Change'. *Aids* 10:327–334.

Lalonde, R. N. and Cameron, J. E. 1994. 'Behavioral Responses To Discrimination: A Focus on Action'. In M. P. Zanna and J. M. Olson (eds). *The Psychology of Prejudice: The Ontario Symposium* (vol. 7). Hillsdale, NJ: Lawrence Erlbaum:257–288.

Lecoeur, S. and Lallemant, M. 1996. 'Pediatric HIV/Aids'. In J. M. Mann and D. J. M. Tarantola (eds). *Aids in the World II: Global Dimensions, Social Roots and Responses*. New York: Oxford University Press:273–277.

Lee, J. 2001. 'Battle To Halt Cyanide Poisoning in Africa: ANU Test To Fight Konzo'. *ANU Reporter* 32:1.

Leibowitz, H.W. and Pick, H. A. 1972. 'Cross-Cultural and Educational Aspects of the Ponzo Perspective Illusion'. *Perception and Psychophysics* 12:430–432.

Leiderman, P. H. and Leiderman, G. F. 1974. 'Familial Influences on Infant Development in an East African Agricultural Community'. In E. J. Anthony and C. Koupernik (eds). *The Child in His Family* (vol. III). New York: John Wiley:305–330.

Leshabari, M. T., Pounds, M. B. and Celentano, D. D. 1988. 'Heterosexual Behavior of Adolescents in Dar-Es-Salaam, Tanzania'. In R. Kulsted (ed.). *Aids 1988: AAAS Symposia Papers*. Washington, DC: American Association For the Advancement of Science:183–190.

Lesthaeghe, R. and Eelens, F.1989. 'The Components of Sub-Saharan Regimes and Their Social and Cultural Determinants: Empirical Evidence'. In R. J. Lesthaeghe (ed.). *Reproduction and Social Organization in Sub-Saharan Africa*. Berkeley, Calif.: University of California Press:60–89.

Lesthaeghe, R., Page, H. J. and Adegbola, O. 1981. 'Child-Spacing and Fertility in Lagos'. In H. J. Page and R. Lesthaeghe (eds). *Child-Spacing in Tropical Africa: Traditions and Change*. London: Academic:147–180.

Lesthaeghe, R., Vanderhoeft, C., Gaisie, S. and Delaine, G. 1989. 'Regional Variation in Components of Child-Spacing: The Role of Women's Education'. In R. J. Lesthaeghe (ed.). *Reproduction and Social Organization in Sub-Saharan Africa*. Berkeley, Calif.: University of California Press:122–166.

Levine, C., Michaels, D. and Back, S. D. 1996. 'Orphans of the HIV/Aids Pandemic'. In J. M. Mann and D. J. M. Tarantola (eds). *Aids in the World II: Global Dimensions, Social Roots and Responses*. New York: Oxford University Press:278–286.

Levine, R. A. 1977. 'Child Rearing as Cultural Adaptation'. In P. H. Leiderman, S. R. Tulkin and A. Rosenfeld (eds). *Culture and Infancy: Variations in the Human Experience*. New York: Academic:15–27.

Levine, R. A., Dixon, S., Levine, S., Richman, A., Leiderman, P. H., Keefer, C. H. and Brazelton, T. B. 1996. *Childcare and Culture: Lessons from Africa*. Cambridge: Cambridge University Press.

Liddell, C. 1997. 'Every Picture Tells A Story – Or Does It? Young South African Children Interpreting Pictures'. *Journal of Cross-Cultural Psychology* 28:266–283.

Lightfoot-Klein, H. 1989. *Prisoners of Ritual: An Odyssey into Female Genital Circumcision in Africa*. New York: Harrington Park.

Lin, C-Y. C. and Fu, V. R. 1990. 'A Comparison of Child-Rearing Practices among Chinese, Immigrant Chinese, and Caucasian-American Parents'. *Child Development* 61:429–433.

Lloyd, B. B. 1970. 'Yoruba Mothers' Reports of Child-Rearing. Some Theoretical and Methodological Considerations: Research Design, Setting and Procedures'. In P. Mayer (ed.). *Socialization: The Approach From Social Anthropology*. London: Tavistock:75–108.

Lloyd, C. B., Mensch, B. S. and Clark, W. H. 2000. 'The Effects of Primary School Quality on School Dropout among Kenyan Girls and Boys'. *Comparative Education Review* 44:113–147.

Lockheed, M. E. and Komenan, A. 1989. 'Teaching Quality and Student Achievement in Africa: The Case of Nigeria and Swaziland'. *Teaching and Teacher Education* 5:93–113.

Lowy, M. J. 1974. 'Me Ko Court: The Impact of Urbanization on Conflict Resolution in a Ghanaian Town'. In G. M. Foster and B. V. Kemper (eds). *Anthropologists in Cities*. Boston: Little, Brown & Co:153–177.

Mabey, D. and Fraser-Hurt, N. 2001. 'Trachoma'. *British Medical Journal* 323:218–221.

Mccallin, M. (ed.), *The Psychological Wellbeing of Refugee Children: Research, Practice and Policy Issues* (2nd ed.). Geneva: International Catholic Child Bureau.

Mccallin, M. and Jareg, E. 1996. 'The Rehabilitation and Social Reintegration of Child Soldiers'. In M. Mccallin (ed.). *The Psychological Wellbeing of Refugee Children: Research, Practice and Policy Issues* (2nd ed.). Geneva: International Catholic Child Bureau:192–217.

Machel, J. Z. 2001. 'Unsafe Sexual Behaviour among Schoolgirls in Mozambique: A Matter of Gender and Class'. *Reproductive Health Matters* 9:82–90.

Macgregor, J. 2000. *Introduction to the Anatomy and Physiology of Children.* London: Routledge.

Mcinerney, D. M. and Mcinerney, V. 1998. *Educational Psychology: Constructing Learning* (2nd ed.). Sydney, Australia: Prentice Hall.

Macintyre, K., Brown, L and Sosler, S. 2001. '"It's Not What You Know, But Who You Know": Examining the Relationship between Behavior Changes and Aids Mortality in Africa'. *Aids Education and Prevention* 13:160–174.

Mackey, W. C. 1981. 'A Cross-Cultural Analysis of Adult-Child Proxemics in relation to the Plowman-Protector Complex: A Preliminary Study'. *Behavior Science Research* 16:187–223.

Maclachlan, M., Chimombo, M. and Mpemba, N. 1997. 'Aids Education for Youth through Active Learning: A School-Based Approach from Malawi'. *International Journal of Educational Development* 17:41–50.

Magnani, R. J., Karim, A. M., Weiss, L. A., Bond, K. C., Lemba, M. and Morgan, G. T. 2002. 'Reproductive Health Risk and Protective Factors among Youth in Lusaka, Zambia'. *Journal of Adolescent Health* 30:76–86.

Makulu, H. F. 1971. *Education, Development and Nation-Building in Independent Africa.* London: SCM.

Malmberg, L-E., Wanner, B., Sumra, S. and Little, T. D. 2001. 'Action-Control Beliefs and School Experiences of Tanzanian Primary School Students'. *Journal of Cross-Cultural Psychology* 32:577–596.

Martorell, R. 1980. 'Interrelationships between Diet, Infectious Disease, and Nutritional Status'. In L. S. Greene and F. E. Johnston (eds). *Social and Biological Predictors of Nutritional Status, Physical Growth and Neurological Development.* New York: Academic:81–108.

Matchinda, B. 1999. 'The Impact of Home Background on the Decision of Children to Run Away: The Case of Yaounde City Street Children in Cameroon'. *Child Abuse and Neglect* 23: 245–255.

Mathews, C., Everett, K., Binedell, J. and Steinberg, M. 1995. 'Learning To Listen: Formative Research in the Development of Aids Education for Secondary School Students'. *Social Science and Medicine* 41:1715–1724.

Mayer, P. and Mayer, I. 1970. 'Socialization By Peers: The Youth Organization of The Red Xhosa'. In P. Mayer (ed.). *Socialization: The Approach from Social Anthropology.* London: Tavistock:159–190.

Mazrui, A. A. 1986. *The Africans: A Triple Heritage.* London: BBC.

Mcgreal, C. 2001. 'Orphans of Aids Face A Lonely Struggle For Life'. *Guardian Weekly* December 6–12:22.

Millar, S. 1968. *The Psychology of Play.* London: Penguin.

Minja, B. M. and Machemba, A. 1996. 'Prevalence of Otitis Media, Hearing Impairment and Cerumen Impaction among School Children in Rural and Urban Dar Es Salaam, Tanzania'. *International Journal of Pediatric Otorhinolaryngology* 37:29–34.

Modiba, M. 1997. 'Distance Teacher Education in South Africa: A Critical Analysis of Pedagogical Assumptions'. *Teaching and Teacher Education* 13:727–739.

Moore, S. M. and Rosenthal, D. A. 1991. 'Condoms and Coitus: Adolescents Attitudes to Aids and Safe Sex Behavior'. *Journal of Adolescence* 14:211–227.

Mouly, G. J. 1982. *Psychology for Teaching*. Boston: Allyn & Bacon.

Mulder, M. B. and Milton, M. 1985. 'Factors Affecting Infant Care in the Kipsigis'. *Journal of Anthropological Research* 41:231–262.

Mulwa, D. 1979. *Master and Servant*. Harlow: Longman.

Munroe, R. L. and Munroe, R. H. 1992. 'Fathers in Children's Environments: A Four Culture Study'. In B. S. Hewlett (ed.). *Father-Child Relations: Cultural and Biosocial Contexts*. New York: Aldine De Gruyter:213–230.

Munroe, R. H. and Munroe, R. L. 1984. 'Infant Experience and Childhood Cognition'. *Ethos* 12:291–305.

Myers, D. 1990. *Social Psychology* (3rd ed.). New York: McGraw-Hill.

Naslund, M. 1997. 'An Investigation of War Related Trauma Experiences and Psychological Symptomatology of Young Refugees'. Unpublished master's thesis, Monash University, Melbourne, Australia.

Ndlovu, R. J. and Sihlangu, R. H. 1992. 'Preferred Sources of Information on Aids among High School Students from Selected Schools in Zimbabwe'. *Journal of Advanced Nursing* 17:507–513.

Network 1993. *Adolescents*. Family International 14(2).

Neubauer, G. and Meltzer, W. 1989. 'The Role of School, Family, and the Peer Group in the Sexual Development of the Adolescent'. In K. Hurrelmann and U. Engel (eds). *The Social World of Adolescents: International Perspectives*. Berlin: Walter De Gruyter:321–338.

Nicholas, L. and Durrheim, K. 1995. 'Religiosity, Aids, and Sexuality Knowledge, Attitudes, Beliefs, and Practices of Black South African First-Year University Students'. *Psychological Reports* 77:1328–1330.

Nobles, W. W. 1995. 'Psychological Research and the Black Self-Concept: A Critical Review'. In N. R. Goldberger and J. B. Veroff (eds). *The Culture and Psychology Reader*. New York: New York University Press:164–183.

Nsamenang, A. B. 1992a. *Human Development in Cultural Context: A Third World Perspective*. Newbury Park, Calif.: Sage.

Nsamenang, B. A. 1992b. 'Perceptions of Parenting among the Nso of Cameroon'. In B. S. Hewlett (ed.). *Father-Child Relations: Cultural and Biosocial Contexts*. New York: Aldine De Gruyter:321–344.

Ntiri, D. W. 1993. 'Experimenting with Family Life Centres in Africa's Development: A Case Study in Somalia, East Africa'. In M. S. Das (ed.). *The Family in Africa*. New Delhi: M. D.:73–88.

Nyanzi, S., Pool, R. and Kinsman, J. 2001. 'The Negotiation of Sexual Relationships among School Pupils in South-Western Uganda'. *Aids Care* 13:83–98.

Nyiti, R. M. 1976. 'The Development of Conservation in The Meru Children of Tanzania'. *Child Development* 47:1122–1129.

Nzioka, C. 2001. 'Perspectives of Adolescent Boys on the Risks of Unwanted Pregnancy and Sexually Transmitted Infections: Kenya'. *Reproductive Health Matters* 9:108–117.

O'Connor, J., Lynch, M., Vitale, S. and West, W. 1999. 'Characteristics of Effective Village Treatment Assistants, The Kwonga Trachoma Project'. *Ophthalmic Epidemiology* 6:257–265.

Ogbu, J. U. 1981. 'Origins of Human Competence: A Cultural-Ecological Perspective'. *Child Development* 52:413–429.

Ogbu, J. U. 1988. 'Cultural Diversity and Human Development'. In D. T. Slaughter (ed.). *Black Children and Poverty: A Developmental Perspective*. (New Directions For Child Development No 42.) San Francisco: Jossey-Bass:11–28.

Okeyo, A. P. 1980. 'Daughters of the Lakes and Rivers: Colonization and the Land Rights of Luo Women'. In M. Etienne and E Leacock (eds). *Women and Colonization: Anthropological Perspectives*. New York: Praeger.

Olasehinde, M. O. 1972. 'An Analytical Study of the Motives of Primary School Teachers For Choosing Teaching As A Career'. *Journal of Teacher Education* 23:207–210.

Omoegun, O. M. 1997. *The Adolescent and You*. Lagos, Nigeria: Mobolak.

Omolulu, A. 1974. 'Nutritional Factors in the Vulnerability of the African Child'. In E. J. Anthony and C. Koupernik (eds). *The Child in his Family* (vol. III). New York: John Wiley:331–336.

Onwuejeogwu, M. A. 1975. *The Social Anthropology of Africa: An Introduction*. London: Heinemann.

Onyango, A., Tucker, K. and Eisemon, T. 1994. 'Household Headship and Child Nutrition: A Case Study in Western Kenya'. *Social Science and Medicine* 39:1633–1639.

Owuamanam, D. O. 1982. 'Adolescent Values in the 80s: Implications for Living in Society'. Unpublished Mimeograph. University of Ife, Nigeria.

Page,. H. J. 1989. 'Childrearing Versus Childbearing: Coresidence of Mother and Child in Sub-Saharan Africa'. In R. J. Lesthaege (ed.). *Reproduction and Social Organization in Sub-Saharan Africa*. Berkeley, Calif.: University of California Press:401–441.

Palmer, N. L. N. 1993. *The Impact of Maternal Education on Infant and Child Mortality and Morbidity in the Cameroon Grasslands*. Ann Arbor, Mich.: University Microfilms International.

Panter-Brick, C. 1998. 'Biological Anthropology and Child Health: Context, Process and Outcome'. In C. Panter-Brick (ed.). *Biosocial Perspectives on Children*. Cambridge: Cambridge University Press:66–101.

Parks, Y. A. and Wharton, B. 1990. 'Iron Deficiency and the Brain: Clinical Significance of Behavioural Changes'. In J. Dobbing (ed.). *Brain, Behaviour, and Iron in the Infant Diet*. London: Springer-Verlag:157–176.

Partington, G. and Mccudden, V. 1992. *Ethnicity and Education*. Wentworth Falls, NSW, Australia: Social Sciences Press.

Pattullo, A. L., Malonza, M., Kimani, G. G., Muthee, A., Otieno, P. A., Odhiambo, K., Moses, S. and Plummer, F. A. 1994. 'Survey of Knowledge, Behaviour and Attitudes Relating To HIV Infection and Aids among Kenyan Secondary School Students'. *Aids Care* 6:173–181.

Pedlow, R., Sanson, A., Prior, M. and Oberklaid, F. 1993. 'Stability of Maternally Reported Temperament From Infancy To 8 Years'. *Developmental Psychology* 29:998–1007.

Pellegrini, A. D. and Smith, P. K. 1998. 'Physical Activity Play: The Nature and Function of a Neglected Aspect of Play'. *Child Development* 69:577–598.

Peltzer, K. 2001. 'Factors Affecting Behaviors That Address HIV Risk among Senior Secondary School Pupils in South Africa'. *Psychological Reports* 89:51–56.

Piaget, J. and Inhelder, B. 1966/1969. *The Psychology of the Child.* London: Routledge & Kegan Paul (original published in French).

Pinxten, R. 1997. 'Applications in the Teaching of Mathematics and the Sciences'. In A. R. Powell and M. Frankenstein (eds). *Ethnomathematics: Challenging Eurocentrism in Mathematics Education.* Albany, N.Y.: State University of New York Press:373–402.

Plotnikoff, N., Murgo, A., Faith, R. and Wybran, J. (eds) 1991. *Stress and Immunity.* Boca Raton, Fla.: CRC.

Pollitt, E. 1990. *Malnutrition and Infection in the Classroom.* Paris: UNESCO.

Ponterotto, J. G. 1991. 'The Nature of Prejudice Revisited: Implications For Counseling Intervention'. *Journal of Counseling and Development* 70:216–224.

Preble, E. A. 1990. 'Impact of HIV/Aids on African Children'. *Social Science and Medicine* 31:671–680.

Prior, M. 1992. *Childhood Temperament. Journal of Child Psychology and Psychiatry* 33:249–279.

Qasem, F. S., Mustafa, A. A., Kazem, N. A. and Shah, N. M. 1998. 'Attitudes of Kuwaiti Parents Toward Physical Punishment of Children'. *Child Abuse and Neglect* 22:1189–1202.

Rabain-Jamin, J. 1989. 'Culture and Early Social Interactions: The Example of Mother-Infant Object Play in African and Native French Families'. *European Journal of Psychology of Education* 4:295–305.

Rama, C. 2001. 'Somalia Suffers in A Book Bind'. *The Canberra Times* June 23 2001:11.

Reed, G. and Leiderman, P. H. 1981. 'Age-Related Changes in Attachment Behavior in Polymatrically Reared Infants: The Kenyan Gusii'. In T. M. Field, A. M. Sostek, P. Vietze and P. H. Leiderman (eds). *Culture and Early Interactions.* Hillsdale, N.J.: Lawrence Erlbaum:215–236.

Reilly, C. 2001. *Give Africa Girl Power.* Guardian Weekly June 28–July 4:11.

Reykowski, J. 1994. 'Individualism and Collectivism As Dimensions of Social Change'. In U. Kim, H. C. Triandis, C. Kagitcibasi, S-C. Choi and G. Yoon (eds). *Individualism and Collectivism: Theory, Methods and Applications.* Thousand Oaks, Calif.: Sage:276–292.

Reynolds, P. 1990. 'The Double Strategy of Children in South Africa'. In P. A. Adler and P. Adler (eds). *Sociological Studies of Child Development: A Research Annual* (vol. 3). Greenwich, Conn.: JAI:113–137.

Richman, A. L., Miller, P. M. and Levine, R. A. 1992. 'Cultural and Educational Variations in Maternal Responsiveness'. *Developmental Psychology* 28:614–621.

Ridley, C. R. 1989. 'Racism in Counseling as an Adverse Behavioral Process'. In P. B. Pedersen, J. G. Draguns, W. J. Lonner and J. E. Trimble (eds). *Counseling across Cultures* (3rd ed.). Honolulu: University of Hawaii Press:55–77.

Robinson, E. 1993. 'The Effects of Family Background on Pupils' Academic Achievement in Mozambique'. *International Journal of Educational Development* 13:289–294.

Rodney, W. 1982. *How Europe Underdeveloped Africa.* Washington: Howard University Press.

Rogoff, B. 1981. 'Schooling and the Development of Cognitive Skills'. In H. C. Triandis and A. Herron (eds). Handbook of Cross-Cultural Psychology (vol. 4): *Developmental Psychology*. Boston: Allyn & Bacon:233–294.

Rohner, R. P. and Pettengill, S. M. 1985. 'Perceived Parental Acceptance-Rejection and Parental Control among Korean Adolescents'. *Child Development* 56:524–528.

Rosenthal, R. and Jacobson, L. 1968. *Pygmalion in the Classroom*. New York: Holt, Rinehart & Winston.

Rossman, B. B. R. 1992. 'School-Age Children's Perceptions of Coping with Distress: Strategies for Emotion Regulation and the Moderation of Adjustment'. *Journal of Child Psychology and Psychiatry* 33:1373–1397.

Ruthven, M. 1991. *Islam in the World*. London: Penguin.

Ryback, D., Sanders, A. L., Lorentz, J. and Koestenblatt, M. 1980. 'Child-Rearing Practices Reported By Students in Six Cultures'. *Journal of Social Psychology* 110:153–162.

Saarni, C. 1988. 'Children's Understanding of the Interpersonal Consequences of Dissemblance of Nonverbal Emotional-Expressive Behavior'. *Journal of Nonverbal Behaviour* 12:275–294.

Sallah, E. D., Grunitzky-Bekele, M., Bassabi, K., Dodzro, K., Sadzo, A., Balogou, A. K., Grunitzky, E. K. and Gaudreau, L. 1999. 'Comportements Sexuels, Connaissances Et Attitudes Des Étudiants De l'Université Du Benin (Togo) Face Au Sida Et Aux Maladies Sexuellement Transmissibles'. *Santé* 9:101–110.

Sarno, L. 1993. *Song from the Forest: My Life among The Ba-Banjelle Pygmies*. New York: Houghton Mifflin.

Save the Children 1990. *Prospects for Africa's Children*. London.

Schmidt, W. H. O. and Nzimande, A. 1970. 'Cultural Differences in Color/Form Preference in Classificatory Behaviour'. *Human Development* 13:140–148.

Schwartz, S. H. 1994. 'Are There Universal Aspects in the Structure and Contents of Human Values?' *Journal of Social Issues* 50(4):19–45.

Schwartz, S. H. 1996. 'Individual and Cultural Value Dimensions: Statistical Improvements Yes: But Conceptually As Confused As Ever'. Paper Presented At The 13th Congress of The International Association For Cross-Cultural Psychology, Montreal, Canada, August 1996.

Scott, J., Williams, J. M. G. and Beck, A. T. 1989. *Cognitive Therapy in Clinical Practice: An Illustrative Casebook*. London: Routledge.

Seboni, N. M. 1993 'Botswana Female Youth Perception of Sexuality and Risk Taking Behaviours'. Unpublished dissertation, UCSA, San Francisco.

Seboni, N. M., Dambe, M. and Abosi, O. 1999. *Socio-Cultural Study of Botswana*. Gaborone, Botswana: UNFPA/Ministry of Education.

Sekgoma, N. 1994. Secondary School Students' *Aids Related Knowledge: Attitude Towards Alcohol Consumption Between Rural and Urban Youth in Botswana*. Gaborone: University of Botswana.

Setumbwe, N. 1995. 'Sighted Lovers and Blind Husbands: Experiences of Blind Women in Uganda'. In B. Ingstad and S. R. Whyte (eds). *Disability and Culture*. Berkeley, Calif.: University of California Press:159–173.

Shaver, P., Schwartz, J., Kirson, D. and O'Connor, C. 1987. 'Emotion Knowledge: Further Exploration of a Prototype Approach'. *Journal of Personality and Social Psychology* 52:1061–1086.

Shaw, J. A. and Harris, J. J. 1994. 'Children of War and Children At War: Child Victims of Terrorism in Mozambique'. In R. J. Ursano, B. G. Mccaughey and C. S. Fullerton (eds). *Individual and Community Responses to Trauma and Disaster: The Structure of Human Chaos*. Cambridge: Cambridge University Press:287–305.

Shelley, J. K. 1985. *Medicines For Misfortune: Diagnosis and Health Care among Southern Turkana Pastoralists of Kenya*. Ann Arbor, Mich.: University Microfilms International.

Shuey, D., Bagarukayo, H., Senkusu, S. and Ryan, K. 1996. 'A Community-Based Progam For Orphans and Vulnerable Children, Luwero District, Uganda: Strategies For Implementation'. In J. M. Mann and D. J. M. Tarantola (eds). *Aids in the World II: Global Dimensions, Social Roots and Responses*. New York: Oxford University Press:283–285.

SIAPAC Aids Unit 1994. *Monitoring Trends in Youth Sexual Behaviour*. Gaborone.

Sigel, E. and Kim, M-I. 1996. 'The Answer Depends on the Question: A Conceptual and Methodological Analysis of A Parent Belief-Behavior Interview Regarding Children's Learning'. In S. Harkness and C. M. Super (eds). *Parents' Cultural Belief Systems: Their Origins, Expressions and Consequences*. New York: Guilford:83–122.

Sigman, M., Neumann, C., Carter, E., Cattle, D. J., C-Souza, S. and Bwibo, N. 1988. 'Home Interactions and the Development of Embu Toddlers in Kenya'. *Child Development* 59:1251–1261.

Sigman, M., Neumann, C., Jansen, A. A. and Bwibo, N. 1989. 'Cognitive Abilities of Kenyan Children in Relation To Nutrition, Family Characteristics, and Education'. *Child Development* 60:1463–1474.

Silverman, P.R. and Worden, J. W. 1993. 'Children's Reactions to the Death of a Parent'. In M. S. Stroebe, W. Stroebe and R. D. Hansson (eds). *Handbook of Bereavement*. Cambridge: Cambridge University Press:300–316.

Simons, J. A., Kalichman, S. and Santrock, J. W. 1994. *Human Adjustment*. Madison, Wis.: Brown & Benchmark.

Smith, K. D. 1995. 'Social Psychological Perspectives on Lay Persons' Theories of Emotion'. In J. A. Russell, J-M Fernandez-Dols, A. S. R. Manstead and J. C. Wellenkamp (eds). *Everday Conceptions of Emotion: An Introduction to the Psychology, Anthropology and Linguistics of Emotion*. Dordrecht, Holland: Kluwer Academic:399–414.

Smith, L C. and Haddad, L. 2000. *Explaining Child Malnutrition in Developing Countries*. Washington, DC: International Food Policy Research Institute.

Smith, P. B. and Bond, M. H. 1993. *Social Psychology across Cultures: Analysis and Perspectives*. Hemel Hempstead, England: Harvester Wheatsheaf.

Solomon, A. W., Akudibillah, J., Abugri, P., Hagan, M., Foster, A., Bailey, R. L. and Mabey, D. C. 2001. 'Pilot Study of the Use of Community Volunteers To Distribute Azithromycin For Trachoma Control in Ghana'. *Bulletin of The World Health Organization* 79:8–14.

Somé, M. P. 1999 *The Healing Wisdom of Africa: Finding Life Purpose Through Nature, Ritual and Community*. London: Thorsons.

Steinberg, L, Lamborn, S. D., Darling, N., Mounts, N. S. and Dornbusch, S. M. 1994. 'Over-Time Changes in Adjustment and Competence among Adolescents from Authoritative, Authoritarian, Indulgent, and Neglectful Families'. *Child Development* 65:754–770.

Stephan, W. G., Diaz-Loving, R. and Duran, A. 2000. 'Integrated Threat Theory and Intercultural Attitudes: Mexico and The United States'. *Journal of Cross-Cultural Psychology* 31:240–249.

Stephens, D. 2000. 'Girls and Basic Education in Ghana: A Cultural Enquiry'. *International Journal of Educational Development* 20:29–47.

Stoppard, M. 2001. *Conception, Pregnancy, and Birth.* Ringwood, Vic., Australia: Dorling Kindersley.

Super, C. M. 1976. 'Environmental Effects on Motor Development: The Case of "African Infant Precocity"'. *Developmental Medicine and Child Neurology* 18:561–567.

Super, C. M. 1981. 'Cross-Cultural Research on Infancy'. In H. C. Triandis and A. Heron (eds). *Hand-Book of Cross-Cultural Psychology: Developmental Psychology* vol. 4. Boston: Allyn & Bacon:17–53.

Super, C. M. 1983. 'Cultural Variations in the Meaning and Uses of Children's "Intelligence"'. In J. B. Deregowski, S. Dziurawiec and R. C. Annis (eds). *Expiscations in Cross-Cultural Psychology: Selected Papers from The Sixth International Conference of The International Association For Cross-Cultural Psychology.* Lisse, Holland: Swets & Zeitlinger.

Super, C. M. and Harkness, S. 1982. 'The Development of Affect in Infancy and Early Childhood'. In D. A. Wagner and H. W. Stevenson (eds). *Cultural Perspectives on Child Development.* San Francisco: W. H. Freeman:1–19.

Super, C. M. and Harkness, S. 1986. 'The Developmental Niche: A Conceptualization at the Interface of Child and Culture'. *International Journal of Behavioral Development* 9:545–569.

Swainson, N. 2000. 'Knowledge and Power: The Design and Implementation of Gender Policies in Education in Malawi'. *International Journal of Educational Development* 20:49–64.

Swart, S. M., Lemmer, R., Parbhoo, J. N. and Prescott, C. A. J. 1995. 'A Survey of Ear and Hearing Disorders amongst a Representative Sample of Grade 1 Schoolchildren in Swaziland'. *International Journal of Pediatric Otorhinolaryngology* 32:23–24.

Swart-Kruger, J. and Richter, L. M. 1997. 'Aids-Related Knowledge, Attitudes and Behaviour among South African Street Youth: *Reflections on Power, Sexuality and the Autonomous Self*'. *Social Science and Medicine* 45:957–966.

Szabo, R. and Short, R. V. 2000. 'How Does Male Circumcision Protect Against HIV Infection?' *British Medical Journal* 320:1592–1594.

Tabulawa, R. 1997. 'Pedagogical Classroom Practice and the Social Context: The Case of Botswana'. *International Journal of Educational Development* 17:189–204.

Taha, T. E. T., Dallabetta, G. A., Canner, J. K., Chiphangwi, J. D., Liomba, G., Hoover, D. R. and Miotti, P. G. 1995. 'The Effect of Human Immunodeficiency Virus Infection on Birthweight, and Infant and Child Mortality in Urban Malawi'. *International Journal of Epidemiology* 24:1022–1029.

Tajfel, H. 1978. *Differentiation between Social Groups.* London: Academic Press.

Talle, A. 1995. 'A Child Is A Child: Disability and Equality among The Kenya Maasai'. In B. Ingstad and S R Whyte (eds). *Disability and Culture*. Berkeley, Calif.: University of California Press:56–72.

Tanner, J. M. 1989. *Foetus Into Man: Physical Growth From Conception To Maturity* (2nd ed.). Ware, Herts: Castlemead.

Thomas, C. L. (ed.). 1988. *Taber's Cyclopedic Medical Dictionary*. Singapore: PG.

Thomas, A., Chess, S. and Birch, H. G. 1968. *Temperament and Behavior Disorders in Children*. New York: New York University Press.

Thomas, D. L. and Carver, C. 1990. 'Religion and Adolescent Competence'. In T. P. Gullotta, G. R. Adams and R. Montemayor (eds). *Developing Social Competency in Adolescence*. Newbury Park, Calif.: Sage:195–219.

Timaeus, I. and Graham, W. 1989. 'Labor Circulation, Marriage, and Fertility in Southern Africa'. In R. J. Lesthaege (ed.). *Reproduction and Social Organization in Sub-Saharan Africa*. Berkeley, Calif.: University of California Press:365–400.

Triandis, H. C. 1995a. 'The Self and Social Behavior'. In N. R. Goldberger and J. B. Veroff (eds). *The Culture and Psychology Reader*. New York: New York University Press:326–365.

Triandis, H. C. 1995b. *Individualism and Collectivism*. Boulder, Colo.: Westview Press.

Tronick, E. Z., Morelli, G. A. and Ivey, P. K. 1992. 'The Efe Forager Infant and Toddler's Pattern of Social Relationships: Multiple and Simultaneous'. *Developmental Psychology* 28:568–577.

Tronick, E. Z., Morelli, G. A. and Winn, S. 1987. 'Multiple Caretaking of Efe (Pygmy) Infants'. *American Anthropologist* 89:96–106.

Tshireletso, L 1997. '"They Are the Government's Children". School and Community Relations in A Remote Area Dweller (Basarwa) Settlement in Kweneng District, Botswana'. *International Journal of Educational Development* 17:172–188.

Ulijaszek, S. J. 1990. 'Nutritional Status and Susceptibility To Infectious Disease'. In G. A. Harrison and J. C. Waterlow (eds). *Diet and Disease in Traditional and Developing Societies*. Cambridge: Cambridge University Press:37–154.

UNAIDS 1998. *A Review of HIV Transmission through Breastfeeding*. Geneva: World Health Organization.

UNICEF 1993. *Planning for People: Strategy for Accelerated Human Development in Botswana*. Gaborone.

UNICEF 1999a. *Breastfeeding: Foundation for a Healthy Future*. New York.

UNICEF 1999b. *Rolling Back Malaria*. New York.

UNICEF 2000a. *The State of the World's Children*. New York.

UNICEF 2000b. *Ending Iodine Deficiency: A Goal Within Our Grasp*. New York.

UNICEF 2002. *The State of the World's Children: Leadership*. New York.

United Nations Development Programme 2000. *Human Development Report 2000*. Oxford: Oxford University Press.

Valsiner, J. and Litvinovic, G. 1996. 'Processes of Generalisation in Parental Reasoning'. In S. Harkness and C. M. Super (eds). *Parents' Cultural Belief Systems: Their Origins, Expressions, and Consequences*. New York: Guilford:56–82.

Volk, J. E. and Koopman, C. 2001. 'Factors Associated With Condom Use in Kenya: A Test of the Health Belief Model'. *Aids Education and Prevention* 13:495–508.

Wagner, D. A. 1981. 'Culture and Memory Development'. In H.C. Triandis and A. Herron (eds). *Handbook of Cross-Cultural Psychology: vol. 4: Developmental Psychology*. Boston: Allyn & Bacon:143–236.

Watkins, D. and Regmi, M. 1996. 'Toward the Cross-Cultural Validation of A Western Model of Student Approaches To Learning'. *Journal of Cross-Cultural Psychology* 27:547–560.

Webb, D. 1997. *HIV and Aids in Africa*. London: Pluto.

Weisner, T. S. 1989. 'Cultural and Universal Aspects of Social Support For Children: Evidence From The Abaluyia of Kenya'. In D. Belle (ed.). *Children's Social Networks and Social Support*. New York: John Wiley:70–89.

Wenger, M. 1989. 'Work, Play and Social Relationships among Children in A Giriama Community'. In D. Belle (ed.). *Children's Social Networks and Social Support*. New York: John Wiley:91–115.

Werner, D. 1993. *Where There Is No Doctor: A Village Health Care Handbook*. London: Macmillan Educational.

Werner, E. E. 1988. 'A Cross-Cultural Perspective on Infancy'. *Journal of Cross-Cultural Psychology* 19:96–113.

Whiting, B. B. and Whiting, J. W. M. 1975. *Children of Six Cultures: A Psycho-Cultural Analysis*. Cambridge, Mass.: Harvard University Press.

Whyte, S. R. 1995. 'Constructing Epilepsy: Images and Contexts in East Africa'. In B. Ingstad and S. R. Whyte (eds). *Disability and Culture*. Berkeley, Calif.: University of California Press:226–245.

Williams, J. M. G. 1992. *The Psychological Treatment of Depression: A Guide To the Theory and Practice of Cognitive Behaviour Therapy* (2nd ed.). London: Routledge.

Williams, R. 1980. *Problems in Materialism and Culture: Selected Essays*. London: NLB.

Wilson, D., Mundy-Castle, A. and Panditji, L. 1998. 'Birth Order and Intellectual Development among Zimbabwean Children'. *Journal of Social Psychology* 130:409–411.

Wing, A. 1997. 'How Can Children Be Taught To Read Differently: Bill's New Frock and the "Hidden Curriculum"'. *Gender and Education* 9:193–204.

Wober, M. 1972. 'Culture and the Concept of Intelligence: A Case Study in Uganda'. *Journal of Cross-Cultural Psychology* 3:327–328.

Wolff, P. H. 1969. 'The Natural History of Crying and Other Vocalizations in Early Infancy'. In B. M. Foss (ed.). *Determinants of Infant Behavior IV*. London: Methuen:81–119.

Worchel, F. F. and Allen, M. 1997. 'Mothers' Ability to Discriminate Cry Types in Low-Birthweight Premature and Full-Term Infants'. *Children's Health Care* 26:183–195.

Worden, J. W. 1996. *Children and Grief: When a Parent Dies*. New York: Guilford.

World Bank 1999. *Confronting Aids: Public Priorities in a Global Epidemic*. New York: Oxford University Press.

World Health Organization 1996. *Fact Sheet No 109: Childhood Diseases in Africa*. New York.

World Health Organization 2000a. *World Health Report 2000: Health Systems: Improving Performance*. New York.

World Health Organization 2000b. *Global Alliance for Vaccines and Immunization: Measles*. New York.

Worthman, C. M. 1999. 'Epidemiology of Human Development'. In C. Panter-Brick and C. M. Worthman (eds). *Hormones, Health and Behavior: A Socio-Ecological and Lifespan Perspective*. Cambridge: Cambridge University Press:17–104.

Wright, J. 1995. 'Recognizing and Understanding Troubled Children'. In P. Kilbourn (ed.). *Healing The Children of War*. Monrovia, Calif.: MARC:31–48.

Wu, D. Y. H. 1996. 'Chinese Childhood Socialization'. In M. H. Bond (ed.). *The Handbook of Chinese Psychology*. Hong Kong: Oxford University Press:143–154.

Yamaguchi, S. 1994. 'Collectivism among the Japanese: A Perspective From the Self'. In U. Kim, H. C. Triandis, C. Kagitcibasi, S-C. Choi and G. Yoon (eds). *Individualism and Collectivism: Theory, Methods and Applications*. Thousand Oaks, Calif.: Sage:175–188.

Young, B. and Papadatou, D. 1997. 'Childhood Death and Bereavement across Cultures'. In C. M. Parkes, P. Lanugani and B. Young (eds). *Death and Bereavement across Cultures*. London: Routledge:191–205.

Youssef, R. M., Attia, M. S-E-D., Kamel, M. I. 1998. 'Children Experiencing Violence II: Prevalence and Determinants of Corporal Punishment in Schools'. *Child Abuse and Neglect* 22:975–985.

Zach, U. and Keller, H. 1999. 'Patterns of Attachment-Exploration Balance of 1-Year-Old Infants From The United States and Northern Germany'. *Journal of Cross-Cultural Psychology* 30:381–388.

Zeskind, P. S. and Marshall, T. R. 1988. 'The Relation between Variations in Pitch and Maternal Perceptions of Infant Crying'. *Child Development* 59:193–196.

Zeitlin, M. 1996. 'My Child Is My Crown: Yoruba Parental Theories and Practices in Early Childhood'. In S. Harkness and C. M. Super (eds). *Parents' Cultural Belief Systems: Their Origins, Expressions and Consequences*. Thousand Oaks, Calif.: Sage:175–188.

Index